Goodman *and* Marshall's
Recognizing *and* Reporting
Red Flags *for the*
Physical Therapist Assistant

Goodman *and* Marshall's
Recognizing *and* Reporting Red Flags *for the* Physical Therapist Assistant

SECOND EDITION

Charlene Marshall, BS, PTA
Director of Rehabilitation
Edgewater Haven Nursing Home
Port Edwards, Wisconsin

ELSEVIER

Elsevier
3251 Riverport Lane
St. Louis, Missouri 63043

GOODMAN AND MARSHALL'S RECOGNIZING AND REPORTING RED FLAGS   ISBN: 978-0-323-87879-1
FOR THE PHYSICAL THERAPIST ASSISTANT

Notice

Practitioners and researchers must always rely on their own experience and knowledge in evaluating and using any information, methods, compounds or experiments described herein. Because of rapid advances in the medical sciences, in particular, independent verification of diagnoses and drug dosages should be made. To the fullest extent of the law, no responsibility is assumed by Elsevier, authors, editors or contributors for any injury and/or damage to persons or property as a matter of products liability, negligence or otherwise, or from any use or operation of any methods, products, instructions, or ideas contained in the material herein.

Executive Content Strategist: Lauren Willis
Senior Content Development Manager: Somodatta Roy Choudhury
Senior Content Development Specialist: Shilpa Kumar
Publishing Services Manager: Deepthi Unni
Senior Project Manager: Manchu Mohan
Design Direction: Ryan Cook

Printed in India.

Last digit is the print number: 9 8 7 6 5 4 3 2 1

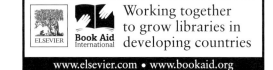

ACKNOWLEDGMENT

First and foremost, I would like to express my sincere gratitude to Catherine C. Goodman. It is because of you that I even have this opportunity! I am so very proud to be a part of your legacy and to call you my friend. You have contributed so much to our profession and we are all better therapists because of you. Every time we talk, I am inspired by your kindness and the level of knowledge that you have for so many things. I truly hope to continue to contribute to the profession of physical therapist assistants in the same way.

To the team at Elsevier—Thank you for all of your hard work and always checking in on me.

Lauren Willis, Executive Content Strategist
Laura Klein, Content Strategist
Shilpa Kumar, Senior Content Development Specialist
Manchu Mohan, Senior Project Manager
Padmavathy Kannabiran, MPS Project Manager

PREFACE

This textbook serves the purpose of preparing the physical therapist assist (PTA) for a role that continues to evolve as the profession of physical therapy and the education of therapists strive to keep up with the healthcare demands of our society. Events in the world of healthcare are moving forward at lightning speed. The integration of digital health care and telehealth services combined with the complexity of health conditions adds challenges that the PTA needs to be prepared for. In addition, there are more active patients with chronic pain conditions and older clients wanting to stay as independent as possible and live at home longer.

The introduction and development of direct access has progressed the education and training of the physical therapist (PT) to be prepared as a primary care provider. For the last three decades the PT's skills in differential diagnosis and screening for medical referral have become even more important. As a result, the PTA needs to progress and be able to safely and accurately recognize yellow or red flags to relay to the PT. We know that early recognition and communication with the PT for follow-up evaluation or referral to a more appropriate health care professional will yield better outcomes for patients.

The PTA profession requires working more autonomously under increasingly stressful situations. Reduced staff, reducing reimbursement rates, more medically complex patients, and intermittent supervision from the PT add additional challenges. The current healthcare environment is unlikely to change, and now more than ever, the PTA must be able to learn new tools to retain the true scope of what physical therapy can provide to the health of the patient as a whole being. With this in mind, the education of the PTA needs to keep up with the demands and education of the PT to foster the best PT/PTA working relationship. The PT needs to be able to rely on the PTA to be smart, capable, intuitive, and prepared to safely treat patients knowing how to recognize and when to report red flag concerns or observations.

The features in this textbook will prepare the PTA to do just that! The PTA Action Plan, Points to Ponder and Picture the Patient in this one-of-a-kind text will bring the PTA up to date with current best practice methods. The clinical decision-making model for recognizing red flags presented in this text apply to all practice settings. In this second edition the instructors will find resources online that include selected images, updated PowerPoint slides, updated review questions and *newly added patient scenarios* to engage the student with a more clinical approach.

We continue to believe that the information provided in this text will not only teach the student PTA, but will also provide crucial knowledge to the working PTA from new graduate to the experienced clinician.

Charlene Marshall, BS, PTA
Catherine C Goodman, MBA, PT

CONTENTS

Goodman *and* Marshall's
Recognizing *and* Reporting
Red Flags *for the*
Physical Therapist Assistant

Introduction to Recognizing and Reporting Red Flags for the Physical Therapist Assistant

INTRODUCTION

The physical therapist's (PT's) responsibility is to make sure that each patient/client is an appropriate candidate for physical therapy. The therapist determines what biomechanical or neuromusculoskeletal (NMS) problem is present, determines a human movement diagnosis, and then treats the problem as specifically as possible. The physical therapist assistant (PTA) follows through by carrying out the plan of care and providing ongoing feedback on the patient's/client's response to the intervention.

As part of the PT's diagnostic process, each patient or client is screened for medical disease. PTs assess for signs and symptoms of systemic disease that can mimic neuromuscular or musculoskeletal (herein referred to as NMS) dysfunction. Peptic ulcers, gallbladder disease, liver disease, and myocardial ischemia are only a few examples of systemic diseases that can cause shoulder or back pain. Other diseases can present as primary neck, upper back, hip, sacroiliac, or low back pain and/or symptoms.

Cancer screening is a major part of the therapist's screening process. Cancer can present as primary neck, shoulder, chest, upper back, hip, groin, pelvic, sacroiliac, or low back pain/symptoms. Whether there is a primary cancer or cancer that has recurred or metastasized, clinical manifestations can mimic NMS dysfunction. The therapist must know how and what to look for to screen for cancer.

The PTA's role is important for performing ongoing assessments and providing information to the PT regarding any red (warning) flags or new or developing signs and/or symptoms. This text is intended to help PTAs become better clinical decision makers in recognizing areas that are beyond the scope of their practice as an assistant under the supervision of the PT. The goal is to provide a step-by-step method for PTAs to identify clients who need further evaluation by the PT or referral or consultation as appropriate with other health care professionals.

Any patient or client can present with red flags requiring reevaluation and at any time—even those individuals who have a clearly identified NMS problem within the scope of the PT/PTA practice—because people often have more than one condition or problem and even many more comorbidities. The methods and clinical decision-making model for recognizing red flags presented in this text apply to all practice settings.

With evidence-based medicine, relying on a red-flag checklist based on the history has proved to be a very safe way to avoid missing the presence of serious disorders. Efforts are being made to validate red flags currently in use. When serious conditions have been missed, it is not for lack of special investigations, but for lack of adequate and thorough attention to clues in the history.[1,2]

Some conditions will be missed even with proper screening by the PT because the condition is early in its presentation and has not progressed enough to be recognizable. In some cases, early recognition makes no difference to the outcome, either because nothing can be done to prevent the progression of the condition or no adequate treatment is available.[1] Most of the time, however, early recognition and reporting by the PTA to the PT with follow-up evaluation by the PT and/or referral to a more appropriate health care professional can yield better outcomes for the patient/client.

TEXTBOOK ELEMENTS

Throughout this text, we have tried to provide helpful elements to guide the PTA and PTA instructor. For example, case examples are provided with each chapter to give the PTA a working understanding of how to recognize the need for additional questions. In addition, information is given concerning the type of questions to ask and when to document and consult with the PT. Each case is based on actual clinical experiences to provide reasonable examples of what the PTA can expect in a variety of inpatient/client and outpatient/client clinical practices.

Picture the Patient is a feature offered to help the student better visualize and understand what to look for when assessing and/or working with patients/clients. Clinical presentation, especially typical red-flag signs, and symptoms of emerging problems are included.

The *PTA Action Plan* gives the PTA student an opportunity to see the clinical application of the text material. These sections include the "how tos" of observing, documenting, and reporting red (or yellow) flags to the PT (or other health care provider when appropriate). Follow-up Questions, Points to Ponder, What to Watch For, and Communication with the Physical Therapist are just a few examples of the components included throughout the text in this section.

The *Case Examples* and *Critical Thinking Activities* provide opportunities for students and instructors to engage in dialog and discussion about the role of the PTA as a team member and in relation to the supervising PT when observing, documenting, and reporting potential red (or yellow) warning/cautionary flags.

YELLOW OR RED FLAGS

The role of the PTA in identifying yellow (caution) or red (warning) flag histories and signs and symptoms is important (Box 1.1). A yellow flag is a cautionary or warning symptom that signals one to "slow down" and think about the need to conduct a more formal observation/assessment. Red flags are features of the individual's medical history and clinical examination thought to be associated with a high risk of serious disorders such as infection, inflammation, cancer, or fracture.[3,4] A red-flag symptom requires immediate attention, either to ask the individual some additional questions and/or bring the information to the attention of the PT.

Listening for yellow- or red-flag symptoms and observing for red-flag signs can be easily incorporated into everyday practice. It is a matter of listening and looking intentionally. The presence of a single yellow or red flag is not usually cause for immediate concern. Each cautionary or warning flag must be viewed in the context of the whole person, given the age, sex, past medical history, known risk factors, medication use, and current clinical presentation of that patient/client.

BOX 1.1 Red Flags

The presence of any one of these symptoms is not usually cause for extreme concern but should raise a red flag for the alert physical therapist assistant (PTA). The therapist will be looking for a pattern that suggests a viscerogenic or systemic origin of pain and/or symptoms. The therapist will proceed with the screening process, depending on which symptoms are grouped together. Often, the next step is to conduct a risk factor assessment and look for associated signs and symptoms. The PTA can assist in this process by reporting any information not previously disclosed to the therapist and/or not documented in the medical record.

Past Medical History (Personal or Family)
- Personal or family history of cancer
- Recent (last 6 weeks) infection (e.g., mononucleosis, upper respiratory infection, urinary tract infection, bacterial such as streptococcal or staphylococcal, viral such as measles or hepatitis), especially when followed by neurologic symptoms 1 to 3 weeks later (Guillain-Barré syndrome), joint pain, or back pain
- Recurrent colds or flu with a cyclical pattern (i.e., the client reports that he or she just cannot shake this cold or the flu, or that it keeps coming back)
- Recent history of trauma, such as motor vehicle accident or fall (fracture, any age), domestic violence, or minor trauma in older adult with osteopenia/osteoporosis
- History of immunosuppression (e.g., steroids, organ transplant, human immunodeficiency virus)
- History of injection drug use (infection)

Risk Factors
Risk factors vary, depending on family history, personal history, and disease, illness, or condition present. For example, risk factors for heart disease will be different from risk factors for osteoporosis or vestibular or balance problems. As with all decision-making variables, a single risk factor may or may not be significant and must be viewed in context of the whole patient/client presentation. This represents only a partial list of all the possible health risk factors.

Substance use/abuse	Alcohol use/abuse
Tobacco use	Sedentary lifestyle
Age	Race/ethnicity
Sex	Domestic violence
Body mass index (BMI)	Hysterectomy/oophorectomy
Exposure to radiation	Occupation

Clinical Presentation
- No known cause, unknown etiology, insidious onset
- Symptoms that are not improved or relieved by physical therapy intervention
- Physical therapy intervention not changing the clinical picture (the client may get worse!)

- Symptoms that get better after physical therapy intervention, but then get worse again—a red flag identifying the need for reevaluation by the therapist
- Significant weight loss or gain without effort (e.g., more than 10% of the client's body weight in 10–21 days)
- Gradual, progressive, or cyclical presentation of symptoms (worse/better/worse)
- Unrelieved by rest or change in position; no position is comfortable
- If relieved by rest, positional change, or application of heat, in time, these relieving factors no longer reduce symptoms
- Symptoms seeming out of proportion to the injury
- Symptoms persisting beyond the expected time for that condition
- Does not fit the expected mechanical or neuromusculoskeletal pattern
- No discernible pattern of symptoms
- A growing mass (painless or painful) considered a tumor until proven otherwise; a hematoma should decrease (not increase) in size with time.
- Postmenopausal vaginal bleeding (bleeding that occurs a year or more after the last period [significance depends on whether the female is on hormone replacement therapy and which regimen is used])
- Bilateral symptoms:

Edema	Clubbing
Numbness, tingling	Nail-bed changes
Skin pigmentation changes	Skin rash

- Change in muscle tone or range of motion (ROM) for individuals with neurologic conditions (e.g., cerebral palsy, spinal cord injury, traumatic brain injury, multiple sclerosis)

Pain Pattern
- Back or shoulder pain (most common location of referred pain; other areas can be affected as well, but these two areas signal a particular need for the therapist's attention)
- Pain accompanied by full and painless ROM
- Night pain (constant and intense; see complete description in Chapter 2)
- Symptoms (especially pain) constant and intense (Remember to ask anyone with "constant" pain: "Are you having this pain right now?")
- Pain made worse by activity and relieved by rest (e.g., intermittent claudication; cardiac: upper quadrant pain with the use of the lower extremities while upper extremities are inactive)
- Pain described as throbbing (vascular), knife-like, boring, or deep aching
- Pain that is poorly localized
- Pattern of pain coming and going like spasms, colicky
- Pain accompanied by signs and symptoms associated with a specific viscera or system (e.g., gastrointestinal, genitourinary, gynecologic, cardiac, pulmonary, endocrine)
- Change in musculoskeletal symptoms with food intake or medication use (immediately or up to several hours later)

BOX 1.1   Red Flags—cont'd

Associated Signs and Symptoms

- Recent report of confusion (or increased confusion); this could be a neurologic sign; it could be drug induced (e.g., nonsteroidal antiinflammary drugs) or a sign of infection; usually, it is a family member who takes the PTA aside to report this concern
- Presence of constitutional symptoms (see Box 1.3) or unusual vital signs (see Chapter 3); body temperature of 100°F (37.8°C) usually indicates a serious illness
- Proximal muscle weakness, especially if accompanied by change in deep tendon reflexes

- Joint pain with skin rashes and nodules (see systemic causes of joint pain, Chapter 2)
- Any cluster of signs and symptoms observed during the Review of Systems that are characteristic of a particular organ system (see Box 4.19)
- Unusual menstrual cycle/symptoms; association between menses and symptoms
- *It is suggested that the PTA ask each patient/client a question at the beginning of each treatment session, such as "Are there any new symptoms or problems anywhere else in your body that have developed in the last 24 hours (or since I saw you last)?"*

⏩ PTA ACTION PLAN

Documenting and Reporting Yellow or Red Flags

Anytime a yellow or red flag is observed or reported, the PTA must document this in the record and report it to the PT. This is true even for single individual flags that may seem inconsequential at the time (remember "Progression of Disease"—what appears benign now may develop into something more significant later; a record of its first appearance can be extremely helpful).

Cases of isolated symptoms will be presented in this text as they occur in clinical practice. Symptoms of any kind that present bilaterally always raise a red flag for concern and further investigation.

Clusters of two or three or more yellow and/or red flags may not represent an emergency but must be documented and reported. Each case is evaluated on its own. Reevaluation by the PT is warranted when risk factors for specific diseases are present that have not been known or both risk factors and red flags are present at the same time.

Even as we write this, the focus on red flags in assessment has been called into question, so this remains an evolving practice.[5,6] It has been reported that in the primary care (medical) setting, some red flags have high false-positive rates and have very little diagnostic value when used by themselves.[7,8] Efforts are being made to identify reliable red flags that are valid based on patient-centered clinical research. Whenever possible, those yellow/red flags are reported in this text.[7,9,10]

Yellow and red flags are only one tool the PTA will monitor. In addition, the PT will review the patient's/client's history, presenting pain pattern, and possible associated signs and symptoms along with results from treatment administered by the PTA in making a decision to modify treatment or consult with other disciplines.

⏩ PTA ACTION PLAN

Key Factors to Consider

Three key factors the PTA should always keep in mind (because these create red-flag signs and symptoms) are as follows:
- Side effects of medications
- Comorbidities
- Visceral pain mechanisms

If the medical diagnosis is delayed, the correct diagnosis is eventually made when:
1. The patient/client does not get better with physical therapy intervention.
2. The patient/client gets better, then worse.
3. Other associated signs and symptoms eventually develop.

At times, a patient/client with NMS complaints is actually experiencing the side effects of medications. In fact, this is probably the most common source of associated signs and symptoms observed in the clinic. Side effects of medication as a cause of associated signs and symptoms, including joint and muscle pain, are discussed more completely in Chapter 2. Visceral pain mechanisms are also discussed in Chapter 2.

As for comorbidities, many patients/clients are affected by other conditions such as depression, diabetes, incontinence, obesity, chemical dependency, hypertension, osteoporosis, and deconditioning, to name just a few. These conditions can contribute to significant morbidity (and mortality) and must be documented as part of the problem list. Physical therapy intervention is often appropriate to address the effects of these comorbidities, but sometimes these problems have not been recognized and addressed yet, so the PTA brings them to the PT's attention as needed.

Finally, consider the fact that some clients with a systemic or viscerogenic origin of NMS symptoms get better with physical therapy intervention. Perhaps there is a placebo effect. Perhaps there is a physiologic effect of movement on the diseased state. The physical therapy intervention may exert a positive influence on the body as it tries to regain a balance of health and homeostasis. You may have experienced this phenomenon yourself when coming down with a cold or symptoms of a virus. You felt much better and even symptom free after exercising.

Movement, physical activity, and moderate exercise aid the body and boost the immune system,[11–16] but sometimes such measures are unable to prevail, especially if other factors are present such as inadequate hydration, poor nutrition, fatigue, depression, immunosuppression, and stress. In such cases the condition will progress to the point that warning signs and symptoms will be observed or reported, and/or the patient's/client's condition will deteriorate. The need for consultation with the PT will become much more evident.

❓ PICTURE THE PATIENT

The PTA must always keep in mind that medical conditions can cause pain, dysfunction, and impairment of the:
- Back/neck
- Shoulder
- Chest/breast/rib
- Hip/groin
- Sacroiliac/sacrum/pelvis

But for the most part the back and shoulder represent the primary areas of referred viscerogenic pain patterns. In essence, anytime a patient or client is being treated for shoulder or back pain, a yellow flag is raised. These two areas are the most commonly affected because the organs are located in the central portion of the body and refer symptoms to the nearby major muscles and joints. This concept will be explained in greater detail in Chapter 2.

▶▶ PTA ACTION PLAN

Monitoring Vital Signs

Monitoring vital signs is a quick and easy way to identify the need for medical conditions that require further evaluation by the PT. Vital signs are discussed more completely in Chapter 4. Asking about the presence of constitutional symptoms is important, especially when the cause is unknown. Constitutional symptoms refer to a constellation of signs and symptoms present whenever the patient/client is experiencing a systemic illness. No matter what system is involved, these core signs and symptoms are often present.

REASONS THAT RED FLAGS POP UP

The practice of physical therapy has changed many times since it was first started with the Reconstruction Aides. Clinical practice, as it was shaped by World War I and then World War II, was eclipsed by the polio epidemic in the 1940s and 1950s. With the widespread use of the live, oral polio vaccine in 1963, polio was eradicated in the United States and clinical practice changed again (Fig. 1.1).

Today, most clients seen by therapists have impairments and disabilities that are clearly related to NMS. Most of the time, the client history and mechanism of injury point to a known cause of movement dysfunction. But changes in technology, the vast amount of information about health problems now available, and the aging of America (and subsequent needs of the older adults) have changed the way health care is delivered and the way PTs function. These factors are making it more important than ever that all health care providers function as a team, observing and reporting any unusual, new, or suspicious signs and/or symptoms.

Because today's health care environment is complex and highly demanding, the PT/PTA team must be alert to red flags of systemic disease at all times. Warning flags may come in the form of reported symptoms or observed signs. It may be a clinical presentation that does not match the recent history. It may be someone who has been given early release from the hospital or transition unit. Specific red and yellow flags are discussed in greater detail later in this chapter, but an understanding of why we must watch out for these may be helpful.

Quicker and Sicker

"Quicker and sicker" is a term used to describe patients/clients in the current health care arena (Fig. 1.2).[17,18] *Quicker* refers to how health care delivery has changed in the last 10 years to combat the rising costs of health care. In the acute care setting the focus is on rapid recovery protocols. As a result, earlier mobility and mobility with more complex patients are allowed.[19-22] Better pharmacologic management of agitation has allowed earlier and safer mobility. Hospital inpatients/clients are discharged much

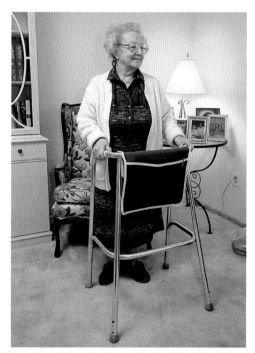

FIG. 1.2 The aging of America from the "traditionalists" (born before 1946) and the Baby Boom generation (born 1946–64) will result in older adults with multiple comorbidities in the care of the physical therapist/ physical therapist assistant team. Even with a known orthopedic and/or neurologic impairment, these clients will require a careful observation for the possibility of other problems, including side effects from medications. (From Sorrentino SA: *Mosby's textbook for nursing assistants*, ed 7, St. Louis, 2008, Mosby.)

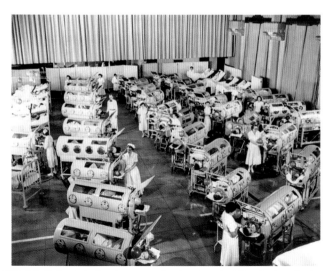

FIG. 1.1 Patients in iron lungs receive treatment at Rancho Los Amigos during the polio epidemic of the 1940s and 1950s. (Courtesy of Rancho Los Amigos National Rehabilitation Center.)

faster today than they were even 10 years ago. Patients are discharged from the intensive care unit (ICU) to rehab, step-down or transition units, or even home. Outpatient/client surgery is much more common, with same-day discharge for procedures that would have required a much longer hospitalization in the past. Patients/clients on the medical-surgical wards of most hospitals today would have been in the ICU 20 years ago.

Sicker refers to the fact that patients/clients in acute care, rehabilitation, or outpatient/client setting with any orthopedic or neurologic problems may have a past medical history of cancer or a current personal history of diabetes, liver disease, thyroid condition, peptic ulcer, and/or other conditions or diseases. Any of these can get worse or spiral out of control—and the first sign of trouble may be one of the many red flags discussed in this text.

The number of people with at least one chronic disease or disability is reaching epidemic proportions. According to the National Institute on Aging,[23] 79% of adults over 70 have at least one of seven potentially disabling chronic conditions (arthritis, hypertension, heart disease, diabetes, respiratory diseases, stroke, and cancer).[24] The presence of multiple comorbidities emphasizes the need to view the whole patient/client and not just the body part in question.

In addition, the number of people who do not have health insurance and who wait longer to seek medical attention are sicker when they access care. This factor, combined with the American lifestyle that leads to chronic conditions such as obesity, hypertension, and diabetes, results in a sicker population base.[24]

Natural History

Improvements in treatment for neurologic and other conditions previously considered fatal (e.g., cancer, cystic fibrosis) are now extending survivorship and life expectancy for many individuals. Improved interventions bring new areas of focus, such as quality-of-life issues. With some conditions (e.g., muscular dystrophy, cerebral palsy), the artificial dichotomy of pediatric versus adult care is gradually being replaced by a lifestyle approach that takes into consideration what is known about the natural history of the condition.

Many individuals with childhood-onset diseases now live well into adulthood. For them, their original pathology or disease process has given way to secondary impairments. These secondary impairments create further limitations and issues as the person ages. For example, a 30-year-old with cerebral palsy may experience chronic pain, changes or limitations in ambulation and endurance, and increased fatigue.

These symptoms result from the atypical movement patterns and musculoskeletal strains caused by chronic increase in tone and muscle imbalances that were originally caused by cerebral palsy. The PTA's assessment may identify signs and symptoms that have developed as a natural result of the primary condition (e.g., cerebral palsy) or long-term effects of treatment for other problems (e.g., chemotherapy, biotherapy, or radiotherapy for cancer).

Signed Prescription

Clients who obtain a signed prescription for physical therapy from their primary care physician or other health care provider, based on similar past complaints of musculoskeletal symptoms, without actually seeing the physician or being examined by the physician will require close observation for red flags.

Medical Specialization

In addition, with the increasing specialization of medicine, clients may be evaluated by a medical specialist who does not immediately recognize the underlying systemic disease, or the specialist may assume that the referring primary care physician has ruled out other causes. This type of situation is a yellow (cautionary) flag, again requiring close observation of the client during the physical therapy intervention.

Progression of Time and Disease

Sometimes in the early presentation, there are no red flags or associated signs and symptoms to suggest an underlying systemic or viscerogenic cause of the client's NMS symptoms or movement dysfunction. But with the passage of enough time, an untreated disease process can eventually progress and get worse (Case Example 1.1). Not until the disease progresses does the clinical picture change enough to raise a red flag. In some cases, exercise stresses the client's physiology enough to tip the scales. Previously unnoticed, unrecognized, or silent symptoms suddenly present more clearly.

Symptoms may become more readily apparent or more easily clustered. In such cases, the alert PTA may be the first to ask the patient/client pertinent questions to determine the presence of underlying symptoms requiring further evaluation by the PT or medical personnel.

The PTA must know what follow-up questions to ask clients to identify the need for reevaluation by the therapist. Knowing what medical conditions can cause signs or symptoms suggestive of NMS involvement (especially in the shoulder, neck, or back) is helpful. Familiarity with risk factors for various diseases, illnesses, and conditions is an important tool for early recognition in the assessment process. All of the components of assessment and follow-up appropriate for the PTA are included in this text.

Patient/Client Disclosure

Finally, sometimes patients/clients tell the PTA things about their current health and social history that are unknown or unreported to the PT or physician. The content of these conversations can reveal red flags and hold important clues to point out a systemic illness or viscerogenic cause of musculoskeletal or neuromuscular impairment.

The PTA may hear the client relate a new onset of symptoms that were not present during the initial examination. Such new information may come forth at any time during the episode of care. If the patient/client does not progress in physical therapy or presents with a new onset of symptoms

---

CASE EXAMPLE 1.1 **Progression of Disease**

A 44-year-old female was referred to the physical therapist (PT) with a complaint of right paraspinal/low thoracic back pain. There was no reported history of trauma or assault and no history of repetitive movement. The past medical history was significant for a kidney infection treated 3 weeks ago with antibiotics. The client stated that her follow-up urinalysis was "clear" and the infection resolved.

The physical therapy examination revealed true paraspinal muscle spasm with an acute presentation of limited movement and exquisite pain in the posterior right middle to low back. Spinal accessory motions were tested following application of a cold modality and were found to be mildly restricted in right side-bending and left rotation of the T8–T12 segments. The PT assessed that this joint motion deficit was still the result of muscle spasm and guarding and not true joint involvement. Prior to the next session, the physical therapist assistant (PTA) initiated face-to-face communication with the PT to discuss details of client status and intervention options.

Result: After three sessions with the PTA in which modalities were used for the acute symptoms, the client was not making observable, reportable, or measurable improvement. Her fourth scheduled appointment was canceled because of the "flu."

Given the recent history of kidney infection, the lack of expected improvement, and the onset of constitutional symptoms (see Box 1.3), the PTA notified the PT of the present concerns. The therapist contacted the client by telephone and suggested that she make a follow-up appointment with her doctor as soon as possible.

As it turned out, this patient's kidney infection had recurred. She recovered from her back sequelae within 24 hours of initiating a second antibiotic treatment. This is not the typical medical picture for a urologically compromised person. Sometimes it is not until the disease progresses that the systemic disorder (masquerading as a musculoskeletal problem) can be clearly differentiated.

Last, sometimes clients do not relay all the necessary or pertinent medical information to their physicians but will confide in the PT or PTA. They may feel intimidated, forget, become unwilling or embarrassed, or fail to recognize the significance of the symptoms and neglect to mention important medical details (see Box 1.1).

Knowing that systemic diseases can mimic NMS dysfunction, the therapist is responsible for identifying, as closely as possible, what NMS pathologic condition is present. It is difficult for a therapist to identify a condition without the timely communication of the competent PTA that is involved with the follow-up treatments.

---

unreported before, the screening process may have to be repeated by the therapist.

DECISION-MAKING PROCESS

This text is designed to help PTAs recognize when it is appropriate to document and report red-flag signs and symptoms. The hallmark of professionalism in any health care practitioner is the ability to understand the limits of his or her professional knowledge. The PTA, either on reaching the limit of his or her knowledge or on reaching the limits prescribed by the client's condition, should not hesitate to consult with the PT. In this way, the PTA will work within the scope of his or her level of skill, knowledge, and practical experience.

Knowing when to consult with the therapist is just as important as carrying out the plan of care. Once the PTA recognizes red-flag histories, risk factors, signs and symptoms, and/or a clinical presentation that do not fit the expected picture for NMS dysfunction, this information must be communicated effectively to the therapist.

▶▶ PTA ACTION PLAN
PT/PTA Team Communication Style

Each PT/PTA team will develop their own unique communication style. With time and experience, the PTA will learn what is appropriate for each situation. One way to maintain a positive, balanced relationship with the PT is to present the situation and then ask:
- How do you want to handle this? or
- How do you want me to handle this?

Unless directed otherwise by the supervising therapist, when providing written documentation, the PTA can include in a note to the therapist (or in the medical record) a short paragraph of findings followed by a list of concerns.

Documentation and Liability

Documentation is any entry into the patient/client record. Documentation may include the PTA's observations and assessment, progress notes, recap of discussions with the therapist or other health care professionals, flow sheets, checklists, objective measurements (e.g., range of motion), and discharge summaries.[25] Various forms are available for use in each clinical setting to aid in collecting data in a standardized fashion. Remember, in all circumstances, in a court of law, if you did not document it, you did not do it (a common catch phrase is "not documented, not done").

Clients with complex medical histories and multiple comorbidities are increasingly common in a PT's practice. Risk management has become an important consideration for many clients. Documentation and communication must reflect this practice.

In cases where the seriousness of the condition can affect the client's outcome, the PTA may need to contact the therapist immediately and directly and describe the problem. The therapist will advise the PTA on what to do if the therapist decides that the client needs medical attention. Good risk management is a proactive process that includes taking action to minimize negative outcomes. If a client is advised to contact his or her physician and fails to do so, the therapist is responsible for calling/contacting the doctor.[26]

Failure on the part of the PTA to properly report on a client's condition or important changes in condition reflects a lack of professional judgment in the management of the client's case. A number of positions and standards of the American Physical Therapy Association (APTA) Board of Directors emphasize the importance of PT communication and collaboration with other health care providers. The APTA also holds the PTA to similar standards of communication and collaboration with the PT, as outlined in the APTA's *Guide for Conduct of the Physical*

Therapist Assistant.[27] This is a key to providing the best possible client care (Case Example 1.2).[28]

Failure to share findings and concerns with the therapist or other appropriate health care provider is a failure to enter into a collaborative team approach. Best practice standards of optimal patient/client care support and encourage interactive exchange.

Prior negative experiences with difficult health care personnel do not exempt the PTA from best practice, which means making every attempt to communicate and document clinical findings and concerns.

The PTA must describe his or her concerns. It may be necessary to explain that the symptoms do not match the expected pattern for a musculoskeletal or neuromuscular problem. It may be appropriate to make a summary statement regarding key objective findings with a follow-up question for the therapist. This may be filed in the client's chart or electronic medical record in the hospital or sent in a letter to the therapist.

For example, after treatment of a person who has not responded to the PTA's treatment, a report to the therapist may include additional information: "Miss Jones reported a skin rash over the backs of her knees 2 weeks before the onset of joint pain and experiences recurrent bouts of sore throat and fever when her knees flare up. These features are not consistent with an athletic injury. Would you please take a look?"

Other useful wording may include "Please advise" or "What do you think?" In this way, the PTA does not suggest a medical cause or attempt to diagnose. Providing a report and stating that the clinical presentation does not follow a typical neuromuscular or musculoskeletal pattern may be all that is needed.

Goodman Model for the Physical Therapist Assistant

The Goodman Screening Model[29] used by PTs in conducting a screening evaluation for any client can be adapted for use by the PTA to aid in recognizing and reporting red flags (Box 1.2).

By using these decision-making tools the PTA will be better able to identify emerging problems that require reporting, identify information that is inconsistent with the presenting complaint, identify noncontributory information, and recognize when consultation with the therapist is indicated.

The recognition process is carried out through the client interview and verified during the physical assessment. The PTA

CASE EXAMPLE 1.2   Failure to Collaborate and Communicate

A 43-year-old female was riding a bicycle when she was struck from behind and thrown to the ground. She was seen at the local walk-in clinic and released with a prescription for painkillers and muscle relaxants. X-rays of her head and neck were unremarkable for obvious injury.

She came to the physical therapy clinic 3 days later with complaints of left shoulder, rib, and wrist pain.

Initial Evaluation: Obvious bruising occurred along the left chest wall and upper abdomen. In fact, the ecchymosis was quite extensive and black, indicating a large area of blood extravasation into the subcutaneous tissues.

She had no other complaints or problems. Shoulder range of motion was full in all planes, although painful and stiff. Ribs 9, 10, and 11 were painful to palpation but without obvious deformity or derangement.

A neurologic screening exam was negative. The client was scheduled for three visits over the next 4 days and started on a program of Codman's exercises, progressing to active shoulder motion.

Intervention: The client was seen by the PTA, experienced some progress, and then reported severe back muscle spasms at the last session.

The client called the clinic and canceled her next appointment (scheduled with the PTA) because she had the flu with fever and vomiting. Up to this point, there has not been any communication between the therapist and the PTA due to varied and busy schedules. When the client returned to the clinic for her fourth visit, the PTA treated her with active exercise, progressing to resistive strengthening according to the plan of care. The client's painful shoulder and back symptoms remained the same, but the client reported that she was "less stiff."

Three weeks after the initial accident, the client collapsed at work and had to be transported to the hospital for emergency surgery. Her spleen had been damaged by the initial trauma with a slow bleed that eventually ruptured.

The client filed a lawsuit in which the therapist and the PTA were named. The complaint against the therapist was that she failed to properly assess the client's condition and failed to refer her to a medical doctor for a condition outside the scope of physical therapy practice.

Did the Physical Therapist Show Questionable Professional Judgment in the Evaluation and Management of this Case?

Did the Physical Therapist Assistant Show Questionable Professional Judgment in the Treatment and Communication of this Case?

Some obvious red-flag signs and symptoms in this case went unreported to a medical doctor as well as signs and symptoms that went unreported to the PT. There was no contact with the physician at any time throughout this client's physical therapy episode of care. The on-call physician at the walk-in clinic did not refer the client to physical therapy—she referred herself.

However, the PT did not send the physician any information about the client's self-referral, physical therapy evaluation, or planned treatment.

Subcutaneous blood extravasation is not uncommon after a significant accident or traumatic impact such as this client experienced. The fact that the physician did not know about this and the PT did not report it demonstrates questionable judgment.

The new onset of muscle spasm and unchanging pain levels with treatment are potential red-flag symptoms. Concomitant constitutional symptoms of fever and vomiting are also red flags, even if the client thought it was the flu.

At no time did the therapist or assistant suggest the client go back to the clinic or see a primary care physician. It is clear that the PTA showed poor communication with the therapist by choosing not to make a phone call or leave written updates for the therapist to follow up on the changing condition. The PTA failed to document and properly report to the therapist when needed and failed to follow the APTA's guidelines governing a PTA's interaction with the PT.

The therapist exercised questionable professional judgment by failing to communicate and collaborate with the attending physician as well as the PTA with whom she works. She did not screen the client for systemic involvement, based on the erroneous thinking that this was a traumatic event with a clear etiology.

She assumed in a case like this where the client was a self-referral that she was "on her own." She failed to properly report on the client's condition, failed to follow the APTA's policies governing a PT's interaction with other health care providers, and was legally liable for mismanagement in this case.

> ### BOX 1.2 Tools Used by the Physical Therapist Assistant to Recognize Red Flags
>
> - Past medical history (including personal and family history)
> - Red-flag risk factors
> - Clinical presentation (including red- or yellow-flag signs and symptoms of systemic disease)
> - Appropriate follow-up questions

listens to the subjective information (what the patient/client tells you) and pays close attention to objective findings (what you find during observation) to identify red- or yellow-flag scenarios.

Given today's time constraints in the clinic, a fast and efficient method of recognizing red flags is essential. Knowledge of common red flags (see Box 1.1), follow-up questions to ask (presented throughout the text as part of the *PTA Action Plan* features), and using the tools outlined in Box 1.2 can guide and streamline the process.

▶▶ PTA ACTION PLAN

Additional Tools to Use When Watching for Red-Flag Signs, Symptoms, or Situations

- Take vital signs
- Use the word "symptom(s)" rather than "pain" during conversations with the client/patient
- Watch for red-flag histories, signs, and symptoms
- Review medications; observe for signs and symptoms that could be a result of drug combinations (polypharmacy) and dual drug dosage (same drug, different names)
- Ask a final, open-ended question such as:
  1. Are you having any other symptoms of any kind anywhere else in your body that you have not discussed with your therapist yet?
  2. Is there anything else you think is important about your condition that we have not discussed yet?

If a young, healthy athlete comes in with a sprained ankle and no other associated signs and symptoms, the PTA is unlikely to see any red-flag problems. However, if that same athlete has an eating disorder, uses anabolic steroids illegally, or is on antidepressants, the clinical picture (and possibly the intervention) changes. Or take, for example, an older adult who presents with hip pain of unknown cause. Two red flags are already present: age and insidious onset. As clients age, the past medical history and risk factor assessment become more important assessment tools. Or, if after ending the interview by asking, "Are there any symptoms of any kind anywhere else in your body that we have not talked about yet?" the client responds with a list of additional symptoms, it may be necessary to document and pass this information on to the therapist.

Past Medical History

Formal past medical history taking (including both family and personal history) is usually carried out by the therapist during the client interview. The client/patient interview is very important because it helps the PT distinguish between problems that he or she can treat and problems that should be referred to a physician (or other appropriate health care professional) for medical diagnosis and intervention.

In fact, the importance of history taking cannot be emphasized enough. Physicians cite a shortage of time as the most common reason to skip the client history, yet history taking is the essential key to a correct diagnosis by the physician (or PT).[30,31] Multiple sources of research over many years continue to recommend performing a detailed *history intake and differential diagnosis* followed by *relevant examination.*[31,32]

The types of data generated from a client history include age, race/ethnicity, sex, and occupation (general demographics). Information about social history, living environment, health status, functional status, and activity level is often important to the patient's/client's clinical presentation and outcomes. Details about the current condition, medical (or other) intervention for the condition, and use of medications are also gathered and considered in the overall evaluation process.

Psychosocial history may provide insight into the client's clinical presentation and overall needs. Age, sex, race/ethnicity, education, occupation, family system, health habits, living environment, medication use, and medical/surgical history are all part of the client history.

Risk Factor Assessment

Greater emphasis has been placed on risk factor assessment in the health care industry recently. Risk factor assessment is an important part of disease prevention.[33] Knowing the various risk factors for different kinds of diseases, illnesses, and conditions is an important part of recognizing red flags (see Box 1.1).

Therapists/PTAs can have an active role in both primary and secondary prevention through education. According to APTA's *Guide*,[25] PTs are involved in primary prevention by preventing a target condition in a susceptible or potentially susceptible population through such specific measures as general health promotion efforts.

In primary care the therapist assesses risk factors, performs screening examinations, and establishes interventions to prevent impairment, dysfunction, and disability. For example, does the client have risk factors for osteoporosis, urinary incontinence, cancer, vestibular or balance problems, obesity, cardiovascular disease, and so on? The PT practice can include routine screening for any of these, as well as other problems. Educating clients about their risk factors is a key element in risk factor reduction.

Convincing people to establish lifelong patterns of exercise and physical activity will continue to be a major focus of the health care industry. As a team, the therapist and the PTA can advocate disease prevention, wellness, and promotion of healthy lifestyles by delivering health care services intended to prevent health problems or maintain health and by offering education about disease prevention.

Clinical Presentation

Observing, recognizing, and reporting red flags observed in the patient's/client's clinical presentation, including pain patterns and pain types, are important parts of the PTA's responsibilities. To assist the PTA in this endeavor, specific pain patterns corresponding to systemic diseases are provided in Chapter 2. Drawings of primary and referred pain patterns are provided in each chapter for quick reference. A summary of key findings associated with systemic illness is listed in Box 1.1.

The presence of any one of these variables is not a cause for extreme concern but should raise a yellow or red flag for the alert PTA. This pattern will not be consistent with what we might expect to see with the neuromuscular or musculoskeletal systems.

The PTA will proceed with appropriate follow-up questions, often asking about associated signs and symptoms. If possible, it is recommended that the PTA discuss appropriate questions with the PT prior to asking the client. Special follow-up questions are provided in sections labeled *PTA Action Plan* to help the PTA know what to ask when gathering information for the therapist.

Associated Signs and Symptoms of Systemic Diseases

The major focus of this text is the recognition of yellow- or red-flag signs and symptoms, either reported by the client subjectively or observed objectively by the PTA. Associated signs and symptoms are actually part of the clinical presentation, but they are usually not typical of musculoskeletal or neuromuscular problems and therefore not reported by the patient/client.

Signs are observable findings easily detected in an objective examination (e.g., unusual skin color, clubbing of the fingers [swelling of the terminal phalanges of the fingers or toes], hematoma [local collection of blood], effusion [fluid]). Signs can be seen, heard, smelled, measured, photographed, shown to someone else, or documented in some other way.

Symptoms are reported indications of disease that are perceived by the client but cannot be observed by someone else. Pain, discomfort, or other complaints, such as numbness, tingling, or "creeping" sensations, are symptoms that are difficult to quantify but are most often reported as the chief complaint.

We include associated signs and symptoms as a component separate from clinical presentation because they are often atypical for the condition being treated. For example, consider the individual with shoulder or back pain caused by intraabdominal bleeding from prolonged nonsteroidal antiinflammatory drugs (NSAIDs) who is having abdominal pain or change in stool color. The person may not think this information is important for the PT to know and therefore does not mention it during the intake interview. Later, as the PTA works with this individual, comments/questions about these symptoms may come up.

Because PTs and PTAs spend a considerable amount of time listening to patients/clients describe and discuss their pain, it is easy to remain focused exclusively on this symptom when other important problems are present but unmentioned. For this reason, the PTA is encouraged to become accustomed to using the word "symptoms" instead of "pain" when talking with the patient/client.

▶▶ PTA ACTION PLAN
Follow-Up Questions

Instead of asking the client, "How are you today?" try asking:
- Are you better, the same, or worse today? (This approach to questioning progress [or lack of progress] may help you see a red-flag pattern sooner than later.)
- What can you do today that you could not do yesterday? (Or last week/last month?)
- Are there any symptoms of any kind anywhere else in your body that we have not talked about yet?
- *Alternatively:* Are there any symptoms or problems anywhere else in your body that may not be related to your current problem?

❓ PICTURE THE PATIENT

The patient/client may not see a connection between shoulder pain and blood in the urine from kidney impairment or blood in the stools from chronic NSAID use. Likewise, the patient/client may not think the diarrhea present is associated with the back pain (GI dysfunction).

The client with temporomandibular joint (TMJ) pain from a cardiac source usually has some other associated symptoms, and in most cases, the client does not see the link. When asked directly, the client may offer additional important information.

Each visceral system has a typical set of core signs and symptoms associated with impairment of that system (see Box 4.19). Systemic signs and symptoms that are listed for each condition should serve as a warning to alert the informed PTA of the need for further questioning and possible consultation with the therapist.

For example, the most common symptoms present with pulmonary pathology are cough, shortness of breath, and pleural pain. Liver impairment is marked by abdominal ascites, right upper quadrant tenderness, jaundice, and skin and nail-bed changes. Signs and symptoms associated with *endocrine* pathology may include changes in body or skin temperature, dry mouth, dizziness, weight change, or excessive sweating.

Perhaps the PTA observes dry skin, brittle nails, cold or heat intolerance, or excessive hair loss and realizes that these signs could be pointing to an endocrine problem. At the very least the PTA recognizes that the clinical presentation is not something associated with the musculoskeletal or neuromuscular systems.

The presence of constitutional symptoms is always a red flag that must be observed carefully (Box 1.3). Being aware of signs

---

BOX 1.3 Constitutional Symptoms

Fever
Diaphoresis (unexplained perspiration)
Sweats (can occur anytime night or day)
Nausea
Vomiting
Diarrhea
Pallor
Dizziness/syncope (fainting)
Fatigue
Weight loss

---

and symptoms associated with each system may help the PTA make an early report back to the therapist. The therapist can use this information to classify groups of signs and symptoms and is, therefore, more likely to recognize a problem outside the scope of physical therapy practice, thus making a timely referral.

SUMMARY

The following is a summary of materials presented in this introductory chapter as well as a sneak preview of information that will be covered in subsequent chapters.

▶▶ PTA ACTION PLAN

Consultation With the Therapist

Experts agree that red flags are important, and ignoring them can result in morbidity and even mortality for some individuals. On the other hand, accepting them uncritically can result in unnecessary referrals.[34] Until the evidence supporting or refuting red flags is complete, the PTA is advised to consider all findings in the context of the total picture.

Consultation with the therapist is advised when:

- Client with anginal pain not relieved in 20 minutes with reduced activity and/or administration of nitroglycerin; angina at rest
- Client with angina has nausea, vomiting, or profuse sweating
- Client presents with bowel/bladder incontinence and/or saddle anesthesia resulting from cauda equina lesion or cervical spine pain concomitant with urinary incontinence
- Client with diabetes appears confused or lethargic or exhibits changes in mental function
- Client shows a sudden worsening of intermittent claudication (which may be due to thromboembolism and must be reported immediately)
- Client has throbbing chest, back, or abdominal pain that increases with exertion, accompanied by a sensation of a heartbeat when lying down and palpable pulsating abdominal mass (which may indicate an aneurysm)
- Lack of expected progress with physical therapy intervention or condition gets worse with treatment[5]
- Development of constitutional symptoms or associated signs and symptoms at any time during the episode of care
- Discovery of significant past medical history unknown to the therapist
- Changes in health status that persist 7 to 10 days beyond the expected time period
- Client who is jaundiced and has not been diagnosed or treated
- Low back, hip, pelvic, groin, or sacroiliac symptoms without known cause in the presence of constitutional symptoms
- Symptoms correlated with menses
- Uterine bleeding after menopause
- For pregnant females:
  - Vaginal bleeding
  - Elevated blood pressure
  - Increased Braxton-Hicks (uterine) contractions in a pregnant female during exercise
- New onset of acute back pain in anyone with a previous history of cancer
- Bone pain, especially on weight bearing, that persists more than 1 week and is worse at night
- Any unexplained bleeding from any area

Report These Findings: Vital Signs
- Persistent rise or fall of blood pressure
- Blood pressure elevation in any female taking birth control pills
- Pulse increase over 20 bpm lasting more than 3 minutes after rest or changing position

- Difference in pulse pressure (between systolic and diastolic measurements) of more than 40 mm Hg
- Persistent low-grade (or higher) fever, especially associated with constitutional symptoms, most commonly sweats
- Any unexplained fever without other systemic symptoms, especially in the person taking corticosteroids

Requires Reevaluation by the Therapist
Cardiac
- More than three sublingual nitroglycerin tablets required to gain relief from angina
- Angina continues to increase in intensity after stimulus (e.g., cold, stress, exertion) has been eliminated
- Changes in pattern of angina
- Abnormally severe chest pain
- Anginal pain radiates to jaw/left arm
- Client has any doubts about his or her condition
- Report of heart or chest palpitations
- Anyone who cannot climb a single flight of stairs without feeling moderately to severely winded or who awakens at night or experiences shortness of breath when lying down should be reevaluated by the therapist
- Anyone with known cardiac involvement who develops progressively worse dyspnea should be reevaluated by the therapist
- Fainting (syncope) without any warning period of lightheadedness, dizziness, or nausea may be a sign of heart valve or arrhythmia problems; unexplained syncope in the presence of heart or circulatory problems(or risk factors for heart attack or stroke) should be reevaluated by the therapist

Pulmonary
- Shoulder pain aggravated by respiratory movements; change in shoulder pain/symptoms with breath holding or the Valsalva maneuver may be a sign of pulmonary or cardiac source of symptoms and requires reevaluation by the therapist
- Shoulder pain that is aggravated by supine positioning; pain that is worse when lying down and improves when sitting up or leaning forward can be pleuritic in origin (abdominal contents push up against diaphragm and, in turn, against parietal pleura); requires reevaluation by the therapist
- Shoulder or chest (thorax) pain that subsides with autosplinting (lying on painful side)
- For the client with asthma: Signs of asthma or abnormal bronchial activity during exercise
- Weak and rapid pulse accompanied by fall in blood pressure (pneumothorax)
- Presence of associated signs and symptoms, such as persistent cough, dyspnea (rest or exertional), or constitutional symptoms (see Box 1.3)

▶▶ PTA ACTION PLAN—cont'd

Consultation With the Therapist

Genitourinary

- Patient/client reports (or PTA observes):
  - Abnormal urinary constituents (e.g., change in color, odor, amount, flow of urine)
  - Any amount of blood in urine
  - Cervical spine pain accompanied by urinary incontinence (unless cervical disk protrusion already has been medically diagnosed)

Gastrointestinal

- New onset (or symptoms previously unreported) of back pain and abdominal pain at the same level, especially when accompanied by constitutional symptoms
- New onset of back pain of unknown cause in a person with a history of cancer
- Back pain or shoulder pain in a person taking NSAIDs, especially when accompanied by gastrointestinal upset or blood in the stools
- Back or shoulder pain associated with meals or back pain relieved by a bowel movement
- Symptoms that seem out of proportion to the injury or symptoms persisting beyond the expected time for the nature of the injury

- Severe or progressive back pain accompanied by constitutional symptoms, especially fever
- New onset of joint pain following surgery with inflammatory signs (warmth, redness, tenderness, swelling)

Precautions/Contraindications to Therapy: Consultation with the Therapist Is Required

- Resting heart rate 120 or 130 bpm[a]
- Resting systolic rate 180 to 200 mm Hg[a]
- Resting diastolic rate 105 to 110 mm Hg[a]
- Moderate dizziness, near syncope
- Marked dyspnea
- Unusual fatigue
- Unsteadiness
- Irregular pulse with symptoms of dizziness, nausea, or shortness of breath or loss of palpable pulse
- Postoperative posterior calf pain
- For the client with diabetes: Unstable blood sugar level (acceptable fasting target glucose range: 60 to 110 mg/dL; precaution: <70 or >250 mg/dL)

[a] Unexplained or poorly tolerated by the client.

REFERENCES

1. Bogduk N: *Evidence-based clinical guidelines for the management of acute low back pain,* The National Musculoskeletal Medicine Initiative, 1999, National Health and Medical Research Council.
2. McGuirk B, King W, Govind J, et al: Safety, efficacy, and cost effectiveness of evidence-based guidelines for the management of acute low back pain in primary care, *Spine* 26(23):2615–2622, 2001.
3. Waddell G, editor: *The back pain revolution* ed 2, Edinburgh, 2004, Churchill Livingstone.
4. Siemionow K, Steinmetz M, Bell G, et al: Identifying serious causes of back pain: cancer, infection, fracture, *Cleve Clin J Med* 75(8):557–566, 2008.
5. Ross MD, Boissonnault WG: Red flags: to screen or not to screen? *JOSPT* 40(11):682–684, 2010.
6. Underwood M: Diagnosing acute nonspecific low back pain: time to lower the red flags? *Arthritis Rheum* 60(10):2855–2857, 2009.
7. Henschke N: Prevalence of and screening for serious spinal pathology in patients presenting to primary care settings with acute low back pain, *Arthritis Rheum* 60(10):3072–3080, 2009.
8. Moffett J, McLean S: The role of physiotherapy in the management of non-specific back pain and neck pain, *Rheumatology* 45(4):371–378, 2006.
9. Henschke N: Screening for malignancy in low back pain patients: a systematic review, *Eur Spine J* 16:1673–1679, 2007.
10. Henschke N: A systematic review identifies five "red flags" to screen for vertebral fractures in patients with low back pain, *J Clin Epidemiol* 61:110–118, 2008.
11. Goodman CC, Kapasi Z: The effect of exercise on the immune system, *Rehab Oncol* 20(1):13–26, 2002.
12. Malm C, Celsing F, Friman G: Immune defense is both stimulated and inhibited by physical activity, *Lakartidningen* 102(11): 867–873, 2005.
13. Kohut ML, Senchina DS: Reversing age-associated immunosenescence via exercise, *Exerc Immunol Rev* 10:6–41, 2004.
14. Radom-Aizik S: Impact of brief exercise on peripheral blood NKk cell gene and microRNA expression in young adults, *J Appl Physiol* 114(5):628–636, 2013.
15. Terra R: Exercise improves the Th1 response by modulating cytokine and NO production in BALB/c mice, *Int J Sports Med* 34(7):661–666, 2013.
16. Ertek S: Impact of physical activity on inflammation: effects on cardiovascular disease risk and other inflammatory conditions, *Arch Med Sci* 8(5):794–804, 2012.
17. Sinnott M: Challenges 2000: Acute care/hospital clinical practice, *PT Magazine* 8(1):43–46, 2000.
18. Qian X: "Quicker and sicker" under Medicare's prospective payment system for hospitals: new evidence on an old issue from a national longitudinal survey, *Bull Econ Res* 63(1):1–27, 2011.
19. Morris PE: Moving our critically ill patients: mobility barriers and benefits, *Crit Care Clin* 23:1–20, 2007.
20. Dammeyer J: Building a protocol to guide mobility in the ICU, *Crit Care Nurs Q* 36(1):37–49, 2013.
21. Pawlik AJ, Kress JP: Issues affecting the delivery of physical therapy services for individuals with critical illness, *Phys Ther* 93(2):256–265, 2013.
22. Drolet A, DeJuilio P, Harkless S, et al: Move to improve: the feasibility of using an early mobility protocol to increase ambulation in the intensive and intermediate care settings, *Phys Ther* 93(2):197–207, 2013.
23. United Nations, Department of Economic and Social Affairs, Population Division: *World Population Ageing 2015. (ST/ESA/SER.A/390),* New York, 2015, United Nations.
24. National Center for Health Statistics: *Health, United States, 2020–2021: annual perspective.* Hyattsville, 2023. https://doi.org/10.15620/cdc:122044.

25. American Physical Therapy Association: *Guide to physical therapist practice*, ed 2 (rev), Alexandria, VA, 2003, APTA.

26. Arriaga R: Stories from the front, Part II: Complex medical history and communication, *PT Magazine* 11(7):23–25, 2003.

27. American Physical Therapy Association: *APTA guide for conduct of the physical therapist assistant*. http://www.apta.org/Ethics/Core/. Accessed July 16, 2023.

28. Management of the individual with pain: I. Physiology and evaluation, *PT Magazine* 4(11):54–63, 1996.

29. Goodman CC, Snyder TE: *Differential diagnosis for physical therapists: screening for referral*, ed 5, Philadelphia, 2013, WB Saunders.

30. Gonzalez-Urzelai V, Palacio-Elua L, Lopez-de-Munain J: Routine primary care management of acute low back pain: adherence to clinical guidelines, *Eur Spine J* 12(6):589–594, 2003.

31. Sandler G: The importance of the history in the medical clinic and cost of unnecessary tests, *Am Heart J* 100:928–931, 1980.

32. Ohm F, Vogel D, Sehner S, Wijnen-Meijer M, Harendza S: Details acquired from medical history and patients' experience of empathy – two sides of the same coin, *BMC Med Educ* 13:67, 2013.

33. Lim SS, Vos T, Flaxman AD, et al: A comparative risk assessment of burden of disease and injury attributable to 67 risk factors and risk factor clusters in 21 regions, 1990-2010: a systematic analysis for the Global Burden of Disease Study 2010, *Lancet* 380(9859):2224–2260, 2013.

34. Moffett J, McLean S: Red flags need more evaluation: reply, *Rheumatology* 45(7):921, 2006.

2

Pain Types and Viscerogenic Pain Patterns

INTRODUCTION

In 2018 the International Association for the Study of Pain formed a task force to evaluate and update both the definition of pain and supportive six key notes related to pain, due to the many advances in our understanding of pain. The updated definition is now stated as "An unpleasant sensory and emotional experience associated with, or resembling that associated with, actual or potential tissue damage."[1] Pain is often the primary symptom the physical therapist assistant (PTA) hears about daily. Pain is now recognized as the "fifth vital sign,"[2–4] along with blood pressure, temperature, pulse, and respiration. Pain assessment is a key feature in the interview and evaluation of physical therapists (PTs).

Recognizing pain patterns that are characteristic of systemic disease is a necessary skill for all health care professionals, including the PTA. Understanding how and when diseased organs can refer pain to the neuromusculoskeletal (NMS) system helps the PTA recognize and report suspicious pain patterns.

This chapter includes a detailed overview of pain patterns that can be used as a foundation for all of the organ systems presented, as well as a discussion of pain types in general and, specifically, viscerogenic (related to the visceral organs) pain patterns. Each section discusses specific pain patterns characteristic of visceral or systemic diseases that can mimic pain from musculoskeletal or neuromuscular disorders.

The PTA must be prepared to listen to information regarding the location, referral pattern, description, frequency, intensity, and duration of systemic pain and must provide accurate and important feedback to the therapist. Knowledge of associated symptoms and relieving and aggravating factors aids the PTA in quickly recognizing what does not fit the expected patient report of current symptoms or response to treatment provided by the PTA.

The back and shoulder are the most common sites of referred pain from a systemic disease process. However, the scapula, upper extremity, pelvis, hip, groin, sacroiliac (SI) joint, and lower extremity can also be affected.

MECHANISMS OF REFERRED VISCERAL PAIN

The neurology of visceral pain is not well understood at this time.[5] Proposed models are based on what is known about the somatic (nonvisceral) sensory system. Scientists have not found actual nerve fibers and specific nociceptors in organs, but rather multiple different pain mechanisms. These mechanisms are beyond the scope of this text but still of interest, such as viscero-visceral convergence; viscero-somatic convergence; hypertonicity of nearby muscles, creating visceral symptoms along with somato-visceral convergence; and central sensitization with expansion of adjacent receptive fields.[6–8]

Research is ongoing to identify the sites and mechanisms of visceral nociception. During inflammation, increased nociceptive input from an inflamed organ can sensitize neurons that receive convergent input from an unaffected organ.[9,10] Mechanisms of viscero-visceral hyperalgesia between organs and referred to soft tissues probably involve sensitization of viscero-viscero-somatic (sensory) convergent neurons.[11]

Viscerosensory fibers ascend the anterolateral system to the thalamus with fibers projecting to several regions of the brain. These regions encode the site of origin of visceral pain, although they do it poorly because of low receptor density, large overlapping receptive fields, and extensive convergence in the ascending pathway. Thus the cortex cannot distinguish the origin of the pain messages.[12,13]

There are a wide number of gastrointestinal (GI) sensations that are conveyed by the afferent nerves to the central nervous system (CNS) ranging from hunger, satiety, fullness, discomfort to pain, urgency, and the need to defecate. The afferent pathway has multiple specialized endings at different levels of the gut that signal these specific sensations to the brain.[14] Studies show that there may be multiple mechanisms operating at different sites to produce the sensation we refer to as "pain." The same symptom can be produced by different mechanisms and a single mechanism may cause different symptoms.

In the case of referred pain patterns of viscera, at least three separate phenomena must be considered from a traditional Western medicine approach:
- Embryologic development
- Multisegmental innervation
- Direct pressure and shared pathways

Embryologic Development

Each system has a bit of its own uniqueness in how pain is referred. For example, the viscera in the abdomen comprise a large percentage of all the organs we have to consider. When a person gives a history of abdominal pain, the location of the pain may not be directly over the involved organ (Fig. 2.1).

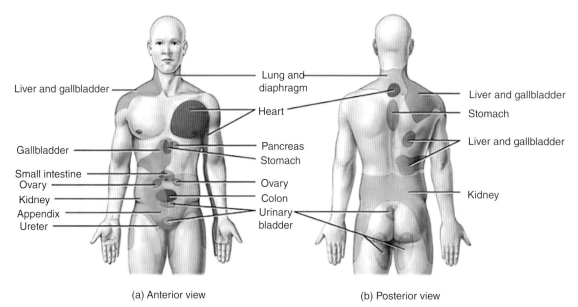

(a) Anterior view   (b) Posterior view

FIG. 2.1 Common sites of referred pain from the abdominal viscera. When a client gives a history of referred pain from the viscera, the pain's location may not be directly over the impaired organ. Visceral embryologic development is the mechanism of the referred pain pattern. Pain is referred to the site where the organ was located in fetal development. (From Orchard Health Clinic (https://www.orchardhealthclinic.com/ohc-truths-11-visceral-referred-pain/.)

Functional magnetic resonance imaging and other neuroimaging methods have shown that the brain has a role in visceral pain patterns.[15–18] However, it is likely that embryologic development has the primary role in referred pain patterns for the viscera. Pain is referred to a site where the organ was located in fetal development. Although the organ migrates during fetal development, its nerves persist in referring sensations from the former location.

Embryologically, the chest is part of the gut. In other words, they are formed from the same tissue in utero. This explains symptoms of intrathoracic organ pathology frequently being referred to the abdomen as a viscero-viscero reflex. For example, it is not unusual for disorders of thoracic viscera, such as pneumonia or pleuritis, to refer pain that is perceived in the abdomen instead of the chest.[19,20] The pericardium around the heart is formed from gut tissue. This explains why myocardial infarction (MI) or pericarditis can also refer pain to the abdomen.[19,20]

The ear and the kidney are two other examples of how embryologic development impacts the viscera and the soma. These two structures have the same shape since they come from the same embryologic tissue (otorenal axis of the mesenchyme) and are formed at the same time (Fig. 2.2).[21]

When a child is born with any anomaly of the ear(s) or even a missing ear, the medical staff knows to look for possible similar changes or absence of the kidney on the same side.

A thorough understanding of fetal embryology is not really necessary to recognize red-flag signs and symptoms of visceral origin. Knowing that it is one of several mechanisms by which the visceral referred pain patterns occur is a helpful start.

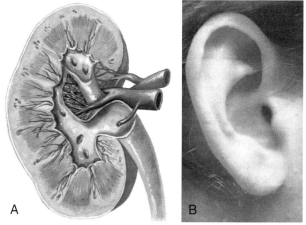

FIG. 2.2 The ear (B) and the kidney (A) have the same shape since they are formed at the same time and from the same embryologic tissue (otorenal axis of the mesenchyme). This is just one example of how fetal development influences form and function. When a child is born with a deformed or missing ear, the medical staff looks for a similarly deformed or missing kidney on the same side. (From Anderson KN: *Mosby's medical, nursing & allied health dictionary*, ed 5, St. Louis, 1988, Mosby, p A-39; Seidel HM, Ball JW, Dains JE, et al.: *Mosby's physical examination handbook*, St. Louis, 2003, Mosby.)

Multisegmental Innervation

Multisegmental innervation is the second mechanism used to explain pain patterns of a viscerogenic source (Fig. 2.3). The autonomic nervous system (ANS) is part of the peripheral nervous system. As shown in this diagram, the viscera have multisegmental innervations. The multiple levels of innervation of the heart, bronchi, stomach, kidneys, intestines, and bladder are demonstrated clearly.

There is new evidence to support referred visceral pain to somatic tissues based on overlapping or same segmental projections of spinal afferent neurons to the spinal dorsal horn. This concept (previously mentioned) is referred to as *visceral-organ cross-sensitization*. The mechanism is likely to be sensitization of viscera-somatic convergent neurons.[11]

For the first time ever, scientists showed that individuals diagnosed with multiple visceral problems obtained relief from pain in all organ systems with overlapping segmental projections when only one visceral area was treated. In other words, nontreated visceral disease significantly decreased when one viscera of the overlapping segments was addressed. For groups of people with no overlapping segments, spontaneous relief of referred pain was not obtained until and unless all involved visceral systems were treated.[11]

? PICTURE THE PATIENT

Pain of a visceral origin can be referred to the corresponding somatic areas. The example of cardiac pain is a good one. Cardiac pain is not felt in the heart but is referred to areas supplied by the corresponding spinal nerves.

Instead of actual physical heart pain, cardiac pain can occur in any structure innervated by C3 to T4 such as the jaw, neck, upper trapezius, shoulder, and arm. Pain of cardiac and diaphragmatic origin is often experienced in the shoulder, in particular, because the C5 spinal segment supplies the heart, respiratory diaphragm, and shoulder.[22]

Direct Pressure and Shared Pathways

A third and final mechanism by which the viscera refer pain to the body (soma) is the concept of direct pressure and shared pathways. As shown in Fig. 2.4, many of the viscera are near the respiratory diaphragm. Any pathologic process that can

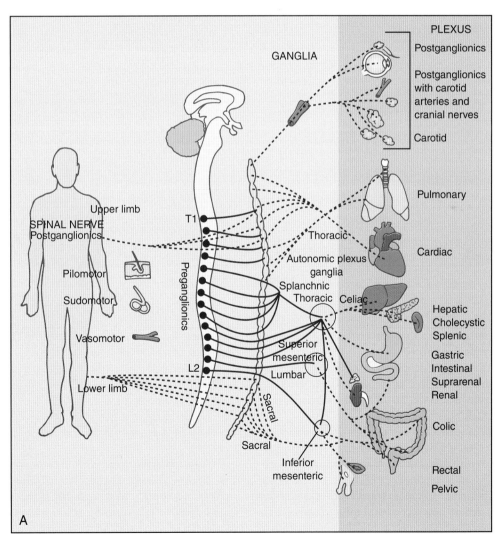

FIG. 2.3 Sympathetic (**A**) and parasympathetic (**B**) divisions of the autonomic nervous system. The visceral afferent fibers mediating pain travel with the sympathetic nerves, except for those from the pelvic organs, which follow the parasympathetics of the pelvic nerve. Major visceral organs have multisegmental innervations overlapping innervations of somatic structures. Visceral pain can be referred to the corresponding somatic area because sensory fibers for the viscera and somatic structures enter the spinal cord at the same levels, converging on the same neurons. (From Levy MN, Koeppen BM: *Berne and Levy principles of physiology*, ed 4, St. Louis, 2006, Mosby.)

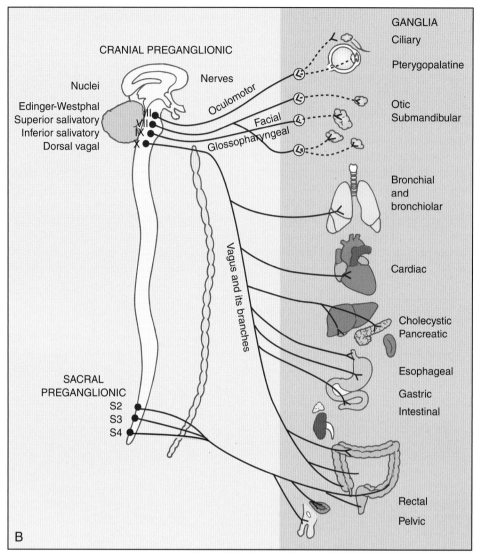

CRANIAL PREGANGLIONIC

Nuclei
Edinger-Westphal
Superior salivatory
Inferior salivatory
Dorsal vagal

VII
IX
X

Nerves
Oculomotor
Facial
Glossopharyngeal

Vagus and its branches

SACRAL
PREGANGLIONIC
S2
S3
S4

B

GANGLIA
Ciliary
Pterygopalatine
Otic
Submandibular
Bronchial
and
bronchiolar
Cardiac
Cholecystic
Pancreatic
Esophageal
Gastric
Intestinal
Rectal
Pelvic

FIG. 2.3, cont'd

inflame, infect, or obstruct the organs can bring them in contact with the respiratory diaphragm.

Anything that impinges the *central diaphragm* can refer pain to the *shoulder*, and anything that impinges the *peripheral diaphragm* can refer pain to the *ipsilateral costal margins* and/or *lumbar region* (Fig. 2.5).

This mechanism of referred pain through shared pathways occurs as a result of ganglions from each neural system gathering and sharing information through the cord to the plexuses. The visceral organs are innervated through the ANS. The ganglions bring in information from around the body; the nerve plexuses decide how to respond to this information (what to do) and give the body finely tuned, local control over responses.

Plexuses originate in the neck, thorax, diaphragm, and abdomen, terminating in the pelvis. The brachial plexus supplies the upper neck and shoulder, whereas the phrenic nerve innervates the respiratory diaphragm. More distally, the celiac plexus supplies the stomach and intestines. The neurologic supply of the

plexuses is from parasympathetic fibers from the vagus and pelvic splanchnic nerves.[22,23]

The plexuses work independently of each other but not independently of the ganglia. The ganglia collect information derived from both the parasympathetic and the sympathetic fibers. The ganglia deliver this information to the plexuses, which in turn provide fine, local control in each of the organ systems.[22]

For example, the lower portion of the heart is in contact with the center of the diaphragm. The spleen on the left side of the body is tucked up under the dome of the diaphragm. The kidneys (on either side) and the pancreas in the center are within easy reach of some portion of the diaphragm.

The body of the pancreas is in the center of the human body. The tail rests on the left side of the body. If an infection, inflammation, or tumor or other obstruction distends the pancreas, it can put pressure on the central part of the diaphragm.

Since the phrenic nerve (C3–5) innervates the central zone of the diaphragm, as well as part of the pericardium, the

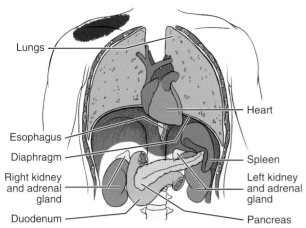

FIG. 2.4 Direct pressure from any inflamed, infected, or obstructed organ in contact with the respiratory diaphragm can refer pain to the ipsilateral shoulder. Note the location of each of the viscera. The spleen is tucked up under the diaphragm on the left side so any impairment of the spleen can cause left shoulder pain. The tail of the pancreas can come in contact with the diaphragm on the left side potentially causing referred pain to the left shoulder. The head of the pancreas can impinge the right side of the diaphragm, causing referred pain to the right side. The gallbladder (not shown) is located up under the liver on the right side with corresponding right referred shoulder pain possible. Other organs that can come in contact with the diaphragm in this way include the heart and the kidneys.

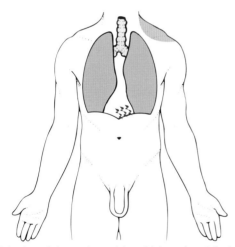

FIG. 2.5 Irritation of the peritoneal (outside) or pleural (inside) surface of the central area of the respiratory diaphragm can refer sharp pain to the upper trapezius muscle, neck, and supraclavicular fossa. The pain pattern is ipsilateral to the area of irritation. Irritation of the peripheral portion of the diaphragm can refer sharp pain to the costal margins and lumbar region (not shown).

gallbladder, and the pancreas, the client with impairment of these viscera can present with signs and symptoms in any of the somatic areas supplied by C3–C5 (e.g., shoulder).[24]

In other words, the person can experience symptoms in the areas innervated by the same nerve pathways. For example, a problem affecting the pancreas can look like a heart problem, a gallbladder problem, or a mid-back/scapular or shoulder problem.

Another example of this same phenomenon occurs with peritonitis or gallbladder inflammation. These conditions can irritate the phrenic endings in the central part of the diaphragmatic peritoneum. The client can experience referred shoulder pain as a result of the root origin shared in common by the phrenic and supraclavicular nerves.

Not only is it true that any structure that touches the diaphragm can refer pain to the shoulder, but even structures adjacent to or in contact with the diaphragm in utero can do the same. Keep in mind that there has to be some impairment of that structure (e.g., obstruction, distention, inflammation) for this to occur (Case Example 2.1).

UNDERSTANDING PAIN AND OTHER SYMPTOMS

The information gathered during the time the PTA is with the patient or client helps provide a description of the individual that is clear, accurate, and comprehensive. The PTA should keep in mind cultural rules and differences in pain perception, intensity, and responses to pain found among various ethnic groups.[25] Pain may also be a factor in levels of physical activity for older adults of various racial/ethnic differences.[26]

To gather a more complete description of symptoms from the client, the PTA may wish to use a term other than *pain* when talking with the person. For example, referring to the client's *symptoms* or using descriptors such as *hurt* or *sore* may be more helpful with some individuals. *Burning, tightness, heaviness, discomfort,* and *aching* are just a few examples of other possible word choices. The use of alternative words to describe a client's symptoms may also aid in refocusing attention away from pain and toward improvement of functional abilities.

Pain in the Older Adult

Pain is an accepted part of the aging process, but we must be careful to take the reports of pain from older persons as serious and very real and not discount the symptoms as part of aging. Well over half (up to 62%) of the older adults in the United States report chronic joint symptoms.[27–29] We are likely to see pain more often as a key feature among older adults as our population continues to age.

The American Geriatrics Society (AGS) reports that the use of over-the-counter (OTC) analgesic medications for pain, aching, and discomfort is common in older adults along with routine use of prescription drugs. Many older adults have taken these medications for 6 months or more.[30,31]

Older adults may avoid giving an accurate accounting of their pain. Some may expect pain with aging or fear that talking about pain will lead to expensive tests or medications with unwanted side effects. Fear of losing one's independence may lead others to underreport pain symptoms.[32] In working with the PTA, the client/patient may let down his or her guard and reveal additional information previously unknown or unreported to the PT or physician.

CASE EXAMPLE 2.1   Mechanism of Referred Pain

A 72-year-old female has come to physical therapy for rehabilitation after cutting her hand and having a flexor tendon repair. She uses a walker to ambulate, reports being short of breath "her whole life," and takes the following prescription and over-the-counter medications:

- Piroxicam (Feldene)
- Celecoxib (Celebrex, a cyclooxygenase-2 [COX-2] inhibitor)
- Lorazepam (Ativan)
- Glucosamine
- Ibuprofen ("on bad days")
- Furosemide
- One other big pill once a week on Sunday ("for my bones")

The physical therapist (PT) reports in the initial evaluation that during the course of evaluating and treating her hand, she reported constant, aching pain in her right shoulder and a sharp, tingling, burning sensation behind her armpit (also on the right side). She does not have any associated bowel or bladder signs and symptoms, but reports excessive fatigue "since the day I was born."

The PT took this opportunity to directly involve the physical therapist assistant (PTA) to provide education on a mechanism of referred pain. The PT told the PTA that he suspects the combination of feldene and ibuprofen along with long-term use of Celebrex may be a problem for this patient. The PT continues the education opportunity by providing the PTA with the following important information regarding his medication concerns.

Even though Celebrex is a COX-2 inhibitor and less likely to cause problems, gastritis and gastrointestinal bleeding are still possible, especially with chronic long-term use of multiple nonsteroidal antiinflammatory drugs (NSAIDs).

Retroperitoneal bleeding from peptic ulcer can cause referred pain to the back at the level of the lesion (T6–10) or right shoulder and/or upper trapezius pain. Shoulder pain may be accompanied by sudomotor changes such as burning, gnawing, or cramping pain along the lateral border of the scapula. The scapular pain can occur alone as the only symptom.

Side effects of NSAIDs can include fatigue, anxiety, depression, paresthesia, fluid retention, tinnitus, nausea, vomiting, dry mouth, and bleeding from the nose, mouth, or under the skin.

The PT describes the mechanism of referred pain pattern pertinent to this patient as the following: if peritoneal bleeding is the cause of her symptoms, the mechanism of pain is blood in the posterior abdominal cavity irritating the diaphragm through direct pressure.

The PT requests that the PTA be sure to take the client's vital signs and observe for significant changes in blood pressure and pulse during the next follow-up treatment. Poor wound healing and edema (sacral, pedal, hands) may be present. The PTA is instructed to ask the patient if the same doctor prescribed each medication and if her physician(s) knows which medications she is taking. It is possible that her medications have not been checked or coordinated from before her hospitalization to the present time.

This case example demonstrates the importance of appropriate direct communication and education that can be provided by the PT to the PTA.

▷▷ PTA ACTION PLAN

Maintain Patient/Client Confidentiality

The PTA needs to keep in mind the role of confidential communication between the PTA and PT. There will be times when the PTA simply needs to explain to the client that there might be things that he or she will need to share with the primary PT. Any time a PTA is working with a client who begins to share information that is important for the safe and effective progression of the physical therapy plan of care, the PTA is responsible for reminding the client that it will be communicated confidentially to the PT in a way that will be professional and directly related to the physical therapy goals.

Sensory and cognitive impairment in older, frail adults can make communication about pain difficult.[30,31] Someone with Alzheimer-type dementia loses short-term memory and cannot always identify the source of recent painful stimuli.[32,33] The PTA can provide helpful information about the frequency, intensity, and duration of the client's discomfort based on the presence of noisy breathing, facial expressions, and overall body language

🛈 PICTURE THE PATIENT

Facial grimacing; nonverbal vocalization such as moans, sighs, or gasps; and verbal comments (e.g., "Ouch," "Stop") are the most frequent behaviors among cognitively impaired older adults during painful movement (Box 2.1). Bracing, holding onto furniture, or clutching the painful area are other behavioral indicators of pain. Alternatively, the client may resist care by others or stay very still to guard against pain caused by movement.[34]

BOX 2.1   Symptoms of Pain in Clients With Cognitive Impairment

- Verbal comments (e.g., "Ouch" or "Stop")
- Nonverbal vocalizations (e.g., moans, sighs, gasps)
- Facial grimacing or frowning
- Audible breathing independent of vocalization (labored, short or long periods of hyperventilation)
- Agitation or increased confusion
- Inability to be consoled or distracted
- Bracing or holding onto furniture
- Decreased mobility
- Lying very still, refusing to move
- Clutching the painful area
- Resisting care provided by others, striking out, pushing others away
- Sleep disturbance
- Weight loss
- Depression

Untreated pain in an older adult with advanced dementia can lead to secondary problems such as sleep disturbances, weight loss, dehydration, and depression. Pain may be manifested as agitation and increased confusion.[35,36]

Older adults are more likely than younger adults to have what is referred to as atypical acute pain. For example, silent acute MI occurs more often in the older adult than in the middle-aged to early senior adult. Likewise, the older adult is more likely to experience appendicitis without any abdominal or pelvic pain.[37]

⟫ PTA ACTION PLAN
Communication With the Physical Therapist

When the PTA prepares to report back to the PT regarding pain patterns in a client who presents with sensory or cognitive impairments, it is important to include behavior changes or visual signs that occur with the onset of pain. The PTA might also do some investigating with family members or nursing staff to find patterns in behavior related to positioning, activity level, or time of day that will be helpful to the PT during the follow-up examination.

Characteristics of Pain

As previously mentioned, patients/clients will share many characteristics of pain with the PTA during their time together. Understanding the following characteristics of visceral and systemic pain patterns will aid the PTA in knowing what to report to the PT:

- Location
- Description of sensation
- Intensity
- Duration
- Frequency
- Pattern

Other additional components are related to factors that aggravate the pain, factors that relieve the pain, and other symptoms that may occur in association with the pain. Specific questions are included in this section for each descriptive component. Keep in mind that an increase in frequency, intensity, or duration of symptoms over time can indicate systemic disease.

Location of Pain

Questions related to the location of pain focus on the client's description as precisely as possible.

⟫ PTA ACTION PLAN
Follow-Up Questions

An opening statement might be as follows:
- Show me exactly where your pain is located.

Follow-up questions may include the following:
- Do you have other pain or symptoms anywhere else?
- If yes, what causes the pain or symptoms to occur in this other area?

If the client points to a small, localized area and the pain does not spread, the cause is likely to be a superficial lesion and is probably not severe. If the client points to a small, localized area but the pain does spread, this is more likely to be a diffuse, segmental, referred pain that may originate in the viscera or deep somatic structure.

The character and location of pain can change and the client may have several pains at once, so repeated pain assessment may be needed.

Description of Pain

To assist in providing the PT with a clear description of pain sensation, it may be helpful to pose the following questions.

⟫ PTA ACTION PLAN
Follow-Up Questions

- What does it feel like?
  After giving the client time to reply, offer some additional choices in potential descriptors. You may want to ask if the pain or symptoms are:
- Knife-like
- Dull
- Boring
- Burning
- Throbbing
- Prickly
- Deep aching
- Sharp

Follow-up questions may include:
- Has the pain changed in quality since it first began?
- Has the pain changed in intensity?
- Has the pain changed in duration (how long it lasts)?

? PICTURE THE PATIENT

When a person describes the pain as knife-like, boring, colicky, coming in waves, or a deep aching feeling, this description may be a signal of a systemic origin of symptoms. Dull, somatic pain of an aching nature can be differentiated from the aching pain of a muscular lesion by squeezing or by pressing the muscle overlying the area of pain.[37] Resisting motion of the limb may also reproduce aching of muscular origin that has no connection to deep somatic aching.

Intensity of Pain

The PTA should assist the patient/client with this assessment by providing a rating scale; depending on the clinical presentation of each client, one or more of these scales can be used. The PTA should show the pain scale to the client and ask the client to choose a number and/or a face that best describes his or her current pain level. This scale can be used to quantify symptoms other than pain, such as stiffness, pressure, soreness, discomfort, cramping, aching, numbness, and tingling. The same scale should always be used for each follow-up assessment.

The visual analog scale (VAS)[38,39] allows the client to choose a point along a 10-cm (100-mm) horizontal line. The left end represents "no pain" and the right end represents "pain as bad as it could possibly be" or "worst possible pain." This same scale can be presented in a vertical orientation for the client who must remain supine and cannot sit up for the assessment. "No pain" is placed at the bottom, and "worst possible pain" is put at the top.

The numeric rating scale allows the client to rate the pain intensity on a scale from 0 ("no pain") to 10 ("worst pain imaginable"). This is probably the most commonly used pain rating scale in both the inpatient and outpatient settings. It is a simple and valid method of measuring pain. The VAS scale is easily combined with the numeric rating scale with possible values ranging from 0 (no pain) to 10 (worst imaginable pain). It can be used to assess current pain, worst pain in the preceding 24 hours, least pain in the past 24 hours, or any combination the clinician finds useful.

Although the scale was tested and standardized using 0 to 10, the plus is used for clients who indicate the pain is "off the scale" or "higher than a 10." Some health care professionals prefer to describe 10 as the "worst pain experienced with this condition" to avoid needing a higher number than 10. This scale is especially helpful for children or cognitively impaired clients. In general, even adults without cognitive impairments may prefer to use this scale.

An alternative method provides a scale of 1 to 5 with word descriptions for each number[40] and asks about the following conditions.

Frequency and Duration of Pain

The frequency of occurrence is related closely to the pattern of the pain, and the client should be asked how often the symptoms occur and whether the pain is constant or intermittent. Duration of pain is a part of this description.

▶▶ PTA ACTION PLAN
Follow-Up Questions

- How long do the symptoms last?
  For example, pain related to systemic disease has been shown to be a constant rather than an intermittent type of pain experience. Clients who indicate that the pain is constant should be asked:
- Do you have this pain right now?
- Did you notice these symptoms this morning immediately when you woke up?

Further responses may reveal that the pain is perceived as being constant but, in fact, is not actually present consistently and/or can be reduced with rest or change in position, which are characteristics more common with pain of musculoskeletal origin. Symptoms that truly do not change throughout the course of the day warrant further attention.

Pattern of Pain

The following sequence of questions may be helpful in further assessing the pattern of pain, especially how the symptoms may change with time.

▶▶ PTA ACTION PLAN
Follow-Up Questions

- Tell me about the pattern of your pain/symptoms.
- *Alternative question:* When does your (name the involved body part) hurt?
- *Alternative question:* Describe your pain/symptoms from first waking up in the morning to going to bed at night. (See special sleep-related questions that follow.)
  Follow-up questions may include:
- Have you ever experienced anything like this before?
- If yes, do these episodes occur more or less often than at first?
- How does your pain/symptom(s) change with time?
- Are your symptoms worse in the morning or evening?

The pattern of pain associated with systemic disease is often a progressive pattern with a cyclical onset (i.e., the client describes

symptoms as being alternately worse, better, and worse over a period of months).

Medications can alter the pain pattern or characteristics of painful symptoms. The PTA should find out how well the client's current medications reduce, control, or relieve pain, and should ask how often medications are needed for breakthrough pain.

When using any of the pain rating scales, the PTA should record the use of any medications that can alter or reduce pain or symptoms, such as antiinflammatory drugs or analgesics, while, at the same time, remembering to look for side effects or adverse reactions to any drugs or drug combinations.

The PTA needs to watch for clients taking nonsteroidal antiinflammatory drugs (NSAIDs) who experience an increase in shoulder, neck, or back pain several hours after taking the medication. Normally, one would expect symptom relief from NSAIDs, so any increase in symptoms may be a red flag.

A client will frequently comment that the pain or symptoms have not changed despite 2 or 3 weeks of physical therapy intervention. This information can be discouraging to both client and PTA; however, when the symptoms are reviewed, a decrease in pain, increase in function, reduced need for medications, or other significant improvement in the pattern of symptoms may be seen.

▶▶ PTA ACTION PLAN
Document Baseline Pain Assessment

The improvement is usually gradual and is best documented through the use of a baseline of pain activity established at an early stage in the episode of care. However, if no improvement in symptoms or function can be demonstrated, the PTA should bring this to the PT's attention.

Aggravating and Relieving Factors

A series of questions addressing aggravating and relieving factors must be included, such as the following.

▶▶ PTA ACTION PLAN
Follow-Up Questions

- What brings on your pain (symptoms)?
- What kinds of things make your pain (symptoms) worse (e.g., eating, exercise, rest, specific positions, excitement, stress)?
  To assess relieving factors, ask:
- What makes the pain better?
  Follow-up questions include:
- How does rest affect the pain/symptoms?
- Are your symptoms aggravated or relieved by any activities? If yes, what?
- How has this problem affected your daily life at work or at home?
- How has this problem affected your ability to care for yourself without assistance (e.g., dress, bathe, cook, drive)?

Systemic pain tends to be relieved minimally, relieved only temporarily, or unrelieved by change in position or by rest. Musculoskeletal pain is often relieved both by a change of position and by rest.

Associated Symptoms

Associated symptoms may occur alone or in conjunction with the pain of systemic disease. They may not be present at the time of the initial evaluation with the PT. Because systemic illness can progress over time, the new onset of any of these additional symptoms requires the PTA's immediate attention. In addition, the client may or may not associate these additional symptoms with the chief complaint and therefore may not mention any new symptoms. The PTA may ask the following.

▶▶ PTA ACTION PLAN

Follow-Up Questions

- What other symptoms have you had that you can associate with this problem?

  If the client denies any additional symptoms, follow up this question with a series of possibilities such as:

Burning	Difficulty in swallowing
Heart palpitations	Nausea
Numbness/tingling	Vomiting
Difficulty in breathing	Dizziness
Hoarseness	Night sweats
Problems with vision	Weakness

Whenever the client says "yes" to such associated symptoms, the PTA should check for the presence of these symptoms bilaterally. In addition, bilateral weakness, either proximally or distally, should serve as a red flag, which may indicate more than a musculoskeletal lesion.

Blurred vision, double vision, scotomas (black spots before the eyes), or temporary blindness may indicate early symptoms of multiple sclerosis[41] or may be warning signs of an impending cerebrovascular accident. The presence of any associated symptoms, such as those mentioned here, should be communicated to the PT, who would likely contact the physician to confirm the physician's knowledge of these symptoms.

In summary, careful and sensitive questioning regarding the individual's pain can bring forth essential information otherwise unknown to the PT that could be used in making a decision regarding treatment or referral. Table 2.1 may help the PTA quickly recognize the difference between the expected musculoskeletal pain pattern and pain from a visceral or systemic cause.

SOURCES OF PAIN

PTAs frequently see clients whose primary complaint is pain that often leads to a loss of function. However, focusing on sources of pain does not always help to identify the causes of tissue irritation. Even so, a careful assessment of pain behavior is invaluable in determining the nature and extent of the

TABLE 2.1 Comparison of Systemic Versus Musculoskeletal Pain Patterns

	Systemic Pain	Musculoskeletal Pain
Onset	• Recent, sudden • Does not present as observed for years without progression of symptoms	May be sudden or gradual, depending on the history **Sudden:** Usually associated with acute overload stress, traumatic event, repetitive motion; can occur as a side effect of some medications (e.g., statins) **Gradual:** Secondary to chronic overload of the affected part; may be present off and on for years
Description	• Knife-like quality of stabbing from the inside out, boring, deep aching • Cutting, gnawing • Throbbing • Bone pain • Unilateral or bilateral	• Usually unilateral • May be stiff after prolonged rest, but painful • Achy, cramping pain level decreases • Local tenderness to pressure
Intensity	• Related to the degree of noxious stimuli; usually unrelated to presence of anxiety • Mild or dull to severe	• May be mild to severe • May depend on the person's anxiety level; the level of pain may increase in a client fearful of a "serious" condition
Duration	• Constant; unchanging; awakens the person	• Duration can be modified by rest or change in position • May be constant but is more likely to be intermittent, depending on the activity or the position

Pattern	• Although constant, may come in waves
	• Gradually progressive, cyclic
	• Night pain
	   • Location: chest/shoulder
	   • Accompanied by shortness of breath, wheezing
	   • Eating alters symptoms
	   • Sitting up relieves symptoms (decreases venous return to the heart: possible pulmonary or cardiovascular etiology)
	• Symptoms unrelieved by rest or change in position
	• Migratory arthralgias: Pain/symptoms last for 1 week in one joint, then resolve and appear in another joint
		• Restriction of active/passive/accessory movement(s) observed
		• One or more particular movements "catch" the client and aggravate the pain

Continued

TABLE 2.1	Comparison of Systemic Versus Musculoskeletal Pain Patterns—cont'd	
	Systemic Pain	**Musculoskeletal Pain**

Aggravating factors	• Cannot alter, provoke, alleviate, eliminate, aggravate the symptoms
	• Organ dependent (examples):
	  • Esophagus—eating or swallowing affects symptoms
	  • Heart—cold, exertion, stress, heavy meal (especially when combined) can bring on symptoms
	  • GI—peristalsis (eating) affects symptoms
		• Altered by movement; pain may become worse with movement, or some myalgia decreases with movement

Relieving factors	• Organ dependent (examples):
	  • Gallbladder—leaning forward may reduce symptoms
	  • Kidney—leaning to the affected side may reduce symptoms
	  • Pancreas—sitting upright or leaning forward
		• Symptoms reduced or relieved by rest or change in position
		• Muscle pain is relieved by short periods of rest without resulting stiffness, except in the case of fibromyalgia; stiffness may be present in older adults
		• Stretching
		• Heat, cold

Associated signs and symptoms	• Fever, chills
	• Sweats (at any time, day or night)
	• Unusual vital signs
	• Warning signs of cancer
	• GI symptoms: Nausea, vomiting, anorexia, unexplained weight loss, diarrhea, constipation
	• Early satiety (feeling full after eating)
	• Bilateral symptoms (e.g., paresthesias, weakness, edema, nail-bed changes, skin rash)
	• Painless weakness of muscles: more often proximal but may occur distally
	• Dyspnea (breathlessness at rest or after mild exertion)
	• Diaphoresis (excessive perspiration)
	• Headaches, dizziness, fainting
	• Visual disturbances
	• Skin lesions, rashes, or itching that the client may not associate with the musculoskeletal symptoms
	• Bowel/bladder symptoms
	  • Hematuria (blood in the urine)
	  • Nocturia
	  • Urgency (sudden need to urinate)
	  • Frequency
	  • Melena (blood in feces)
	  • Fecal or urinary incontinence
	  • Bowel smears
		• Usually none, although stimulation of trigger points may cause sweating, nausea, or blanching

GI, Gastrointestinal.

underlying pathology, and this is something the PTA can help provide. From an observation perspective, the PTA should be aware of possible *sources* of pain and *types* of pain. When listening to the client's description of pain, consider the following possible sources of pain (Box 2.2). (Types of pain will be discussed next.)

- Cutaneous
- Somatic
- Visceral
- Neuropathic
- Referred

Cutaneous Sources of Pain

Cutaneous pain (related to the skin) includes superficial somatic structures located in the skin and subcutaneous tissue. The pain is well localized because the client can point directly to the area that "hurts." Pain from a cutaneous source can usually be localized with one finger. Skin pain or tenderness can be associated with referred pain from the viscera or referred from deep somatic structures.

Impairment of any organ can result in sudomotor changes that present as trophic changes such as itching, dysesthesia, skin temperature changes, or dry skin.[42] The difficulty is that biomechanical dysfunction can also result in these same changes, which is why the PT may need to conduct a more careful evaluation of soft tissue structures and a screening examination for systemic disease when the PTA reports suspicious findings.

Somatic Sources of Pain

Somatic pain can be superficial or deep. Somatic pain is labeled according to its source as deep somatic, somato-visceral, somato-emotional (also referred to as *psychosomatic*), or viscero-somatic.

BOX 2.2   Sources of Pain, Pain Types, and Pain Patterns

Sources
- Cutaneous
- Deep somatic
- Visceral
- Neuropathic
- Referred

Types
- Tension
- Inflammatory
- Ischemic
- Myofascial pain
  - Muscle tension
  - Muscle spasm
  - Trigger points
  - Muscle deficiency (weakness and stiffness)
  - Muscle trauma
- Joint pain
  - Drug induced
  - Chemical exposure
  - Inflammatory bowel disease
  - Septic arthritis

- Reactive arthritis
- Musculoskeletal/spondylotic
- Radicular pain
- Arterial, pleural, tracheal
- Gastrointestinal pain
- Pain at rest
- Night pain
- Pain with activity
- Diffuse pain
- Chronic pain

Characteristics/Patterns
- Client describes:
  - Location/onset
  - Description
  - Frequency
  - Duration
  - Intensity
- Therapist recognizes the pattern:
  - Vascular
  - Neurogenic

Most of what the therapist treats is part of the somatic system, whether it is called the neuromuscular system, the musculoskeletal system, or the NMS system. When psychological disorders present as somatic dysfunction, we refer to these conditions as psychophysiologic disorders.

Superficial somatic structures involve the skin, superficial fasciae, tendon sheaths, and periosteum. *Deep somatic pain* comes from pathologic conditions of the periosteum and cancellous (spongy) bone, nerves, muscles, tendons, ligaments, and blood vessels. Deep somatic structures also include deep fasciae and joint capsules. Somatic referred pain does not involve stimulation of nerve roots; it is produced by stimulation of nerve endings within the superficial and deep somatic structures just mentioned.[43]

Somatic referred pain is usually reported as dull, aching, or gnawing or is described as an expanding pressure too diffuse to localize. No neurologic signs are associated with somatic referred pain since this type of pain is considered nociceptive and is not caused by compression of spinal nerves or nerve roots. It is possible to have combinations of pain and neurologic findings when more than one pathway is disturbed.[44-47]

Deep somatic pain is poorly localized and may be referred to the body surface, becoming cutaneous pain. It can be associated with an autonomic phenomenon, such as sweating, pallor, or changes in pulse and blood pressure, and it is commonly accompanied by a subjective feeling of nausea and faintness.[48,49]

Pain associated with deep somatic lesions follows patterns that relate to the embryologic development of the musculoskeletal system. This explains why such pain may not be perceived directly over the involved organ[50] (see Fig. 2.1).

Parietal pain (related to the wall of the chest or abdominal cavity) is also considered deep somatic. The visceral pleura (the membrane enveloping the organs) is insensitive to pain, but the parietal pleura is well supplied with pain nerve endings. For this reason, it is possible for a client to have extensive visceral disease (e.g., heart, lungs) without pain until the disease progresses enough to involve the parietal pleura.

Visceral Sources of Pain

Visceral sources of pain include the internal organs and the heart muscle. This source of pain includes all body organs located in the trunk or abdomen, such as those of the respiratory, digestive, urogenital, and endocrine systems, as well as the spleen, the heart, and the great vessels.

Visceral pain is not well localized for two reasons[22]:
1. Innervation of the viscera is multisegmental.
2. There are few nerve receptors in these structures (see Fig. 2.3). The pain tends to be poorly localized and diffuse.

Visceral pain is well known for its ability to produce referred pain (i.e., pain perceived in an area other than the site of the stimuli). Referred pain occurs because visceral fibers synapse at the level of the spinal cord close to fibers supplying specific somatic structures. In other words, visceral pain corresponds to dermatomes from which the organ receives its innervations, which may be the same innervations for somatic structures.

For example, the heart is innervated by the C3–T4 spinal nerves. Pain of a cardiac source can affect any part of the soma (body) also innervated by these levels. This is one reason why someone having a heart attack can experience jaw, neck, shoulder, mid-back, arm, or chest pain and accounts for the many and varied clinical pictures of MI. More specifically, the pericardium (the sac around the entire heart) is adjacent to the diaphragm. Pain of cardiac and diaphragmatic origin is often experienced in the shoulder because the C5–C6 spinal segment (innervation for the shoulder) also supplies the heart and the diaphragm.[22]

As mentioned earlier, diseases of internal organs can be accompanied by cutaneous hypersensitivity to touch, pressure, and temperature. This viscerocutaneous reflex occurs during the acute phase of the disease and disappears with its recovery.

The neurology of visceral pain is not well understood. There is not a known central processing system unique to visceral pain. In the early stage of visceral disease, sympathetic reflexes arising from afferent impulses of the internal viscera may be expressed first as sensory, motor, and/ or trophic changes in the skin, subcutaneous tissues, and/ or muscles. As mentioned earlier, this can present as itching, dysesthesia, skin temperature changes, or dry skin. The viscera do not perceive pain, but the sensory side is trying to get the message out that something is wrong by creating sympathetic sudomotor changes.[51]

It appears that there is not one specific group of spinal neurons that respond only to visceral inputs. Since messages from the soma and viscera come into the cord at the same level (and sometimes visceral afferents converge over several segments of the spinal cord), the nervous system has trouble deciding whether the message is somatic or visceral. It sends efferent information back out to the plexus for change or reaction, but the input results in an unclear impulse at the cord level.

The body may receive skin or somatic responses, such as muscle pain or aching periosteum, or it may tell a viscus innervated at the same level to take action (e.g., the stomach increases its acid content). This also explains how sympathetic signals from the liver to the spinal cord can result in itching or other sudomotor responses in the area embryologically related to the liver.[52]

Pain and symptoms of a visceral source are usually accompanied by an ANS response such as a change in vital signs, unexplained perspiration (diaphoresis), and/or skin pallor. Signs and symptoms associated with the involved organ system may also be present. We call these *associated signs and symptoms*, and they serve as red flags to document and report to the PT.

Neuropathic Pain

Neuropathic or neurogenic pain results from damage to or pathophysiologic changes of the peripheral nervous system or CNS.[53,54] Neuropathic pain can occur as a result of injury or destruction to the peripheral nerves, pathways in the spinal cord, or neurons located in the brain. This type of pain can be acute or chronic, depending on the time frame.

Neuropathic pain is not elicited by the stimulation of nociceptors or kinesthetic pathways as a result of tissue damage, but rather by malfunction of the nervous system itself.[55] Disruptions[56] in the transmission of afferent and efferent impulses in the peripheral nervous system, spinal cord, and brain can give rise to alterations in sensory modalities (e.g., touch, pressure, temperature) and sometimes motor dysfunction.

It can be drug induced, metabolic based, or brought on by trauma to the sensory neurons or pathways in either the peripheral nervous system or CNS. It appears to be idiosyncratic; not all individuals with the same lesion will have pain.[57] Some examples are listed in Table 2.2.

TABLE 2.2	Causes of Neuropathic Pain
Type	**Causes**
Central neuropathic pain	Multiple sclerosis Headache (migraine) Stroke Traumatic brain injury Parkinson disease Spinal cord injury (incomplete)
Peripheral neuropathic pain	Trigeminal neuralgia (tic douloureux) Poorly controlled diabetes mellitus (metabolic induced) Vincristine (Oncovin) (drug induced, used in cancer treatment) Isoniazid (drug induced, used to treat tuberculosis) Amputation (trauma) Crush injury/brachial avulsion (trauma) Herpes zoster (shingles, postherpetic neuralgia) Complex regional pain syndrome (causalgia) Nerve compression syndromes (e.g., carpel tunnel syndrome, thoracic outlet syndrome) Paraneoplastic neuropathy (cancer induced) Cancer (tumor infiltration/compression of the nerve) Liver or biliary impairment (e.g., liver cancer, cirrhosis, primary biliary cirrhosis) Leprosy Congenital neuropathy (e.g., porphyria) Guillain-Barré syndrome

❓ PICTURE THE PATIENT

Neuropathic pain is usually described as sharp, shooting, burning, tingling, or producing an electric shock sensation. The pain is steady or evoked by some stimulus that is not normally considered noxious (e.g., light touch, cold). Some affected individuals report aching pain. Muscle spasm does not occur in pure neurogenic pain.[55] Acute nerve root irritation tends to be severe and described as burning, shooting, and constant. Chronic nerve root pain is more often described as annoying or nagging.

Neuropathic pain is not alleviated by opiates or narcotics, although local anesthesia can provide temporary relief. Medications used to treat neuropathic pain include antidepressants, anticonvulsants, antispasmodics, adrenergics, and anesthetics. Many clients have a combination of neuropathic and somatic pain, making it more difficult to identify the underlying pathology.

Referred Pain

By definition, referred pain is felt in an area far from the site of the lesion but supplied by the same or adjacent neural segments. Referred pain occurs by way of shared central pathways for afferent neurons and can originate from any somatic or visceral source. (Primary cutaneous pain is not usually referred to other parts of the body.[50])

Referred pain is usually well localized (i.e., the person can point directly to the area that hurts), but it does not have sharply defined borders and can spread or radiate from its point of origin. Local tenderness is present in the tissue of the referred pain area, but there is no objective sensory deficit. Referred pain is often accompanied by muscle hypertonus over the referred area of pain.[50]

TABLE 2.3   Risk Factors for Rhabdomyolysis

Risk Factors for Rhabdomyolysis	Examples	Signs and Symptoms
Trauma	Crush injury Electric shock Severe burns Extended mobility	Profound muscle weakness Pain Swelling Stiffness and cramping Associated signs and symptoms: • Reddish-brown urine (myoglobin) • Decreased urine output • Malaise • Fever • Sinus tachycardia • Nausea, vomiting • Agitation, confusion
Extreme muscular activity	Strenuous exercise Status epilepticus Severe dystonia	
Toxic effects	Ethanol Ethylene glycol Isopropanol Methanol Heroin Barbiturates Methadone Cocaine Tetanus Ecstasy (street drug) Carbon monoxide Snake venom Amphetamines	
Metabolic abnormalities	Hypothyroidism Hyperthyroidism Diabetic ketoacidosis	
Medication induced	Inadvertent intravenous infiltration (e.g., amphotericin B, azathioprine, cyclosporine) Cholesterol-lowering statins (e.g., simvastatin [Zocor], atorvastatin [Lipitor], rosuvastatin calcium [Crestor])	

(From Fort CW: How to combat 3 deadly trauma complications, *Nursing* 33(5):58–64, 2003.)

Visceral disorders can refer pain to somatic tissue (Table 2.3). On the other hand, as mentioned in the earlier topic on visceral sources of pain, some somatic impairments can refer pain to visceral locations or mimic known visceral pain patterns. Finding the original source of referred pain can be quite a challenge.

Differentiating Sources of Pain

Sometimes it can be very difficult to tell when a person is experiencing somatic versus visceral pain. That is one reason why clients end up in physical therapy even though there is a viscerogenic source of the pain and/or symptomatic presentation.

▶▶ PTA ACTION PLAN

Follow-Up Questions

When you think it is appropriate, ask one or both of these two additional questions:
• Are you having any pain anywhere else in your body?
• Are you having symptoms of any other kind that may or may not be related to your main problem?

？ PICTURE THE PATIENT

The quality of superficial somatic pain tends to be sharp and more localized. Deep somatic pain is more likely to be a dull or deep aching that responds to rest or a non–weight-bearing position. Deep somatic pain is often poorly localized and can be referred from some other site.

Pain of a deep somatic nature increases after movement. Sometimes the client can find a comfortable spot, but after moving the extremity or joint, cannot find that comfortable spot again. This is in contrast to visceral pain, which usually is not reproduced with movement, but rather tends to hurt all the time or with all movements.[22]

Pain from a visceral source can also be dull and aching but usually does not feel better after rest or recumbency. Keep in mind that pathologic processes occurring within somatic structures (e.g., metastasis, primary tumor, infection) may produce localized pain that can be mechanically irritated. This is why movement in general (rather than specific motions) can make it worse. Back pain from metastasis to the spine can become quite severe before any radiologic changes are seen.[22]

Visceral diseases of the abdomen and pelvis are more likely to refer pain to the back, whereas intrathoracic disease refers pain to the shoulder(s). Visceral pain rarely occurs without associated signs and symptoms, although the client may not recognize the correlation. Careful questioning will usually elicit a systemic pattern of symptoms.

TYPES OF PAIN

It may be helpful to consider some specific types of pain patterns. Not all pain types can be discussed here, but some of the most commonly encountered in the rehab setting are included.

Tension Pain

Organ distention, such as that occurs with bowel obstruction, constipation, or the passing of a kidney stone, can cause tension pain. Tension pain can also be caused by blood pooling from trauma and pus or fluid accumulation from infection or other underlying causes. In the bowel, tension pain may be described as "colicky" with waves of pain and tension occurring intermittently as peristaltic contractile force moves irritating substances through the GI system. Tension pain makes it difficult to find a comfortable position.

Inflammatory Pain

Inflammation of the viscera or parietal peritoneum (e.g., acute appendicitis) may cause pain that is described as deep or boring. If the visceral peritoneum is involved, the pain is usually poorly localized. If the parietal peritoneum is the primary area affected, the pain pattern may become more localized (i.e., the affected individual can point to it with one or two fingers). Pain arising from inflammation causes people to seek positions of quiet with little movement.

Ischemic Pain

Ischemia denotes a loss of blood supply. Any area without adequate perfusion will quickly die. Ischemic pain of the viscera is sudden, intense, constant, and progressive in severity or intensity. It is not typically relieved by analgesics, and no position is comfortable. The person usually avoids movement or change in positions.

Myofascial Pain

Myalgia, or muscle pain, can be a symptom of an underlying systemic disorder. Cancer, renal failure, hepatic disease, and endocrine disorders are only a few possible systemic sources of muscle involvement.

For example, muscle weakness, atrophy, myalgia, and fatigue that persist despite rest may be early manifestations of thyroid or parathyroid disease, acromegaly, diabetes, Cushing syndrome, or osteomalacia.

Myalgia can be present in anxiety and depressive disorders. Muscle weakness and myalgia can occur as a side effect of drugs. Prolonged use of systemic corticosteroids and immunosuppressive drugs has known adverse effects on the musculoskeletal system, including degenerative myopathy with muscle wasting and tendon rupture.

Infective endocarditis caused by acute bacterial infection can present with myalgia and no other manifestation of endocarditis. The early onset of joint pain and myalgia as the first sign of endocarditis is more likely if the person is older and has had a previously diagnosed heart murmur.[58]

Polymyalgia rheumatica (PR), which literally means "pain in many muscles," is a disorder marked by diffuse pain and stiffness that primarily affects muscles of the shoulder and pelvic girdles. With PR, symptoms are vague and difficult to diagnose, resulting in delay in medical treatment. The person may wake up one morning with muscle pain and stiffness for no apparent reason, or the symptoms may come on gradually over several days or weeks. Adults over age 50 years are affected most often (White females have the highest incidence); most cases occur after age 70 years.[59]

Temporal arteritis occurs in 25% of all cases of PR. PTAs should watch for headache, visual changes (blurred or double vision), intermittent jaw pain (claudication), and cranial nerve involvement. The temporal artery may be prominent and painful to touch, and the temporal pulse absent.[59]

Many types of muscle-related pain can occur, such as tension, spasm, weakness, trauma, inflammation, infection, neurologic impairment, and trigger points (TrPs) (see Box 2.2). The clinical presentation most common with systemic disease is presented here.

Muscle Tension

Muscle tension, or sustained muscle tone, occurs when prolonged muscular contraction (or *cocontraction*) results in local ischemia, increased cellular metabolites, and subsequent pain. Ischemia as a factor in muscle pain remains controversial. Interruption of blood flow in a resting extremity does not cause pain unless the muscle contracts during the ischemic condition.[60]

Muscle tension can also occur with physical stress and fatigue. Muscle tension and the subsequent ischemia may occur as a result of faulty ergonomics, prolonged work positions (e.g., as with computer or telephone operators), or repetitive motion. Take, for example, the person sitting at a keyboard for hours each day. Constant typing with muscle cocontraction does not allow for the normal contract-relax sequence. Muscle ischemia results in greater release of substance P, a pain neurotransmitter (neuropeptide). Increased substance P levels increase pain sensitivity. Increased pain perception results in more muscle spasm as a splinting or protective guarding mechanism, and thus the pain-spasm cycle is perpetuated. This is a somatic-somatic response.[61]

Muscle tension from a visceral-somatic response can occur when pain from a visceral source results in increased muscle tension and even muscle spasm. For example, the pain from any inflammatory or infectious process affecting the abdomen (e.g., appendicitis, diverticulitis, pelvic inflammatory disease) can cause increased tension in the abdominal muscles.

Given enough time and combined with overuse and repetitive use or infectious or inflammatory disease, muscle tension can turn into muscle spasm. When opposing muscles such as the flexors and extensors contract together for long periods (cocontraction), muscle tension and then muscle spasm can occur.

Muscle Spasm

Muscle spasm is a sudden involuntary contraction of a muscle or group of muscles, usually occurring as a result of overuse or injury of the adjoining NMS or musculotendinous attachments. A person with a painful musculoskeletal problem may also have a varying degree of reflex muscle spasm to protect the joint(s) involved (a somatic-somatic response). A client with painful visceral disease can have muscle spasm of the overlying musculature (a viscero-somatic response).[62]

Spasm pain cannot be attributed to transient increased muscle tension because the intramuscular pressure is insufficiently elevated. Pain with muscle spasm may occur from prolonged contraction under an ischemic situation. An increase in the partial pressure of oxygen has been documented inside the muscle in spasm under these circumstances.[63]

Muscle Trauma

Muscle trauma can occur with acute trauma, burns, crush injuries, or unaccustomed intensity or duration of muscle contraction, especially eccentric contractions. Muscle pain occurs as broken fibers leak potassium into the interstitial fluid. Blood extravasation (seeping into the soft tissues) results from damaged blood vessels, setting off a cascade of chemical reactions within the muscle.[60]

When disintegration of muscle tissues occurs with release of their contents (e.g., oxygen-transporting pigment myoglobin) into the bloodstream, a potentially fatal muscle toxicity called *rhabdomyolysis* can occur. Risk factors and clinical signs and symptoms are listed in Table 2.4. Immediate medical attention is required (Case Example 2.2).

Muscle Deficiency

Muscle deficiency (weakness and stiffness) is a common problem as we age and even among younger unconditioned adults. Connective tissue changes may occur as small amounts of fibrinogen (produced in the liver and normally converted to fibrin to serve as a clotting factor) leak from the vasculature into the intracellular spaces, adhering to cellular structures.

The resulting microfibrinous adhesions among the cells of muscle and fascia cause increased muscular stiffness. Activity and movement normally break these adhesions; however, with the aging process, production of fewer and less efficient macrophages combined with immobility for any reason results in reduced lysis of these adhesions.[64]

Other possible causes of aggravated stiffness include increased collagen fibers from reduced collagen turnover, increased crosslinks of aged collagen fibers, changes in the mechanical properties of connective tissues, and structural and functional changes in the collagen protein. Tendons and ligaments also have less water content, resulting in increased stiffness.[65]

When muscular stiffness occurs as a result of aging, increased physical activity and movement can reduce associated muscular pain. As part of the diagnostic evaluation, consider a general conditioning program for the older adult reporting generalized muscle pain. Even 10 minutes a day on a stationary bike, on a treadmill, or in an aquatics program can bring dramatic and fast relief of painful symptoms caused by muscle deficiency.

TABLE 2.4   Common Patterns of Pain Referral

Pain Mechanism	Lesion Site	Referral Site
Somatic	C7, T1–5 vertebrae	Interscapular area, posterior
	Shoulder	Neck, upper back
	L1, L2 vertebrae	SI joint and hip
	Hip joint	SI hip and knee
	Pharynx	Ipsilateral ear
	TMJ	Head, neck, heart
Visceral	Diaphragmatic irritation	Shoulder, lumbar spine
	Heart	Shoulder, neck, upper back, TMJ
	Urothelial tract	Back, inguinal region, anterior thigh, genitalia
	Pancreas, liver, spleen, gallbladder	Shoulder, midthoracic or low back
	Peritoneal or abdominal cavity	Hip pain from abscess of psoas or obturator muscle
Neuropathic	Nerve or plexus	Anywhere in distribution of a peripheral nerve
	Nerve root	Anywhere in corresponding dermatome
	Central nervous system	Anywhere in region of body innervated by damaged structure

SI, Sacroiliac; *TMJ*, temporomandibular joint.

CASE EXAMPLE 2.2   Military Rhabdomyolysis

A 20-year-old soldier reported to the military physical therapy clinic with bilateral shoulder pain and weakness. He was unable to perform his regular duties as a result of these symptoms. He attributed this to doing many push-ups during physical training 2 days ago.

When asked if there were any other symptoms of any kind to report, the client said that he noticed his urine was a dark color yesterday (the day after the push-up exercises).

The soldier had shoulder active range of motion (ROM) to 90 degrees accompanied by an abnormal scapulohumeral rhythm with excessive scapular elevation on both sides. Passive shoulder ROM was full but painful. Elbow active and passive ROM was also restricted to 90 degrees of flexion second to pain in the triceps muscles.

The client was unable to handle manual muscle testing with pain on palpation to the pectoral, triceps, and infraspinatus muscles, bilaterally. The rotator cuff tendon appeared to be intact.

What are the Red Flags in This Case?
- Bilateral symptoms (pain and weakness)
- Age (for cancer, too young [under 25 years old] or too old [over 50 years] is a red-flag sign)
- Change in urine color

Result: The soldier had actually done hundreds of different types of push-ups, including regular, wide-arm, and diamond push-ups. Although the soldier was not in any apparent distress, laboratory studies were ordered. Serum creatine kinase level was measured as 9600U/L (normal range: 55–170U/L).

The results were consistent with acute exertional rhabdomyolysis, and the soldier was hospitalized. Early recognition of a potentially serious problem may have prevented serious complications possible with this condition.

Physical therapy intervention for muscle soreness without adequate hydration could have led to acute renal failure. He returned to physical therapy for a recovery program following hospitalization.

(Data from Baxter RE, Moore JH: Diagnosis and treatment of acute exertional rhabdomyolysis, *J Orthop Sports Phys Ther* 33(3):104–108, 2003.)

Trigger Points

TrPs, sometimes referred to as *myofascial TrPs*, are hyperirritable spots within a taut band of skeletal muscle or in the fascia. Taut bands are rope-like indurations palpated in the muscle fiber. These areas are very tender to palpation and are referred to as *local tenderness*.[66] There is often a history of immobility (e.g., cast immobilization after fracture or injury), prolonged or vigorous activity such as bending or lifting, or forceful abdominal breathing such as in marathon running.

TrPs are reproduced with palpation or resisted motions. Pressing on the TrP may elicit a "jump sign." Some people say the jump sign is a local twitch response of muscle fibers to TrP stimulation, but this is an erroneous use of the term.[61]

The *jump sign* is a general pain response as the client physically withdraws from the pressure on the point and may even cry out or wince in pain. The *local twitch response* is the visible contraction of tense muscle fibers in response to stimulation. When TrPs are compressed, local tenderness with possible referred pain results. In other words, pain that arises from the TrP is felt at a distance, often remote from its source.

The referred pain pattern is characteristic and specific for every muscle. Knowing the TrP's locations and its referred pain patterns is helpful. By knowing the pain patterns, you can go to the site of origin and confirm (or rule out) the presence of the TrP. The distribution of referred TrP pain rarely coincides entirely with the distribution of a peripheral nerve or dermatomal segment.[61]

TrPs can be categorized as active, latent, key, or satellite. *Active* TrPs refer pain locally or to another location and can cause pain at rest. *Latent* TrPs do not cause spontaneous pain but generate referred pain when the affected muscle(s) are put under pressure, palpated, or strained. *Key* TrPs have a pain-referral pattern along nerve pathways, and *satellite* TrPs are set off by key TrPs.

The PT will eliminate TrPs as part of the process to rule out systemic pathology as a cause of muscle pain. If the therapist has

BOX 2.3   Systemic Causes of Joint Pain

Infectious and noninfectious systemic causes of joint pain can include but are not limited to:
- Allergic reactions (e.g., medications such as antibiotics)
- Side effects of other medications such as statins, prolonged use of corticosteroids, aromatase inhibitors
- Delayed reaction to chemicals or environmental factors
- Sexually transmitted infections (e.g., human immunodeficiency virus, syphilis, chlamydia, gonorrhea)
- Infectious arthritis
- Infective endocarditis
- Recent dental surgery
- Lyme disease
- Rheumatoid arthritis
- Other autoimmune disorders (e.g., systemic lupus erythematosus, mixed connective tissue disease, scleroderma, polymyositis)
- Leukemia
- Tuberculosis
- Acute rheumatic fever
- Chronic liver disease (hepatic osteodystrophy affecting wrists and ankles; hepatitis causing arthralgias)
- Inflammatory bowel disease (e.g., Crohn's disease or regional enteritis)
- Anxiety or depression (major depressive disorder)
- Fibromyalgia
- Artificial sweeteners

included instruction in this area for the PTA, the PTA should consider a client failing to respond to TrP therapy as a yellow flag. It is *not* necessarily a red flag that suggests the need for further screening for systemic or other causes of muscle pain. Muscle recovery from TrPs is not always so simple.

Joint Pain

Noninflammatory joint pain (no redness, warmth, or swelling) of unknown etiology can be caused by a wide range of pathologic conditions (Box 2.3). Fibromyalgia, leukemia, sexually transmitted infections, artificial sweeteners,[67–70] Crohn disease (CD, also known as *regional enteritis*), postmenopausal status or low estrogen levels, and infectious arthritis are all possible causes of joint pain. Joint pain in the presence of fatigue may be a red flag for anxiety, depression, or cancer.

One of the major differences between systemic versus musculoskeletal causes of joint pain is in the area of associated signs and symptoms (Table 2.5). Joint pain of a systemic or visceral origin usually has additional signs or symptoms present. The client may not realize there is a connection, or the condition may not have progressed enough for associated signs and symptoms to develop.

? PICTURE THE PATIENT

Joint pain from a systemic cause is more likely to be constant and present with all movements. Rest may help at first, but over time even this relieving factor will not alter the symptoms. The client with osteoarthritis (OA), in comparison, often feels better after rest (although stiffness may remain). Morning joint pain associated with OA is less than joint pain at the end of the day after using the joint(s) all day. On the other hand, muscle pain may be worse in the morning and gradually improve as the client stretches and moves about during the day.

TABLE 2.5 Joint Pain: Systemic or Musculoskeletal?

	Systemic	Musculoskeletal
Clinical presentation	Awakens at night Deep aching, throbbing Reduced by pressure[a] Constant or waves/spasm Cyclic, progressive symptoms	Decreases with rest Sharp Reduced by change in position Reduced or eliminated when stressful action is stopped Restriction of A/PROM Restriction of accessory motions One or more movements "catch," reproducing or aggravating pain/symptoms
Past medical history	Recent history of infection: Hepatitis, bacterial infection from Staphylococcus or Streptococcus (e.g., cellulitis), mononucleosis, measles, URI, UTI, gonorrhea, osteomyelitis, cellulitis History of bone fracture, joint replacement, or arthroscopy History of human bite Sore throat, headache with fever in the last 3 weeks, or family/household member with recently diagnosed strep throat Skin rash (infection, medications) Recent medications (in last 6 weeks); any drug but especially statins (cholesterol lowering), antibiotics, aromatase inhibitors, chemotherapy Hormone associated (postmenopausal status, low estrogen levels) History of injection drug use/abuse History of allergic reactions History of GI symptoms Recent history of enteric or venereal infection Presence of extensor surface nodule	Repetitive motion Arthritis Static postures (prolonged) Trauma (including domestic violence)
Associated signs and symptoms	Jaundice Migratory arthralgia Skin rash/lesions Nodules (extensor surfaces) Fatigue Weight loss Low-grade fever Suspicious or aberrant lymph nodes Presence of GI symptoms Cyclic, progressive symptoms Proximal muscle weakness	Usually none Check for TrPs TrPs may be accompanied by some minimal ANS phenomenon (e.g., nausea, sweating)

[a]This is actually a cutaneous or somatic response because the pressure provides a counter irritant; it does not really affect the viscera directly.
ANS, Autonomic nervous system; A/PROM, active/passive range of motion; GI, gastrointestinal; TrPs, trigger points; URI, upper respiratory infection; UTI, urinary tract infection.

PTA ACTION PLAN
Communication With the Physical Therapist

The PTA should document and report any joint pain of unknown cause or with an unusual presentation or history. Joint pain and symptoms that do not fit the expected pattern for injury, overuse, or aging will require further evaluation by the PT.

Drug-Induced Pain

Joint pain as an allergic response, sometimes referred to as *serum sickness*, can occur up to 6 weeks after taking a prescription drug (especially antibiotics).[60,71] Joint pain is also a potential side effect of statins (e.g., Lipitor, Zocor), which are cholesterol-lowering agents.

Musculoskeletal symptoms (e.g., morning stiffness, bone pain, arthralgia, arthritis) are a well-known side effect of chemotherapy and aromatase inhibitors used in the treatment of breast cancer. Low estrogen concentrations and postmenopausal status are linked with these symptoms. Risk factors for developing joint symptoms may include previous hormone replacement therapy, hormone-receptor positivity, previous chemotherapy, obesity, and treatment with the aromatase inhibitor anastrozole (Arimidex).[72]

PICTURE THE PATIENT

Noninflammatory joint pain is typical of a delayed allergic reaction. The client may report fever, skin rash, and fatigue that go away when the drug is stopped. Joint pain may persist weeks to months after the drug has been discontinued.

Radicular Pain

Radicular pain results from direct irritation of axons of a spinal nerve or neurons in the dorsal root ganglion and is experienced in the musculoskeletal system in a dermatome, sclerotome, or myotome.

Radicular, radiating, and referred pain are not the same, although a client can have radicular pain that radiates. *Radiating* means the pain spreads or fans out from the originating point of pain. Whereas radicular pain is caused by nerve root compression, referred pain results from activation of nociceptive free nerve endings (nociceptors) of the nervous system in somatic or visceral tissue. The physiologic basis for referred pain is convergence of afferent neurons onto common neurons within the CNS.

The term *sciatica* is outdated and reflects our previous (limited) understanding of referred pain. Regional pain anywhere near, around, or along the pathway of the sciatic nerve was automatically attributed to irritation of the sciatic nerve and labeled "sciatica." The International Association for the Study of Pain recommends replacing the term *sciatica* with radicular pain.[44]

Radiculopathy is another symptom that is separate from radicular pain. Radiculopathy describes a neurologic state in which conduction along a spinal nerve or its roots is blocked.

Instead of pain, numbness (when sensory fibers are blocked) or weakness (when there is a motor block) is the primary symptom. The numbness will be in a dermatomal pattern, whereas the weakness will present in a myotomal distribution. Radiculopathy is determined by these objective neurologic signs and symptoms rather than by pain. It is possible to have radiculopathy and radicular symptoms at the same time. Radiculopathy can occur alone (no pain) and radicular pain can occur without radiculopathy.[44]

Differentiating between radicular (pain from the peripheral nervous system) and referred pain from the ANS can be difficult. Both can start at one point and radiate outward, and both can cause pain distal to the site of pathology.

Remember that referred pain occurs most often far away from the site of pathologic origin of symptoms. On the other hand, radicular pain does not skip myotomes, dermatomes, or sclerotomes associated with the affected peripheral nerves.

Physical disease can localize pain in dermatomal or myotomal patterns. If the experienced PTA sees a client who describes pain that does not match a dermatomal or myotomal pattern, the PT should be notified. (*Note*: This is not entry-level knowledge.) This is neither referred visceral pain from ANS involvement nor irritation of a spinal nerve. For example, the client who describes whole leg pain or whole leg numbness may be experiencing *inappropriate illness behavior*. Inappropriate illness behavior is recognized clinically as illness behavior that is out of proportion to the underlying physical disease and is related more to associated psychological disturbances than to actual physical disease.[73]

PTA ACTION PLAN
Communication With the Physical Therapist

If the PTA recognizes this behavioral component to pain, it should be immediately reported to the therapist.

Arterial, Pleural, and Tracheal Pain

PICTURE THE PATIENT

Pain arising from arteries, as with arteritis (inflammation of an artery), migraine, and vascular headaches, increases with systolic impulse so that any process associated with increased systolic pressure, such as exercise, fever, alcohol consumption, or bending over, may intensify the already throbbing pain.

PTA ACTION PLAN
What to Document and Report

Pain from the pleura, as well as the trachea, correlates with respiratory movements. Look for associated signs and symptoms of the cardiac or pulmonary systems. Listen for a description of pain that is "throbbing" (vascular) or sharp and increases with respiratory movements such as breathing, laughing, or coughing. Palpation and resisted movements will not reproduce the symptoms, which may get worse with recumbency, especially at night or while sleeping. Document and report all findings of this type.

Gastrointestinal Pain

Pain arising from the GI tract tends to increase with peristaltic activity, particularly if there is any obstruction to forward progress of the food bolus. The pain increases with ingestion and may lessen with fasting or after emptying the involved segment (vomiting or bowel movement).

On the other hand, pain may occur as a result of the effect of gastric acid on the esophagus, stomach, or duodenum. This pain is relieved by the presence of food or by other neutralizing material in the stomach, and the pain is intensified when the stomach is empty and secreting acid.

▶▶ PTA ACTION PLAN

Follow-Up Questions

In these cases, it is important to ask the client about the effect of eating on musculoskeletal pain. Does the pain increase, decrease, or stay the same immediately after eating and 1 to 3 hours later?

❓ PICTURE THE PATIENT

When hollow viscera, such as the liver, kidneys, spleen, and pancreas, are distended, body positions or movements that increase intraabdominal pressure may intensify the pain, whereas positions that reduce pressure or support the structure may ease the pain.

The client with an acutely distended gallbladder may slightly flex the trunk. With pain arising from a tense, swollen kidney (or distended renal pelvis), the client flexes the trunk and tilts toward the involved side; with pancreatic pain, the client may sit up and lean forward or lie down with the knees drawn up to the chest.

Inflammatory Bowel Disease

Ulcerative colitis (UC) and regional enteritis (CD) are accompanied by an arthritic component and skin rash in about 55% of all people affected by this inflammatory bowel condition.[70,74] The person may have a known diagnosis of inflammatory bowel disease (IBD) but may not know that new onset of joint symptoms can be part of this condition. See further discussion in Chapter 4, "Arthralgia" section.

❓ PICTURE THE PATIENT

Peripheral joint disease associated with IBD involves the large joints, most often a single hip or knee. Joint symptoms often occur simultaneously with UC but less often at the same time as CD. Ankylosing spondylitis (AS) is also possible with either form of IBD. As with typical AS, symptoms affect the low back, sacrum, or SI joint first. The most common symptoms are intermittent low back pain with decreased low back motion. The course of AS associated with IBD is the same as without the bowel component.

Pain at Rest

Pain at rest may arise from ischemia in a wide variety of tissues (e.g., vascular disease or tumor growth). The acute onset of severe unilateral extremity involvement accompanied by the "five Ps"—pain, pallor, pulselessness, paresthesia, and paralysis—signifies acute arterial occlusion (peripheral vascular disease).[75] Pain in this situation is usually described by the client as burning or shooting and may be accompanied by paresthesia.

Pain related to ischemia of the skin and subcutaneous tissues is characterized by the client as burning and boring. All these occlusive causes of pain are usually worse at night and are relieved to some degree by dangling the affected extremity over the side of the bed and by frequent massaging of the extremity.

Pain at rest that is caused by neoplasm usually occurs at night. Although neoplasms are highly vascularized (a process called *angiogenesis*), the host organ's vascular supply and nutrients may be compromised simultaneously, causing ischemia of the local tissue. The pain awakens the client from sleep and prevents the person from going back to sleep, despite all efforts to do so. See the next section, "Night Pain."

The client may describe pain noted on weightbearing or bone pain that may be mild and intermittent in the initial stages, becoming progressively more severe and more constant.

Night Pain

Whenever the PTA hears the client describing his or her pain, it is important to ask about night pain (Box 2.4). The PT evaluates pain responses to identify where the client might be on the continuum from acute to subacute to chronic. This information helps guide the treatment plan and intervention.

BOX 2.4   Follow-up Questions for Night Pain

When attempting to obtain more information for the physical therapist from someone with night pain, some possible questions are:
- Tell me about the pattern of your symptoms at night (open-ended question).
- Can you lie on that side? For how long?
  - (Alternative question): Does the pain wake you up when you roll onto that side?
- How are you feeling in general when you wake up?
- Do you have any other symptoms when the pain wakes you up? (Give the client time to answer before prompting with choices such as coughing, wheezing, shortness of breath, nausea, need to go to the bathroom, or night sweats.) Always ask the client reporting night pain of any kind (not just bone pain) the following questions:
  - What makes it better/worse?
  - What happens to your pain when you sit up? (Upright posture reduces venous return to the heart; decreased pain when sitting up may indicate a cardiopulmonary cause.)
  - How does taking aspirin affect your pain symptoms? (Disproportionate pain relief can occur using aspirin in the presence of bone cancer.)
  - How does eating or drinking affect your pain/symptoms (for shoulder, neck, back, hip, pelvis, gastrointestinal system)?
  - Does taking an antacid such as Tums change your pain/symptoms? (Some females with pain of a cardiac nature experience pain relief much like males do with nitroglycerin. This would likely be a female who is postmenopausal, possibly with a personal and/or family history of heart disease, so check vital signs.)

The client who cannot even lie on the involved side is probably fairly acute. The physical therapy plan of care will likely focus on pain relief first. Modalities and cryotherapy may be most effective. On the other hand, the client who can roll onto the involved side and stay there for 30 minutes to an hour may be more in the subacute phase. A combination of modalities, hands-on treatment, and exercise may be prescribed by the therapist.

The client who can lie on the involved side for up to 2 hours is more likely in the chronic phase of the musculoskeletal condition. Tissue ischemia brings on painful symptoms after prolonged static positioning. A more aggressive approach can usually be taken in these cases. These comments all apply to pain of an NMS origin.

⏩ PTA ACTION PLAN

Communication With the Physical Therapist

The PTA will provide feedback to the therapist about the client's sleeping patterns and changes in condition at night. The new information will be used by the PT to progress or modify the plan of care.

Night Pain and Cancer

Pain at night is a classic red-flag symptom of cancer, but it does not mean that all pain at night is caused by cancer or that all people with cancer will have night pain.[76] For example, the person who lies down at night and has not even fallen asleep who reports increased pain may just be experiencing the first moment in the day without distractions. Suddenly, his or her focus is on nothing but the pain, so the client may report the pain as much worse at night.

Bone pain at night is the most highly suspicious symptom, especially in the presence of a previous history of cancer. Neoplasms are highly vascularized at the expense of the host. This produces local ischemia and pain.

⏩ PTA ACTION PLAN

Communication With the Physical Therapist

Always report deep pain reported on weightbearing (or the inability to bear weight on the limb). The therapist may want to perform additional tests and measures. Keep in mind for the older adult that pain on weightbearing may be a symptom of a hip fracture. It is not uncommon for an older adult to fall and have hip pain and the x-rays are initially negative. If the pain persists, new x-rays or additional imaging may be needed.

Pain With Activity

Pain with activity from a systemic or disease process is most often caused by vascular compromise. In this context, activity pain of the upper quadrant is known as *angina* when the heart muscle is compromised and *intermittent vascular claudication* in the case of peripheral vascular compromise (lower quadrant).

Pain from an ischemic muscle (including heart muscle) builds up with the use of the muscle and subsides with rest.

With vascular-induced pain, there is usually a delay or lag time between the beginning of activity and the onset of symptoms.

? PICTURE THE PATIENT

The client complains that pain occurs after walking a certain distance, after a certain level of increased physical activity, or after a fixed amount of usage of the extremity.

⏩ PTA ACTION PLAN

Communication With the Physical Therapist

By documenting and reporting the timing of symptom onset, the PTA offers the therapist valuable screening clues for determining when symptoms are caused by musculoskeletal impairment or by vascular compromise.

The PTA can look for immediate pain or symptoms (especially when these can be reproduced with palpation, resistance to movement, and/or a change in position) versus symptoms 5 to 10 minutes after activity begins. Document and report the onset of pain with activity that occurs several minutes after the start of the activity or exercise.

Chronic Pain

Chronic pain persists past the expected physiologic time of healing. This may be less than 1 month or, more often, longer than 6 months. An underlying pathology is no longer identifiable and may never have been present.[77] The International Association for the Study of Pain has fixed 3 months as the most convenient point of division between acute and chronic pain.[78]

Chronic pain syndrome is characterized by a constellation of life changes that produce altered behavior in the individual and persist even after the cause of the pain has been eradicated. This syndrome is a complex multidimensional phenomenon that requires a focus toward maximizing functional abilities rather than treatment of pain.

In acute pain, the pain is proportional and appropriate to the problem and is treated as a symptom. In the chronic pain syndrome, uncontrolled and prolonged pain alters both the peripheral nervous system and CNS through processes of neural plasticity and central sensitization. Thus pain becomes a disease itself.[79,80]

⏩ PTA ACTION PLAN

Points to Ponder

Always keep in mind that painful symptoms that are out of proportion to the injury or are not consistent with the objective findings may be a red flag indicating systemic disease and should be documented and reported.

Catastrophizing and Fear Avoidance

Catastrophizing. Catastrophizing is an overreaction with a tendency to express negative thoughts and emotions, exaggerate the impact of painful experiences, and view the situation as hopeless (and the person in the situation as helpless) and expect the worst to happen. Catastrophizing boosts anxiety and worry and increases the risk for the development of chronic pain.[81–83]

PTA ACTION PLAN

Communication With the Physical Therapist

Identifying catastrophizing pain can help the PT make appropriate referral for behavioral therapy and coordinate rehabilitative efforts. The PTA should discuss with the therapist any observations that might suggest overreactions or catastrophizing pain and pain experiences.

Risk factors for persistent postsurgical pain include pain in other areas of the body before the operation, high levels of psychosocial distress (e.g., anxiety, depression, panic disorder), tobacco use, sleep disturbance (e.g., insomnia, sleep disruption), and chronic use of opioids. It may be helpful to report observations that might indicate opioid misuse.

Fear-Avoidance Behavior. Fear-avoidance behavior (FAB) can also be a part of disability from chronic pain.[84] The concept is based on studies that show a person's fear of pain (and not physical impairments) is the most important factor in how he or she responds to persistent musculoskeletal pain.[85-88]

❓ PICTURE THE PATIENT

FABs refer to ways people with chronic pain change their behavior, actions, movements, and activities. These changes are based on the fear that their pain will increase or that their actions will cause re-injury. Thoughts and emotions rule their behaviors because of concerns, worries, and fears that further harm will come to them.

For the most part, these fears are unfounded and become an obstacle to recovery. Patients put much more importance on pain and assume the pain means the injured body part is weak and vulnerable. The individual may be anxious, depressed, and inactive. They may start using more and more medications and become more like a "sick" person. Watch for (and report) multiple complaints, excessive preoccupation with pain, and ingestion of more pain relievers or narcotics than prescribed.

Elevated fear-avoidance beliefs are not indicative of a red flag for serious medical pathology. They are indicative of someone who has a poorer prognosis for rehabilitation (e.g., poor clinical outcomes, elevated pain symptoms, development of depressive symptoms, greater physical impairments, continued disability).[89] They are more accurately considered a yellow flag indicating psychosocial involvement and provide insight into the prognosis. Such a yellow flag signals the need for the PT to modify intervention and consider the need for referral to a psychologist or behavioral counselor.

PTA ACTION PLAN

Chronic Pain Assessment

- All older clients should be assessed for signs of chronic pain during the initial evaluation as well as on a consistent basis during therapy sessions. The PTA will need to be proactive in communicating accurate observations to the PT. The AGS recommends that the following techniques be used in clinic[90]:
  - Use alternative words for pain when asking the older client for a description (e.g., burning, discomfort, aching, sore, heavy feeling, tightness).
  - Contact caregiver for pain assessment in adults with cognitive or language impairments.
  - Clients with cognitive or language impairments should be observed for nonverbal pain behaviors, recent changes in function, and vocalizations to suggest

pain (e.g., irritability, agitation, withdrawal, gait changes, tone changes, nonverbal but vocal utterances such as groaning, crying, or moaning).
- The PT will follow the AGS guidelines for comprehensive pain assessment, including:
  - Medical history
  - Medication history, including current and previously used prescription and OTC drugs, as well as any nutraceuticals (e.g., natural products, "remedies")
  - Physical examination
  - Review of pertinent laboratory results and diagnostic tests (look for clues to the sequence of events leading to present pain complaint)
  - Assess characteristics of pain (frequency, intensity, duration, pattern, description, aggravating and relieving factors); use a standard pain scale such as the VAS

The PTA should take special note of the specific information just discussed from the initial evaluation report and from direct communication or instruction from the PT.
- The PTA should also be able to observe NMS system for:
  - Neurologic impairments
  - Weakness
  - Hyperalgesia; hyperpathia (exaggerated response to pain stimulus)
  - Allodynia (skin pain to nonnoxious stimulus)
  - Numbness, paresthesia
  - Tenderness, TrPs
  - Inflammation
  - Deformity

COMPARISON OF SYSTEMIC VERSUS MUSCULOSKELETAL PAIN PATTERNS

Table 2.1 provides a comparison of the clinical signs and symptoms of systemic pain versus musculoskeletal pain using the typical categories described earlier. Table 2.3 provides a review of pain mechanisms as they relate to the lesion site and the corresponding referred musculoskeletal pain patterns. The PTA must be very familiar with the information contained within these tables and communicate with the PT any time pain characteristics appear to fall more into the category of systemic pain than musculoskeletal pain.

The PTA is not expected to identify the underlying pathology, but it is imperative to recognize when the clinical presentation does not fit the expected pattern for NMS impairment.

❓ PICTURE THE PATIENT

Watch for a sudden or recent change in the clinical presentation and/or when the client develops constitutional symptoms or signs and symptoms commonly associated with an organ system. Pay attention any time someone uses words such as knife-like, boring, deep, or throbbing to describe the symptoms. These descriptors are more common with pain of a systemic nature.

PTA ACTION PLAN

Recognizing and Reporting Aberrant Patterns of Pain

Symptoms of an NMS origin can usually be altered, provoked, alleviated, eliminated, or aggravated. If this is not the case, the PTA will communicate this information to the therapist. For example, chest pain, neck pain, or upper back pain from a problem with the esophagus will likely get worse when the client is swallowing or eating.

The PTA must be alert for males over 50 years or postmenopausal females with a significant family history of heart disease, who are borderline hypertensive. New onset or reproduction of back, neck, temporomandibular joint, shoulder, or arm pain brought on by exertion with arms raised overhead or by starting a new exercise program is a reportable red flag.

Pain with activity is immediate when the NMS system is involved. There may be a delayed increase in symptoms after the initiation of activity with a systemic (vascular) cause. Aggravating and relieving factors associated with NMS impairment often involve a change in position.

Back, shoulder, pelvic, or sacral pain that is made better or worse by eating, passing gas, or having a bowel movement is a red flag and should be reported. Painful symptoms that start 3 to 5 minutes after initiating an activity and go away when the client stops the activity suggest pain of a vascular nature. This is especially true when the client uses the word "throbbing," which is a descriptor of a vascular origin.

Leaning forward or assuming a hands-and-knees position sometimes lessens gallbladder pain. This position moves the distended or inflamed gallbladder away from its position under the liver. Leaning or side bending toward the painful side sometimes ameliorates kidney pain. Again, for some people, this may move the kidney enough to take the pressure off during early onset of an infectious or inflammatory process.

Finally, notice the long list of potential signs and symptoms associated with systemic conditions (see Table 2.1). At the same time, note the *lack* of associated signs and symptoms listed on the musculoskeletal side of the table. Except for the possibility of some ANS responses with the stimulation of TrPs, there are no comparable constitutional or systemic signs and symptoms associated with the NMS system.

Characteristics of Viscerogenic Pain

Some characteristics of viscerogenic pain can occur regardless of which organ system is involved. For example, whether the individual is experiencing a urinary tract infection (renal/urologic system), pneumonia (respiratory system), or heart attack (cardiac system), the same symptoms can develop, such as a change in blood pressure, nausea, vomiting, and/or unexplained perspiration. Any of these individually is cause for suspicion and careful listening and watching. They often occur together in clusters of two or three. Watch for any of the following components of the pain pattern:

- Pain or other symptoms are progressive and cyclical pain (pain comes and goes over time but often stays longer with less time between episodes); the difference between an NMS pattern of pain and symptoms and a visceral pattern is that the NMS problem gradually improves over time, whereas the systemic condition gets worse.
- Constant, intense pain in a client with a previous personal history of cancer and/or in the presence of other associated signs and symptoms raises a red flag.
- Reports of sleep disturbance. Cancer pain wakes the client up from a sound sleep. An actual record of being awake and up for hours at night or awakened repeatedly is significant. See the discussion on "Night Pain" earlier in this chapter.
- Physical therapy intervention "fails" or the client does not get better with treatment. The lack of progression in treatment could very well be a red-flag symptom, as could the client reporting improvement in the early intervention phase but later taking a turn for the worse.

- Pain does not fit the expected pattern.
- Pain that is constant and intense, which should raise a red flag. There is a logical and important first question to ask anyone who says the pain is "constant," as indicated in the following PTA Action Plan.

▶▶ PTA ACTION PLAN

Follow-Up Questions

- Do you have that pain right now?
  It is surprising how often the client will answer negatively to this question. Although pain of an NMS origin can be constant, there is usually some way to make it better or worse.

RECOGNIZING EMOTIONAL AND PSYCHOLOGICAL SYMPTOMS

Pain, emotions, and pain behavior are all integral parts of the pain experience. There is no disease, illness, or state of pain without an accompanying psychological component.[22] This does not mean the client's pain is not real or does not exist on a physical level; in fact, clients with behavioral changes may also have significant underlying injury.[91] Physical pain and emotional changes are two sides of the same coin.[92]

Pain is not just a physical sensation that passes up to consciousness and then produces secondary emotional effects. Rather, the neurophysiology of pain and emotions are closely linked throughout the higher levels of the CNS. Sensory and emotional changes occur simultaneously and influence each other.[93]

The PTA often works with individuals who have personality disorders, who may be malingering, or who have other psychophysiologic disorders. Psychophysiologic disorders (also known as *psychosomatic* disorders) are any conditions in which the physical symptoms may be caused or made worse by psychological factors.

▶▶ PTA ACTION PLAN

Recognizing and Reporting Psychological Symptoms

Recognizing somatic signs of any psychophysiologic disorder is an important part of the PTA's observations for the PT. Behavioral, psychological, or medical treatment may be indicated. The PTA can describe the symptoms and relay that information to the therapist for further consideration.

❓ PICTURE THE PATIENT

Psychophysiologic disorders are generally characterized by subjective complaints that exceed objective findings, symptom development in the presence of psychosocial stresses, and physical symptoms involving one or more organ systems. Psychological factors, such as emotional stress and conflicts leading to anxiety, depression, and panic disorder, play an important role in the client's experience of physical symptoms. It will be helpful if the PTA can recognize anxiety, depression, and panic disorder (Table 2.6).

TABLE 2.6 Symptoms of Anxiety and Panic

Type	Symptoms
Physical	Increased sighing respirations
	Increased blood pressure
	Tachycardia
	Muscle tension
	Dizziness
	Lump in throat
	Shortness of breath
	Lump in throat
	Clammy hands
	Dry mouth
	Diarrhea
	Nausea
	Muscle tension
	Profuse sweating
	Restlessness, pacing, irritability, difficulty concentrating
	Chest pain[a]
	Headache
	Low back pain
	Myalgia (muscle pain, tension, or tenderness)
	Arthralgia (joint pain)
	Abdominal (stomach) distress
	Irritable bowel syndrome
Behavioral	Hyperalertness
	Irritability
	Uncertainty
	Apprehension
	Difficulty with memory or concentration
	Sleep disturbance
Cognitive	Fear of losing mind
	Fear of losing control
Psychological	Phobias
	Obsessive-compulsive behavior

[a]Chest pain associated with anxiety accounts for more than half of all emergency department admissions for chest pain. The pain is a substernal, dull ache that does not radiate and is not aggravated by respiratory movements but is associated with hyperventilation and claustrophobia.

Anxiety

Anxiety intensifies physical symptoms, much like an amplifier on a sound system. The amplifier does not change the sound but rather increases the power to make it louder. The tendency to amplify a broad range of bodily sensations may be an important factor in experiencing, reporting, and functioning with an acute and relatively mild medical illness.[94]

Anxiety increases muscle tension, thereby reducing blood flow and oxygen to the tissues and resulting in reports of sore muscles, back pain, headache, or fatigue. Anxiety-caused tension can produce heightened sensitivity to pain.

💡 PICTURE THE PATIENT

Anxious people have a reduced ability to tolerate painful stimulation, noticing it more or interpreting it as more significant than do nonanxious people. This leads to further complaining about pain and to more disability and pain behavior such as limping, grimacing, or medication seeking.

A known organic condition, such as a pulmonary embolus or chronic obstructive pulmonary disease (COPD), can cause fear and anxiety in older persons, especially if the client views the condition as unpredictable, variable, and disabling.

Depression

Once defined as a deep and unrelenting sadness lasting 2 weeks or more, depression is no longer viewed in such simplistic terms. As an understanding of this condition has evolved, scientists have come to speak of the *depressive illnesses*. This term gives a better idea of the breadth of the disorder, encompassing several conditions, including depression, dysthymia, bipolar disorder, and seasonal affective disorders.

The most common clinical signs and symptoms of depression include the following:

- Persistent sadness, low mood, or feelings of emptiness
- Frequent or unexplained crying spells
- A sense of hopelessness
- Feelings of guilt or worthlessness
- Problems in sleeping
- Loss of interest or pleasure in ordinary activities or loss of libido
- Fatigue or decreased energy
- Appetite loss (or overeating)
- Difficulty in concentrating, remembering, and making decisions
- Irritability
- Persistent joint pain
- Headache
- Chronic back pain
- Bilateral neurologic symptoms of unknown cause (e.g., numbness, dizziness, weakness)
- Thoughts of death or suicide
- Pacing and fidgeting
- Chest pain and palpitations

Although these conditions can differ among individuals, each includes some of the symptoms listed. Often the classic signs of depression are not as easy to recognize in people older than 65, and many people attribute such symptoms simply to "getting older" and ignore them.

Anyone can be affected by depression at any time. There are, in fact, many underlying physical and medical causes of depression (Box 2.5), including medications used for Parkinson disease, arthritis, cancer, hypertension, and heart disease (Box 2.6). The PTA should be familiar with these.

💡 PICTURE THE PATIENT

About one-third of the clinically depressed clients treated do not feel sad or blue. Instead, they report somatic symptoms such as fatigue, joint pain, headaches, or chronic back pain (or any chronic, recurrent pain present in multiple places). Many of the common GI disorders (e.g., esophageal motility disorder, nonulcer dyspepsia, irritable bowel syndrome) are associated with depressive or anxiety disorders.[95–98]

BOX 2.5 Physical Conditions Commonly Associated With Depression

Cardiovascular
Atherosclerosis
Hypertension
Myocardial infarction
Angioplasty or bypass surgery

Central Nervous System
Parkinson disease
Huntington disease
Cerebral arteriosclerosis
Stroke
Alzheimer disease
Temporal lobe epilepsy
Postconcussion injury
Multiple sclerosis
Miscellaneous focal lesions

Endocrine, Metabolic
Hyperthyroidism
Hypothyroidism
Addison disease
Cushing disease
Hypoglycemia
Hyperglycemia
Hyperparathyroidism
Hyponatremia
Diabetes mellitus
Pregnancy (postpartum)

Viral
Acquired immunodeficiency syndrome
Hepatitis

Pneumonia
Influenza

Nutritional
Folic acid deficiency
Vitamin B_6 deficiency
Vitamin B_{12} deficiency

Immune
Fibromyalgia
Chronic fatigue syndrome
Systemic lupus erythematosus
Sjögren syndrome
Rheumatoid arthritis
Immunosuppression (e.g., corticosteroid treatment)

Cancer
Pancreatic
Bronchogenic
Renal
Ovarian

Miscellaneous
Pancreatitis
Sarcoidosis
Syphilis
Porphyria
Corticosteroid treatment

(From Goodman CC: Biopsychosocial-spiritual concepts related to health care. In Goodman CC, Fuller K, editors: *Pathology: implications for the physical therapist*, ed 4, Philadelphia, 2014, WB Saunders.)

BOX 2.6 Drugs Commonly Associated With Depression

- Antianxiety medications (e.g., Valium, Xanax)
- Illegal drugs (e.g., cocaine, crack)
- Antihypertensive drugs (e.g., beta blockers, antiadrenergics)
- Cardiovascular medications (e.g., digitoxin, digoxin)
- Antineoplastic agents (e.g., vinblastine)
- Opiate analgesics (e.g., morphine, Demerol, Darvon)
- Anticonvulsants (e.g., Dilantin, phenobarbital)
- Corticosteroids (e.g., prednisone, cortisone, dexamethasone)
- Nonsteroidal antiinflammatory drugs (e.g., indomethacin)
- Alcohol

Depression is not a normal part of the aging process, but it is a normal response to pain or disability and may influence the client's ability to cope. Whereas anxiety is more apparent in acute pain episodes, depression occurs more often in clients with chronic pain.

Anxiety and depressive disorders occur at a higher rate in clients with COPD, obesity, diabetes, asthma, arthritis, cancer, and cardiovascular disease.[99,100] Other risk factors for depression

include lifestyle choices such as tobacco use, physical inactivity and sedentary lifestyle, and binge drinking.[101]

Another red flag for depression is any condition associated with smooth muscle spasm such as asthma, irritable or overactive bladder, Raynaud disease, and hypertension. Neurologic symptoms with no apparent cause such as paresthesias, dizziness, and weakness may actually be symptoms of depression. This is particularly true if the neurologic symptoms are symmetric or not anatomic.[102]

▶▶ PTA ACTION PLAN

Communication With the Physical Therapist

Systemic effects of depression are wide ranging; the PTA may be the first to recognize telltale signs of a problem and bring this to the PT's attention. The therapist may want to screen for psychosocial factors, such as depression, that influence physical rehabilitation outcomes, especially when a client demonstrates acute pain that persists for more than 6 to 8 weeks. Screening is also important because depression is an indicator of poor prognosis.[95]

In the primary care setting the PT has a key role in identifying comorbidities that may have an impact on physical therapy intervention. Depression has been clearly identified as a factor that delays recovery for clients with low back pain.

The longer depression is undetected, the greater the likelihood of prolonged physical therapy intervention and increased disability.[95,103]

Tests can be administered by the therapist to obtain baseline information that may be useful in determining the need for a medical referral. In the acute care setting the PTA may see results of the testing for depression in the medical record. Communication with the PT to find out more about the individual's needs and ways to incorporate education and treatment into the plan of care may be helpful.

Drugs, Depression, or Dementia?

The older adult often presents with such a mixed clinical presentation that it is difficult to know what is a primary musculoskeletal problem and what could be caused by drugs or depression (Case Example 2.3).

> ## ▶ PTA ACTION PLAN
>
> ### *Observation and Reporting*
>
> Family members confuse signs and symptoms of depression with dementia, and they may ask the PTA questions about this. In situations like this, it is always best to refer the family to the PT or physician. The PTA may be able to provide observational clues to the therapist by noting any of the following[104]:
> - Mental function: declines more rapidly with depression
> - Disorientation: present only in dementia

- Difficulty concentrating: depression
- Difficulty with short-term memory: dementia
- Writing, speaking, and motor impairments: dementia
- Memory loss: people with depression notice and comment, people with dementia are indifferent to the changes

Panic Disorders

Persons with panic disorders have episodes of sudden, unprovoked feelings of terror or impending doom with associated physical symptoms such as racing or pounding heartbeat, breathlessness, nausea, sweating, and dizziness. During an attack, people may fear that they are gravely ill, going to die, or going crazy.

The fear of another attack can itself become debilitating so that these individuals avoid situations and places that they believe will trigger the episodes, thus affecting their work, their relationships, and their ability to take care of everyday tasks.

Initial panic attacks may occur when people are under considerable stress, such as an overload of work or loss of a family member or close friend. The attacks may follow surgery, a serious accident, illness, or childbirth. The use of alcohol or drugs to mitigate these symptoms could make the panic disorder worse.[105]

CASE EXAMPLE 2.3   After Total Knee Replacement

A 71-year-old female has been referred for home health following a left total knee replacement. The initial evaluation and plan of care have been completed by the PT and the PTA is now providing the second treatment session. The client's surgery was 6 weeks ago, and she has had severe pain, swelling, and loss of motion. She has had numerous previous surgeries, including right shoulder arthroplasty, removal of the right eye (macular degeneration), rotator cuff repair on the left, hysterectomy, two cesarean sections, and several inner ear surgeries. In all, she proudly tells the PTA she has had 21 operations in 21 years.

Her family states, "She is taking Percocet prescribed by the orthopedic surgeon and Darvon left over from a previous surgery." They estimate that she takes at least 10 to 12 pills every day. They are concerned because she complains of constant pain and sleeps 18 hours a day.

They are hoping that physical therapy will "do something to help her constant pain."

How should the PTA approach working with this patient?

Take some time to listen to the client's pain description and concerns. Find out what her goals are and what would help her to reach those goals. This will be helpful information for the PT to follow-up on when reevaluating the client's progress later.

It will be important to be observant of any emotional overlay behaviors that you will want to report to the PT. With a long history of medical care, she may be dependent on the attention she gets for each operation. Addiction to pain-relieving drugs can occur, but it is more likely that she has become dependent on them because of a cycle of pain spasm/inactivity/pain spasm and so on.

Physical therapy intervention may help reduce some of this and change her pain pattern.

Depression may be a key factor in this case. Review the possible signs and symptoms of depression with the client. Keep in mind that it may not be necessary to tell the client ahead of time that these signs and symptoms are typical of

depression. Read the list and ask her to let you know if she is experiencing any of them. See how many she reports at this time. Afterward, ask her if she may be depressed and see how she responds to the question. Document this information to report back to the PT.

Medical referral for review of her medications and possible psychological evaluation may be in her best interest. You will want to communicate this to the PT for possible contact with the physician with the concerns and/or suggest the family report their concerns as well.

Keep in mind that exercise is a key intervention strategy for depression. As part of the physical therapy plan of care, you may be able to "do something" by including a general conditioning program in addition to her specific knee exercises.

The most common signs and symptoms associated with panic disorder include:
- Racing or pounding heartbeat
- Chest pains and/or palpitations
- Dizziness, lightheadedness, nausea
- Headaches
- Difficulty in breathing
- Bilateral numbness or tingling in nose, cheeks, lips, fingers, or toes
- Sweats or chills
- Hand wringing
- Dreamlike sensations or perceptual distortions
- Sense of terror
- Extreme fear of losing control
- Fear of dying

PICTURE THE PATIENT

The symptoms of a panic attack can mimic those of other medical conditions, such as respiratory or heart problems. Anxiety or panic is a leading cause of chest pain mimicking a heart attack. Residual sore muscles are a consistent finding after the panic attack and can also occur in individuals with social phobias. Panic disorder is characterized by a period of sudden, unprovoked, intense anxiety with associated physical symptoms lasting a few minutes up to a few hours. Dizziness, paresthesia, headaches, and palpitations are common.

People suffering from these attacks may be afraid or embarrassed to report their symptoms to the physician but may mention them to the PTA, who can then communicate this information to the therapist.

 PTA ACTION PLAN

Follow-Up Questions

The client may be aware of the symptoms but not know that these problems can be caused by depression, anxiety, or panic disorder. Besides observing for signs and symptoms of psychophysiologic disorders, the PTA can ask a few of the following questions to gather important information for the PT[1]:
- Do you have trouble sleeping at night?
- Do you have trouble focusing during the day?
- Do you worry about finances, work, or life in general?
- Do you feel a sense of dread or worry without cause?
- Do you ever feel happy?
- Do you have a fear of being in groups of people? Fear of flying? Public speaking?
- Do you have a racing heart, unexplained dizziness, or unexpected tingling in your face or fingers?
- Do you wake up in the morning with your jaw clenched or feeling sore muscles and joints?
- Are you irritable or jumpy most of the time?

OTHER CONSIDERATIONS

There are many different ways the PTA may recognize something that does not fit the expected pattern, whether it is something the patient says or does or perhaps reports as a change in symptoms or whether it is a new onset of sign or symptom. Physical, emotional, psychological, and spiritual stress or distress can manifest in many different ways. The educated and alert PTA may recognize and report red flags earlier, potentially reducing patient morbidity.

 PTA ACTION PLAN

Recognizing Red Flags of Distress

In all cases of pain the PTA can compile a list of behavioral signs and identify how the client is reacting to pain and report this to the therapist. Watch for the client who reports any of the following red-flag symptoms:
- Symptoms are out of proportion to the injury.
- Symptoms persist beyond the expected time for physiologic healing.
- No position is comfortable.
- Dramatization of complaints, leading to overtreatment and overmedication.
- Progressive dysfunction, leading to decreased physical activity and often compounding preexisting musculoskeletal or circulatory dysfunction.

- Drug misuse.
- Progressive dependency on others, including health care professionals, leading to overuse of the health care system.

These symptoms reflect both the possibility of emotional or psychological factors, as well as the possibility of a more serious underlying systemic disorder (including domestic violence or cancer).

 PTA ACTION PLAN

Recognizing Functional Outcomes

In these situations in which pain becomes too much of the focus during the treatment session, the therapist may direct the PTA to inquire about functional outcomes, instead of asking whether the client's symptoms are "better, the same, or worse." For example, it may be more appropriate to ask what the client can accomplish at home that she or he was unable to attempt at the beginning of treatment, last week, or even yesterday.

 PTA ACTION PLAN

Points to Ponder

We must keep in mind that pain from a disease process or viscerogenic source is often a late symptom rather than a reliable danger signal. For this reason the PTA must remain alert to other signs and symptoms that may be present but unreported. Pain with the following features raises a red flag to alert the PTA of the need to take a closer look and report back to the primary therapist:
- Pain of unknown cause.
- Pain that persists beyond the expected time for physiologic healing.
- Pain that is out of proportion to the injury.
- Pain that is unrelieved by rest or change in position.
- Pain pattern that does not fit the expected clinical presentation for a neuromuscular or musculoskeletal impairment.
- Pain that cannot be altered, aggravated, provoked, reduced, eliminated, or alleviated.
- There are some positions of comfort for various organs (e.g., leaning forward for the gallbladder or side bending for the kidney), but with progression of disease the client will obtain less and less relief of symptoms over time.
- Pain, symptoms, or dysfunction not improved or altered by physical therapy intervention.
- Pain that is poorly localized (patient cannot point to the exact spot and may indicate a more generalized area).
- Pain accompanied by signs and symptoms associated with a specific viscera (e.g., GI, genitourinary, gynecologic, cardiac, pulmonary, endocrine).
- Pain that is constant and intense no matter what position is tried and despite rest, eating, or abstaining from food; a previous history of cancer in this client is an even greater red flag necessitating further evaluation.
- Listen to the client's choice of words to describe pain. Systemic or viscerogenic pain can be described as deep, sharp, boring, knife-like, stabbing, throbbing, colicky, or intermittent (comes and goes in waves).
- Pain accompanied by full and normal ROM.

Recognizing clients whose symptoms are the direct result of organic dysfunction helps us in coping with clients who are hostile, ungrateful, noncompliant, negative, or adversarial. Patience is a vital tool for the PTA when working with clients who are having difficulty adjusting to the stress of illness and disability or the client who has a psychological disorder. The PTA can discuss with the therapist ways to cope when working with clients who have chronic illnesses or psychological disturbances.

REFERENCES

1. Raja SN, Carr DB, Cohen M, et al: The revised International Association for the Study of Pain definition of pain: concepts, challenges, and compromises, *Pain* 161(9):1976–1982, 2020.
2. Flaherty JH: Who's taking your fifth vital sign? *J Gerontol A Biol Sci Med Sci* 56:M397–M399, 2001.
3. Neale KL: The fifth vital sign: chronic pain assessment of the adolescent oncology patient, *J Pediatr Oncol Nurs* 29(4):185–198, 2012.
4. Casey G: Pain—the fifth vital sign, *Nurs N Z* 17(5):24–29, 2011.
5. Janig W: Visceral pain—still an enigma [commentary], *Pain* 151(2):239–240, 2010.
6. Brumovsky PR, Gebhart GF: Visceral organ cross-sensitization—an integrated perspective, *Auton Neurosci* 153(1–2):106–115, 2010.
7. Hoffman D: Understanding multisymptom presentations in chronic pelvic pain: the inter-relationships between the viscera and myofascial pelvic floor dysfunction, *Curr Pain Headache Rep* 15(5):343–346, 2011.
8. Woolf C: Central sensitization: implications for the diagnosis and treatment of pain, *Pain* 152(3S):S2–S15, 2011.
9. Chaban VV: Peripheral sensitization of sensory neurons, *Ethn Dis* 20(1 Suppl 1):S1–S6, 2010.
10. Fornasari D: Pain mechanisms in patients with chronic pain, *Clin Drug Investig* 32(Suppl 1):45–52, 2012.
11. Giamberardino MA: Viscero-visceral hyperalgesia: characterization in different clinical models, *Pain* 151(2):307–322, 2010.
12. Squire LR: *Fundamental neuroscience*, ed 4, Burlington, 2012, Academic Press.
13. Saladin KS: *Human anatomy & physiology II*, ed 5, New York, 2010, McGraw-Hill.
14. De Winter BY, Deiteren A, De Man JG: Novel nervous system mechanisms in visceral pain, *Neurogastroenterol Motil* 28:309–315, 2016.
15. Tanaka Y, Kanazawa M, Fukudo S, Drossman DA: Biopsychosocial model of irritable bowel syndrome, *J Neurogastroenterol Motil* 17(2):131–139, 2011.
16. Larauche M, Mulak A, Taché Y: Stress and visceral pain: from animal models to clinical therapies, *Exp Neurol* 233(1):49–67, 2012.
17. Rosenberger C, Elsenbruch S, Scholle A, et al: Effects of psychological stress on the cerebral processing of visceral stimuli in healthy women, *Neurogastroenterol Motil* 21(7):740–e45, 2009.
18. Aziz Q, Schnitzler A, Enck P: Functional neuroimaging of visceral sensation, *J Clin Neurophysiol* 17(6):604–612, 2000.
19. Pezone I, Iezzi ML, Leone S: Retrocardiac pneumonia mimicking acute abdomen: a diagnostic challenge, *Pediatr Emerg Care* 28(11):1230–1231, 2012.
20. Paul SP, Banks T, Fitz-John L: Abdominal pain in children with pneumonia, *Nurs Times* 108(14-15):21, 2012.
21. Sadler TW: *Langman's medical embryology*, ed 12, Philadelphia, 2011, Lippincott, Williams & Wilkins.
22. Hall JE: *Guyton and Hall textbook of medical physiology*, ed 12, Philadelphia, 2010, Saunders.
23. Söyüncü S, Bekta F, Cete Y: Traditional Kehr's sign: left shoulder pain related to splenic abscess, *Ulus Travma Acil Cerrahi Derg* 18(1):87–88, 2012.
24. Di Massa A, Avella R, Gentili C: Respiratory dysfunction related to diaphragmatic shoulder pain after abdominal and pelvic laparoscopy, *Minerva Anestesiol* 62(5):171–176, 1996.
25. Leavitt RL: Developing cultural competence in a multicultural world. Part II, *PT Magazine* 11(1):56–70, 2003.
26. Grubert E, Baker TA, McGeever K, Shaw BA: The role of pain in understanding racial/ethnic differences in the frequency of physical activity among older adults, *J Aging Health* 25(3):405–421, 2013.
27. American Geriatrics Society (AGS): Chronic pain in older persons, *J Am Geriatr Soc* 57(8):1331–1346, 2009.
28. Laslett LL, Stephen JQ, Tania MW, et al: A prospective study of the impact of musculoskeletal pain and radiographic osteoarthritis on health related quality of life in community dwelling older people, *BMC Musculoskelet Disord* 13:168, 2012.
29. Strauss VY, Carter P, Ong BN, et al: Public priorities for joint pain research: results from a general population survey, *Rheumatology (Oxford)* 51(11):2075–2082, 2012.
30. American Geriatrics Society Panel on Persistent Pain in Older Persons: The management of persistent pain in older persons, *J Am Geriatr Soc* 50(6 Suppl):S205–S224, 2002.
31. American Geriatrics Society Panel on Pharmacological Management of Persistent Pain in Older Persons: Pharmacological management of persistent pain in older persons, *J Am Geriatr Soc* 57(8):1331–1346, 2009.
32. Monroe TB, Herr KA, Mion LC, Cowan RL: Ethical and legal issues in pain research in cognitively impaired older adults, *Int J Nurs Stud* 50(9):1283–1287, 2013.
33. O'Connor L: Case report: a patient with dementia presenting with hip fracture in the emergency department—challenges of acute pain assessment, *Int Emerg Nurs* 20(4):255–260, 2012.
34. Feldt K: The checklist of nonverbal pain indicators (CNPI), *Pain Manag Nurs* 1(1):13–21, 2000.
35. Barr J, Fraser GL, Puntillo K, et al: Clinical practice guidelines for the management of pain, agitation, and delirium in adult patients in the intensive care unit, *Crit Care Med* 41(1):278–280, 2013.
36. Scherder EJ, Plooij B: Assessment and management of pain, with particular emphasis on central neuropathic pain, in moderate to severe dementia, *Drugs Aging* 29(9):701–706, 2012.
37. McCaffery M: *Pain: clinical manual*, ed 3, St. Louis, 2012, Mosby.
38. Huskinson EC: Measurement of pain, *Lancet* 2:1127–1131, 1974.
39. Carlsson AM: Assessment of chronic pain: aspects of the reliability and validity of the visual analog scale, *Pain* 16:87–101, 1983.
40. Melzack R: The McGill Pain Questionnaire: major properties and scoring methods, *Pain* 1:277, 1975.
41. Andreoli TE: *Andreoli and Carpenter's Cecil essentials of medicine*, ed 8, Philadelphia, 2010, Saunders.
42. DeLee JC, Drez D Jr., Miller MD: *Delee & Drez's orthopaedic sports medicine: principles and practice*, ed 3, Philadelphia, 2009, Saunders.
43. Melzack DC: *Handbook of pain assessment*, ed 3, New York, 2010, Guilford Press.
44. Bogduk N: On the definitions and physiology of back pain, referred pain, and radicular pain, *Pain* 147(1–3):17–19, 2009.
45. International Association for the Study of Pain: Classification of chronic pain. In *IASP pain terminology*, ed 2, 1994 (updated 2011). Available at: http://www.iasp-pain.org/PublicationsNews/Content.aspx?ItemNumber=1673. Accessed January 30, 2014.
46. Schaible HG: Joint pain, *Exp Brain Res* 196:153–162, 2009.
47. Schaible HG: Mechanisms of chronic pain in osteoarthritis, *Curr Rheumatol Rep* 14(6):549–556, 2012.
48. Duthie EH: *Practice of geriatrics*, ed 4, Philadelphia, 2007, Saunders.

49. Firestein GS: *Kelley's textbook of rheumatology*, ed 9, Philadelphia, 2012, Saunders.

50. Gerwin RD: Myofascial and visceral pain syndromes: Visceral-somatic pain representations, *J Musculoskel Pain* 10(1-2):165–175, 2002.

51. Daroff RB: *Bradley's neurology in clinical practice*, ed 6, Philadelphia, 2012, Saunders.

52. Rex L: *Evaluation and treatment of somatovisceral dysfunction of the gastrointestinal system*, Edmonds, 2012, URSA Foundation.

53. McMahon S, Koltzenburg M, editors: *Wall and Melzack's textbook of pain*, ed 6, New York, 2013, Churchill Livingstone.

54. Bouhassira D, Attal N: Diagnosis and assessment of neuropathic pain: the saga of clinical tools, *Pain* 152(3S):S74–S83, 2011.

55. Wells PE, Frampton V, Bowsher D: *Pain management in physical therapy*, ed 2, Oxford, 1994, Butterworth- Heinemann.

56. Stannard C: *Evidence-based chronic pain management*, West Sussex, 2010, Wiley-Blackwell.

57. Tasker RR: Spinal cord injury and central pain. In Aronoff GM, editor: *Evaluation and treatment of chronic pain*, ed 3, Philadelphia, 1999, Lippincott, Williams & Wilkins, pp 131–146.

58. Mandell GL: *Mandell, Douglas, and Bennett's principles and practice of infectious diseases*, ed 7, Philadelphia, 2009, Churchill Livingstone.

59. Bope ET, Kellerman RD: *Conn's current therapy 2013*, Philadelphia, 2012, Saunders.

60. Cailliet R: *Low back pain syndrome*, ed 5, Philadelphia, 1995, FA Davis.

61. Simons D, Travell J: *Myofascial pain and dysfunction: the trigger point manual*, ed 2, vols 1 and 2, Baltimore, 1999, Williams & Wilkins.

62. Jarrell J, Giamberardino MA, Robert M, Nasr-Esfahani M: Bedside testing for chronic pelvic pain: discriminating visceral from somatic pain, *Pain Res Treat* 2011:692102, 2011.

63. Emre M, Mathies H: *Muscle spasms and pain*, Park Ridge, 1988, Parthenon.

64. Plowden J, Renshaw-Hoelscher M, Engleman C, et al: Innate immunity in aging: impact on macrophage function, *Aging Cell* 3(4):161–167, 2004.

65. Potter JF: The older orthopaedic patient: general considerations, *Clin Orthop Relat Res* 425:44–49, 2004.

66. Myburgh C, Larsen AH, Hartvigsen J: A systematic, critical review of manual palpation for identifying myofascial trigger points: evidence and clinical significance, *Arch Phys Med Rehabil* 89(6):1169–1176, 2008.

67. Blaylock RL: *Excitotoxins: the taste that kills*, New Mexico, 1996, Health Press. Available at: http://www.russellblaylockmd.com/. Accessed January 30, 2014.

68. Roberts HJ: *Aspartame disease: the ignored epidemic*, West Palm Beach, 2001, Sunshine Sentinel Press.

69. Roberts HJ: *Defense against Alzheimer's disease*, West Palm Beach, 2001, Sunshine Sentinel Press.

70. Brakenhoff LK, van der Heijde DM, Hommes DW, et al: The joint-gut axis in inflammatory bowel disease, *J Crohns Colitis* 4(3):257–268, 2010.

71. Habif TP: *Clinical dermatology: a color guide to diagnosis and therapy*, ed 5, St. Louis, 2010, Mosby.

72. Sestak I, Cuzick J, Sapunar F: Risk factors for joint symptoms in patients enrolled in the ATAC trial: a retrospective, exploratory analysis, *Lancet Oncol* 9(9):866–872, 2008.

73. Waddell G, Bircher M, Finlayson D, et al: Symptoms and signs: physical disease or illness behavior? *Br Med J (Clin Res Ed)* 289:739–741, 1984.

74. Huang V, Mishra R, Thanabalan R, Nguyen GC: Patient awareness of extraintestinal manifestations of inflammatory bowel disease, *J Crohns Colitis* 7(8):e318–e324, 2013.

75. Jarvis C: *Physical examination and health assessment*, ed 5, Philadelphia, 2008, WB Saunders.

76. Slipman CW: Epidemiology of spine tumors presenting to musculoskeletal physiatrists, *Arch Phys Med Rehabil* 84:492–495, 2003.

77. Management of the individual with pain: Part 1—Physiology and evaluation, *PT Magazine* 4(11):54–63, 1996.

78. Turk DC, Melzack R, editors: *Handbook of pain assessment*, ed 3, New York, 2010, Guilford Press.

79. Simmonds MJ: Pain, mind, and movement—an expanded, updated, and integrated conceptualization, *Clin J Pain* 24(4):279–280, 2008.

80. Berna C: Induction of depressed mood disrupts emotion regulation neurocircuitry enhances pain unpleasantness, *Biol Psychiatry* 67(11):1038–1090, 2010.

81. Celestin J: Pretreatment psychosocial variables as predictors of outcomes following lumbar surgery and spinal cord stimulation: a systematic review and literature synthesis, *Pain Med* 10(4):639–653, 2009.

82. Wood BM, Nicholas MK, Blyth F, et al: Catastrophizing mediates the relationship between pain intensity and depressed mood in older adults with persistent pain, *J Pain* 14(2):149–157, 2013.

83. Pincus T, Vogel S, Burton AK, et al: Fear avoidance and prognosis in back pain: a systematic review and synthesis of current evidence, *Arthritis Rheum* 54(12):3999–4010, 2006.

84. Lethem J, Slade PD, Troup JDG, et al: Outline of a fear-avoidance model of exaggerated pain perception. I, *Behav Res Ther* 21(4):401–408, 1983.

85. Slade PD, Troup JDG, Lethem J, et al: The fear-avoidance model of exaggerated pain perception. II, *Behav Res Ther* 21(4):409–416, 1983.

86. George SZ, Valencia C, Beneciuk JM: A psychometric investigation of fear-avoidance model measures in patients with chronic low back pain, *J Orthop Sports Phys Ther* 40(4):197–205, 2010.

87. Calley D, Jackson S, Collins H, George SZ: Identifying patient fear-avoidance beliefs by physical therapists managing patients with low back pain, *J Orthop Sports Phys Ther* 40(12):774–783, 2010.

88. Leeuw M: The fear-avoidance model of musculoskeletal pain: current state of scientific evidence, *J Behav Med* 30(1):77–94, 2007.

89. American Geriatrics Society (AGS) Panel on Chronic Pain in Older Persons: Clinical practice guidelines, *J Am Geriatr Soc* 46:635–651, 1998.

90. Connelly C: Managing low back pain and psychosocial overlie, *J Musculoskelet Med* 21(8):409–419, 2004.

91. Main CJ, Waddell G: Behavioral responses to examination: a reappraisal of the interpretation of "nonorganic signs", *Spine (Phila Pa 1976)* 23(21):2367–2371, 1998.

92. Waddell G: *The back pain revolution*, ed 2, Philadelphia, 2004, Churchill Livingstone.

93. Crofford LJ: Chronic pain: where the body meets the brain, *Trans Am Clin Climatol Assoc* 126:167–183, 2015.

94. Haggman S, Maher CG, Refshauge KM: Screening for symptoms of depression by physical therapists managing low back pain, *Phys Ther* 84(12):1157–1166, 2004.

95. Bravo JA, Julio-Pieper M, Forsythe P, et al: Communication between gastrointestinal bacteria and the nervous system, *Curr Opin Pharmacol* 12(6):667–672, 2012.

96. Banerjee A, Sarkhel S, Sarkar R, et al: Anxiety and depression in irritable bowel syndrome, *Indian J Psychol Med* 39:741–745, 2017.

97. Bouchoucha M, Hejnar M, Devroede G, et al: Anxiety and depression as markers of multiplicity of sites of functional gastrointestinal disorders: a gender issue? *Clin Res Hepatol Gastroenterol* 37(4):422–430, 2013.

98. Brenes GA: Anxiety and chronic obstructive pulmonary disease: prevalence, impact, and treatment, *Psychosom Med* 65(6):963–970, 2003.

99. Gonzalez O: Current depression among adults in the United States, *MMWR Morb Mortal Wkly Rep* 59(38):1229–1235, 2010.

100. Strine TW: Depression and anxiety in the United States: findings from the 2006 Behavioral Risk Factor Surveillance System, *Psychiatr Serv* 59:1383–1390, 2008.

101. Smith NL: *The effects of depression and anxiety on medical illness*, Sandy, 2002, University of Utah, Stress Medicine Clinic.

102. Sartorius N, Ustun T, Lecrubier Y, et al: Depression comorbid with anxiety: results from the WHO study on psychological disorders in primary health care, *Br J Psychiatry* 168:38–40, 1996.

103. Rubin R: Exploring the relationship between depression and dementia, *JAMA* 320(10):961–962, 2018.

104. Jacobson JL: *Psychiatric secrets*, ed 2, Philadelphia, 2001, Hanley and Belfus.

105. Smith JP, Book SW: Anxiety and substance use disorders: a review, *Psychiatr Times* 25(10):19–23, 2008.

3

Recognizing, Documenting, and Reporting Red Flags

In the medical model, clients are often assessed from head to toe. The doctor, physician assistant, nurse, or nurse practitioner starts with inspection, followed by percussion and palpation, and finally by auscultation.

In a screening assessment, the physical therapist (PT) may not need to perform a complete head-to-toe physical assessment. If the initial observations, client history, screening questions, and screening tests are negative, a thorough examination may not be necessary.

In most situations, the therapist will assess one system above and below the area of complaint based on evidence supporting a regional-interdependence model of musculoskeletal impairments (i.e., symptoms present may be caused by musculoskeletal impairments proximal or distal to the site of presenting symptoms distinct from the phenomenon of referred pain).[1]

If the situation changes and the patient/client presents with changing, new, or different clinical signs and/or symptoms, the physical therapist assistant (PTA) may be the first one to hear about or observe these changes. With progression of disease or new onset of comorbidities, what the PTA observes may differ from what the PT described in the initial evaluation. During a general survey, the PTA must remain alert for any changes from the expected norm as well as changes from the client's baseline measurements.

In the normal course of a PTA's practice the initial evaluation is read with an eye toward areas that will require the PTA's attention (e.g., balance, posture, range of motion). During each treatment session, the PTA must remain alert to the presence of any red-flag clinical presentations affecting any of the systems.

In the next two chapters, we will help the PTA identify red-flag findings by making general observations (in this chapter) and by recognizing red flags suggestive of each body system (e.g., hematologic system, cardiovascular system, pulmonary system). The PTA will gain an understanding of when to consult with the PT (or nurse), how much information to collect and share, and how much information to collect and communicate is too much or too little.

⏩ PTA ACTION PLAN

Points to Ponder

Having trouble deciding who to report your abnormal observations to? Ask yourself:
- Who is responsible for the immediate care of the individual according to the type of setting you are working in?
- Does the change require further assessment or examination by the PT, registered nurse, or physician?
- Is the change a medical emergency?

GENERAL SURVEY

The general survey begins the moment the PTA meets the client and can observe body size and type and facial expressions, assess self-care, and note anything unusual in appearance or presentation. As the PTA makes a general survey of each client, it is also possible to observe posture, movement patterns and gait, balance, and coordination (Box 3.1). For more involved clients, the first impression may be based on level of consciousness, respiratory and vascular function, or nutritional status.

Observations of the head and neck provide information about oral health and the general health of multiple systems, including integumentary, neurologic, respiratory, endocrine, hepatic, and gastrointestinal (GI).

The head, hair, scalp, and face are observed for size, shape, symmetry, cleanliness, and presence of infection. The head should be positioned over the spine and in the midline. Because the head and neck have a large blood supply, infection from the mouth can quickly spread throughout the body, increasing the risk of osteomyelitis, pneumonia, and septicemia in critically ill patients. Evidence of gum disease (e.g., bright red, enlarged, spongy, or bleeding) should be medically evaluated. Ulcerations on the tongue, lips, or gums also require further medical/dental evaluation.

The eyes can be observed for changes in shape, motor function, and color (conjunctiva and sclera). Conducting an assessment of cranial nerves II, III, and IV will also help screen for visual problems. The PTA should be aware that there are changes in the way older adults perceive color. This kind of change can affect function and safety; for example, some older adults are unable to tell when floor tiles end and the bathtub begins in a bathroom. Stumbling and loss of balance can occur at boundary changes.

Headaches are common and often the result of specific foods, stress, muscle tension, hormonal fluctuations, nerve compression, or cervical spine or temporomandibular joint dysfunction. Most headaches are acute and self-limited. Headaches can be a symptom of a serious medical condition and should be documented and reported to the PT.

In an acute care or trauma setting the PTA may be using vital signs and the ABCDE (*a*irway, *b*reathing, *c*irculation, *d*isability, *e*xposure) method of quick assessment. A common strategy for history taking in the trauma unit is the mnemonic AMPLE: *a*llergies, *m*edications, *p*ast medical history, *l*ast meal, and *e*vents of injury.

BOX 3.1   Guide To Physical Assessment

- Level of consciousness
- Mental and emotional status
- Vision and hearing
- Speech
- General appearance
- Nutritional status
- Level of self-care
- Body size and type (body mass index)
- Obvious deformities
- Muscle atrophy
- Posture
- Body and breath odors
- Movement patterns and gait
- Use of assistive devices or mobility aids
- Balance and coordination
- Skin, hair, and nails
- Vital signs

BOX 3.2   Risk Factors for Iatrogenic or Postoperative Delirium

- Stress, trauma, pain, infection
- Hospitalization (for hip fracture, serious illness, or trauma including surgery) or change in residence
- Older age (65 years or older)
- Anesthesia
- Hip or knee joint replacement
- Poor cognitive function, underlying dementia, previous cognitive impairment
- Vision or hearing deficits
- Decreased physical function
- History of alcohol abuse
- Medications (e.g., benzodiazepine, narcotics, nonsteroidal antiinflammatory drugs, anticholinergics prescribed for sleep, psychoactive drugs/antidepressants/antipsychotics, dopamine agents, analgesics, sedative agents for pain and anxiety after surgery)*
- Dehydration
- Urinary retention, fecal impaction, diarrhea
- Sleep deprivation
- Postoperative low hemoglobin, abnormal fluid and/or electrolytes, low oxygen saturation
- Malnutrition, vitamin B_{12}/folate deficiency, low albumin

* Higher risk medications are commonly associated with delirium; lower risk medications associated with delirium include some cardiovascular agents (e.g., antiarrhythmics, beta blockers, clonidine, digoxin), antimicrobials (e.g., fluoroquinolones, penicillins, sulfonamides, acyclovir), anticonvulsants, and medications for gastroesophageal reflux or nausea. (From Alfonso DT: Nonsurgical complications after total hip and total knee arthroplasty, *Am J Orthop* 35(11):503–510, 2006; Short M, Winstead PS: Delirium dilemma: pharmacology update, *Orthopedics* 30(4):273–277, 2007.)

In any setting, knowing the client's personal health history will also help guide and direct the PTA's attention and observations. The PT will be screening for medical diseases masquerading as neuromusculoskeletal (NMS) problems. Many physical illnesses, diseases, and medical conditions directly impact the NMS system and must be taken into account. The PTA assists in this endeavor as well by reporting any unusual, suspicious, or new findings. A working knowledge of what to look for is essential in this process.

PICTURE THE PATIENT

Inspection of the integument, limb inspection, and screening of the peripheral vascular system, to list some examples, is important for someone at risk for lymphedema. For someone with diabetes, observing neurologic function, balance, reflexes, and peripheral circulation may be important. Peripheral neuropathy is common in this population group, often making walking more difficult and increasing the risk of other problems developing.

Mental Status

Level of consciousness, orientation, and ability to communicate are all part of every health care professional's assessment of a client's mental status. Orientation refers to the client's ability to correctly answer questions about time, place, and person. A healthy individual with normal mental status will be alert, speak coherently, and be aware of the date, day, and time of day.

The PTA must be aware of any factor that can affect a client's current mental status. Shock, head injury, stroke, hospitalization, surgery (use of anesthesia), medications, age, and the use of substances and/or alcohol can cause impaired consciousness.

Other factors affecting mental status may include malnutrition, exposure to chemicals, and hypothermia or hyperthermia. Depression and anxiety can also affect a client's functioning, mood, memory, ability to concentrate, judgment, and thought processes. Educational and socioeconomic background along with communication skills (e.g., English as a second language, aphasia) can affect mental status and function.

In a hospital, transition unit, or extended care facility, mental status is often evaluated and documented by the social worker or nursing service. It is always a good idea for the PTA to review the client's chart or electronic record regarding this information before meeting with the client.

Risk Factors for Delirium

It is not uncommon for older adults to experience a change in mental status or go through a stage of confusion about 24 hours after hospitalization for a serious illness or trauma, including surgery under a general anesthetic. Physicians may refer to this as *iatrogenic delirium, anesthesia-induced dementia*, or *postoperative delirium*. It is usually temporary but can last several hours to several weeks.

The cause of deterioration in mental ability is unknown. In some cases, delirium/dementia appears to be triggered by the shock to the body from anesthesia and surgery.[2] It may be a passing phase with complete recovery by the client, although this can take weeks to months. The likelihood of delirium associated with hospitalization is much higher with hip fractures and hip and knee joint replacements,[3–7] possibly attributed to older age, slower metabolism, and polypharmacy (more than four prescribed drugs at admission).[8]

The PTA should pay attention to factors for dementia (Box 3.2) and watch out for any of the signs or symptoms of delirium. The general survey should include vital signs with oxygen concentration measured and surveillance for signs of infection. A medical diagnosis is needed to make the distinction between postoperative delirium (also known as postoperative cognitive dysfunction), baseline dementia, depression, and withdrawal from drugs and alcohol.[9-11] Look for this type of diagnostic information in the medical record.

❓ PICTURE THE PATIENT

These are clinical signs and symptoms of iatrogenic delirium:

Cognitive Impairment
- Unable to concentrate during conversations
- Easily distracted or inattentive
- Switches topics often
- Unable to complete simple math or spell simple words backward

Impaired Orientation
- Unable to remember familiar concepts (e.g., say the days of the week, unable to tell time)
- Does not know who he is or where he is
- Unable to recognize family or close friends without help

Impaired Speech
- Speech is difficult to understand
- Unable to speak in full sentences; sentences do not make sense

Psychological Impairment
- Anxious and afraid; requires frequent reassurance
- Suspicious of others, paranoid
- Irritable, jumpy, or in constant motion
- Experiencing delusions and hallucinations (e.g., sees objects or people who are not there; smells scents that are not present)

▶▶ PTA ACTION PLAN

Reporting Potential Red Flags of Delirium

Report any new or emerging clinical signs and/or symptoms. Any observed change in level of consciousness, orientation, judgment, communication or speech pattern, or memory should be documented and reported. The PTA may be the first to notice increased lethargy, slowed motor responses, or disorientation or confusion.

Confusion is not a normal change with aging and must be reported and documented. Confusion is often associated with various systemic conditions (Table 3.1). Increased confusion in a client with any form of dementia can be a symptom of infection (e.g., pneumonia, urinary tract infection), electrolyte imbalance, or delirium. Likewise, a sudden change in muscle tone (usually increased tone) in the client with a neurologic disorder (adult or child) can signal an infectious process.

Nutritional Status

Nutrition is an important part of growth and development and recovery from infection, illness, wounds, and surgery. Clients can exhibit signs of malnutrition or overnutrition (obesity).

TABLE 3.1 Systemic Conditions Associated With Confusional States

System	Impairment/Condition
Endocrine	Hypothyroidism, hyperthyroidism; Perimenopause, menopause
Metabolic	Severe anemia; Fluid and/or electrolyte imbalances; dehydration; Wilson disease (copper disorder); Porphyria (inherited disorder)
Immune/Infectious	AIDS; Cerebral amebiasis, toxoplasmosis, or malaria; Fungal or tuberculosis meningitis; Lyme disease; Neurosyphilis
Cardiovascular	CHF
Cerebrovascular	Cerebral insufficiency (TIA, CVA); Postanoxic encephalopathy
Pulmonary	COPD; Hypercapnia (increased CO_2); Hypoxemia (decreased arterial O_2)
Renal	Renal failure, uremia; Urinary tract infection
Neurologic	Encephalopathy (hepatic, hypertensive); Head trauma; Cancer; CVA; stroke
Other	Chronic drug and/or alcohol use; Medication (e.g., anticonvulsants, antidepressants, antiemetics, antihistamines, antipsychotics, benzodiazepines, narcotics, sedative-hypnotics, Zantac, Tagamet); Postoperative; Severe anemia; Cancer metastasized to the brain sarcoidosis; Sleep apnea; Vasculitis (e.g., SLE); Vitamin deficiencies (B_{12}, folate, niacin, thiamine); Whipple disease (severe intestinal disorder)

(From Dains JE, Baumann LC, Scheibel P: *Advanced health assessment & clinical diagnosis in primary care*, ed 4, St. Louis, 2011, Mosby.) *AIDS*, Acquired immunodeficiency syndrome; *CHF*, congestive heart failure; *COPD*, chronic obstructive pulmonary disease; *CVA*, cerebrovascular accident; *SLE*, systemic lupus erythematosus; *TIA*, transient ischemic attack.

❓ PICTURE THE PATIENT

These are clinical signs and symptoms of undernutrition or malnutrition:
- Muscle wasting
- Alopecia (hair loss)
- Dermatitis; dry, flaking skin
- Chapped lips, lesions at corners of mouth
- Brittle nails
- Abdominal distention
- Decreased physical activity/energy level; fatigue, lethargy
- Peripheral edema
- Bruising

▶▶ PTA ACTION PLAN
Nutritional Status

Be aware in the health history of any risk factors for nutritional deficiencies (Box 3.3). Remember that some medications can cause appetite changes and that psychosocial factors such as depression, eating disorders, drug or alcohol addictions, and economic variables can affect nutritional status.

It may be necessary to determine the client's ideal body weight by calculating the body mass index (BMI).[12,13] Several websites are available to help anyone make this calculation. The National Center for Chronic Disease Prevention and Health Promotion sponsors a separate website for children and teens.[14]

Whenever nutritional deficiencies are suspected, the PTA should notify the PT, who may request a referral to a registered dietitian.

Body and Breath Odors

Odors may provide some significant clues to overall health status. For example, a fruity (sweet) breath odor (detectable by some but not all health care professionals) may be a symptom of diabetic ketoacidosis. Bad breath (halitosis) can be a symptom of dental decay, lung abscess, throat or sinus infection, or GI disturbances from food intolerances, *Helicobacter pylori* bacteria, or bowel obstruction. Keep in mind that ethnic foods and alcohol can affect breath and body odor.

Clients who are incontinent (bowel or bladder) may smell of urine, ammonia, or feces. It is important to ask the client about any unusual odors. It may be best to offer an introductory explanation with some follow-up questions, as follows.

BOX 3.3   **Risk Factors for Nutritional Deficiency**

- Economic status
- Living alone
- Older age (metabolic rate slows in older adults; altered sense of taste and smell affects appetite)
- Depression, anxiety
- Eating disorders
- Lactose intolerance (common in Mexican Americans, African Americans, Asians, Native Americans)
- Alcohol/drug addiction
- Chronic diarrhea
- Nausea
- Gastrointestinal impairment (e.g., bowel resection, gastric bypass, pancreatitis, Crohn's disease, pernicious anemia)
- Chronic endocrine or metabolic disorders (e.g., diabetes mellitus, celiac sprue)
- Liver disease
- Dialysis
- Medications (e.g., captopril, chemotherapy, steroids, insulin, lithium), including over-the-counter drugs (e.g., laxatives)
- Chronic disability affecting activities of daily living (e.g., problems with balance, mobility, food preparation)
- Burns
- Difficulty chewing or swallowing (dental problems, stroke, or other neurologic impairment)

▶▶ PTA ACTION PLAN
Follow-Up Questions

- Are you being treated by anyone for any other problems? (Wait for a response, but add prompts as needed: chiropractor? acupuncturist? naturopath?)
- [If you suspect urinary incontinence]: Are you having any trouble with leaking urine or making it to the bathroom on time? (Ask appropriate follow-up questions about cause, frequency, severity, triggers, etc.)
- [If you suspect fecal incontinence]: Do you have trouble getting to the toilet on time for a bowel movement? Do you have trouble wiping yourself clean after a bowel movement? (Ask appropriate follow-up questions about cause, frequency, severity, triggers, etc.)
- [If you detect unusual breath odor]: I notice an unusual smell on your breath. Do you know what might be causing this? (Ask appropriate follow-up questions depending on the type of smell you perceive.)
- Report any concerning information obtained from the follow-up questions to the primary PT for further evaluation.
- Document pertinent information and plan follow-through with the PT.

Vital Signs

The need for all health care professionals to assess vital signs, especially pulse and blood pressure (BP), is increasing.[15,16] Without the benefit of laboratory values, physical assessment becomes much more important. Vital signs, observations, and reported associated signs and symptoms are among the best observational tools available.

Vital sign assessment is an important tool because high BP is a serious concern in the United States. Many people are unaware they have high BP and are asymptomatic.[17] Primary orthopedic clients often have secondary cardiovascular disease.[18,19]

PTAs practicing in a primary care setting will especially need to know when and how to assess vital signs. The *Guide to Physical Therapist Practice*[20] recommends that heart rate (pulse) and blood pressure measurements be included in the examination of new clients. Exercise professionals are strongly encouraged to measure BP during each visit.[21]

Taking a client's vital signs remains the single easiest, most economic, and fastest way to quickly identify the presence of many systemic illnesses. If the PTA does not conduct any other screening physical assessment, vital signs should be assessed for a baseline value and then monitored.

All the vital signs are important (Box 3.4); temperature and BP have the greatest utility as early screening tools for systemic illness or disease, whereas pulse, BP, and oxygen (O_2) saturation levels offer valuable information about the cardiovascular/pulmonary systems.

BOX 3.4   **Vital Signs**

- Pulse (beats per minute)
- Blood pressure
- Core body temperature (oral or ear)
- Respirations
- Pulse oximetry (oxygen [O_2] saturation)
- Pain (now called the fifth vital sign)
- Walking speed (the sixth vital sign)[22]

▶▶ PTA ACTION PLAN

Using Vital Signs

Using vital signs is an easy yet effective way to document outcomes. In today's evidence-based practice, the PTA can use something as simple as pulse or BP to document changes that occur with intervention. These documented changes in the client's activity tolerance can provide crucial information to the PT regarding appropriate modifications needed in the plan of care.

For example, if ambulating with a client in the morning and afternoon results in no change in ease of ambulation, speed, or distance, consider taking BP, pulse, and O_2 saturation levels before and after each session. Improvement in O_2 saturation levels or a faster return to normal heart rate after exercise are just two examples of how vital signs can become an important part of outcome documentation.

Assessment of baseline vital signs should be a part of the initial data collected so that correlations and comparisons with future values are available when necessary. The PTA compares measurements taken against normal values and compares future measurements to the baseline units to identify significant changes (normalizing values or moving toward abnormal findings) for each client.

❓ PICTURE THE PATIENT

Normal ranges of values for the vital signs are provided for your convenience (Table 3.2). However, these ranges can be exceeded by a client and still represent normal for that person. Keep in mind that many factors can affect vital signs, especially pulse and blood pressure (3.5 mm Hg). Substances, such as alcohol, caffeine, nicotine, and cocaine/cocaine derivatives, as well as pain and stress/anxiety can cause fluctuations in blood pressure. Adults who monitor their own blood pressure may report wide fluctuations without making the association between these and other factors listed. It is the unusual vital sign in combination with other signs and symptoms, medications, and medical status that gives clinical meaning to the pulse rate, blood pressure, and temperature.

Pulse Rate

The pulse reveals important information about the client's heart rate and heart rhythm. A resting pulse rate (normal range: 60–100 beats per minute [bpm]) taken at the carotid artery or radial artery pulse point (preferred sites) should be available for comparison with the pulse rate taken during treatment or after exercise. A pulse rate above 100 bpm indicates tachycardia; a rate below 60 bpm indicates bradycardia.

Pulse oximeter devices cannot be relied on for pulse rate because these units often take a sample pulse rate that reflects a mean average and may not reveal dysrhythmias (e.g., a regular irregular pulse rate associated with atrial fibrillation). It is recommended that the pulse always be checked in two places: in older adults and in anyone with diabetes. Pulse strength (amplitude) can be graded as follows:

0	Absent, not palpable
1+	Pulse diminished, barely palpable
2+	Easily palpable, normal
3+	Full pulse, increased strength
4+	Bounding, too strong to obliterate

Keep in mind that taking the pulse measures the peripheral arterial wave propagation generated by the heart's contraction; it is not the same as measuring the true heart rate (and should not be recorded as heart rate when measured by palpation). A true measure of heart rate requires auscultation or electrocardiographic recording of the electrical impulses of the heart. The distinction between pulse rate and heart rate becomes a matter of concern in documentation liability and even greater importance for individuals with dysrhythmias. In such cases, the output of blood by some beats may be insufficient to produce

TABLE 3.2 Classification of Blood Pressure (BP)*

	Systolic Blood Pressure	Diastolic Blood Pressure
For Adults†		
Normal (mm Hg)	<120	<80
Prehypertension	120–139	80–89
Stage 1 hypertension	140–159	90–99
Stage 2 hypertension	≥160	≥100
For Children and Adolescents‡		
Normal	<90th percentile; 50th percentile is the midpoint of the normal range	
Prehypertension	90th–95th percentile or if BP is greater than 120/80 mm Hg (even if this figure is <90th percentile)	
Stage 1 Hypertension	95th–99th percentile + 5 mm Hg	
Stage 2 Hypertension	>99th percentile + 5 mm Hg	

*The relationship between BP and risk of coronary vascular disease (CVD) events is continuous, consistent, and independent of other risk factors. The higher the BP, the greater the chance of heart attack, heart failure, stroke, and kidney disease. For individuals 40 to 70 years of age, each 20 mm Hg incremental increase in systolic BP (SBP) or 10 mm Hg in diastolic BP (DBP) doubles the risk of CVD across the entire BP range from 115/75 to 185/115 mm Hg.

†From the Seventh Report of the Joint National Committee on Prevention, Detection, Evaluation, and Treatment of High Blood Pressure, NIH Publication No. 03-5233, May 2003. National Heart, Lung, and Blood Institute (NHLBI). Available at: www.nhlbi.nih.gov/.

‡From National Heart, Lung, and Blood Institute (NHLBI): Fourth report on the diagnosis, evaluation, and treatment of high blood pressure in children and *adolescents, Pediatrics* 114(2):555–576, 2004.

a detectable pulse wave that would be discernible with an electrocardiogram.[24]

Pulse amplitude (weak or bounding quality of the pulse) gives an indication of the circulating blood volume and the strength of left ventricle ejection. Normally, the pulse increases slightly with inspiration and decreases with expiration. This slight change is not considered significant.

Pulse amplitude that fades with inspiration instead of strengthening and strengthens with expiration instead of fading is paradoxic and should be reported to the physician. Paradoxic pulse occurs most commonly in clients with chronic obstructive pulmonary disease (COPD) but is also observed in clients with constrictive pericarditis.[25]

Constriction or compression around the heart from pericardial effusion, tension pneumothorax, pericarditis with fluid, or pericardial tamponade may be associated with paradoxical pulse. When the person breathes in, the increased mechanical pressure of inspiration added to the physiologic compression from the underlying disease prevents the heart from contracting fully and results in a reduced pulse. When the person breathes out, the pressure from chest expansion is reduced, and the pulse increases.

▶▶ PTA ACTION PLAN

Measuring and Reporting Pulse Rate

A pulse increase with activity of more than 20 bpm lasting for more than 3 minutes after rest or changing position should be reported. Other pulse abnormalities are listed in Box 3.6.

The resting pulse may be higher than normal with fever, anemia, infections, some medications, hyperthyroidism, anxiety, or pain. A low pulse rate (below 60 bpm) is not uncommon among trained athletes. Medications such as beta blockers and calcium channel blockers can also prevent the normal rise in pulse rate that usually occurs during exercise. In such cases, the PTA must monitor rates of perceived exertion (RPE) instead of pulse rate.

When taking the resting pulse or pulse during exercise, it is always best to palpate the pulse for a full minute. Longer pulse counts give more reliable information and provide more time for the detection of some dysrhythmias (Box 3.7).[21]

Respiration

Try to assess the client's breathing without drawing attention to what is being done. This measure can be taken right after counting the pulse while still holding the client's wrist.

Count respirations for 1 minute unless respirations are unlabored and regular, in which case the count can be taken for 30 seconds and multiplied by 2. The rise and fall of the chest equals 1 cycle. The normal rate is between 12 and 20 breaths per minute.

▶▶ PICTURE THE PATIENT

When assessing rate it is important to observe excursion (shallow or normal or deep), effort (gasping, straining or relaxed), and pattern. Note any use of accessory muscles and whether breathing is silent or noisy. Watch for puffed cheeks, pursed lips, nasal flaring, or asymmetric chest expansion. Changes in the rate, depth, effort, or pattern of a client's respirations can be early signs of neurologic, pulmonary, or cardiovascular impairment.

Pulse Oximetry

Oxygen saturation on hemoglobin (SaO_2) and pulse rate can be measured simultaneously using pulse oximetry (SpO_2). This is a noninvasive, photoelectric device with a sensor that can be attached to a well-perfused finger, the bridge of the nose, toe, forehead, or ear lobe. Digital readings are less accurate with clients who are anemic, undergoing chemotherapy, or using fingernail polish or nail acrylics. In such cases, attach the sensor to one of the other accessible body parts.

The sensor probe emits red and infrared light, which is transmitted to the capillaries. When in contact with the skin, the probe measures transmitted light passing through the vascular bed and detects the relative amount of color absorbed by the arterial blood. The SaO_2 level is calculated from this information.

The normal SpO_2 range at rest and during exercise is 95% to 100%. The exception to this normal range is for clients with a history of tobacco use and/or COPD. Some individuals with COPD tend to retain carbon dioxide (CO_2) and can become apneic if the O_2 levels are too high. For this reason, SpO_2 levels are normally kept lower for this population.

The drive to breathe in a healthy person results from an increase in the arterial carbon dioxide level ($PaCO_2$). In the normal adult, increased CO_2 levels stimulate chemoreceptors in the brainstem to increase the respiratory rate. With some chronic lung disorders these central chemoreceptors may become desensitized to $PaCO_2$ changes, resulting in a dependence on the peripheral chemoreceptors to detect a fall in arterial oxygen levels (PaO_2) to stimulate the respiratory drive. Too much O_2 delivered as a treatment can depress the respiratory drive in those individuals with COPD who have a dampening of the CO_2 drive. Monitoring respiratory rate, level of O_2 administered by nasal cannula, and SaO_2 levels is very important in this client population.

▶▶ PTA ACTION PLAN

Observing and Reporting on SaO_2 Levels

Any condition that restricts blood flow (including cold hands) can result in inaccurate SpO_2 readings. Relaxation and physiologic quieting techniques can be used to help restore more normal temperatures in the distal extremities. Do not apply a pulse oximetry sensor too tightly or to an extremity with an automatic BP cuff.[26]

Hemoglobin levels can be affected by positioning, which can affect a person's ability to breathe. Upright sitting in individuals with low muscle tone or kyphosis can cause forward flexion of the thoracic spine, compromising O_2 intake. Tilting the person back slightly can open the trunk, ease ventilation, and improve SpO_2 levels.[27] Using SpO_2 levels may be a good way to document outcomes of positioning programs for clients with impaired ventilation.

Other factors affecting pulse oximeter readings can include nail polish and nail coverings, irregular heart rhythms, hyperemia (increased blood flow to the area), motion artifact, pressure on the sensor, electrical interference, and venous congestion.[24,26]

In addition to SpO_2 levels, assess other vital signs, skin and nail bed color and tissue perfusion, mental status, breath sounds, and respiratory pattern for all clients using pulse oximetry. If the client cannot talk easily, whether at rest or while exercising, SpO_2 levels are likely to be inadequate. Referral for further evaluation is advised when resting saturation levels fall below 90%.

BOX 3.5 Factors Affecting Pulse and Blood Pressure

Pulse	Blood Pressure*
Age	Age
Anemia	Alcohol
Autonomic dysfunction (diabetes, spinal cord injury)	Anxiety
Caffeine	Blood vessel size
Dehydration (decreased blood volume increases heart rate)	Blood viscosity
Conditioned/deconditioned state	Caffeine
Cardiac muscle dysfunction	Cocaine and cocaine derivatives
Exercise	Diet
Fear	Distended urinary bladder
Fever, heat	Force of heart contraction
Hyperthyroidism	Living at higher altitudes
Infection	Medications
Medications	• Adrenergic inhibitors (lower pressure)
• Antidysrhythmic (slows rate)	• Angiotensin-converting enzyme inhibitors (lowers pressure)
• Atropine (increases rate)	• Beta blockers (lower pressure)
• Beta blocker (slows rate)	• Diuretics (lower pressure)
• Digitalis (slows rate)	• Narcotic analgesics (lower pressure)
Sleep disorders or sleep deprivation	Nicotine
Stress (emotional or psychological)	Pain
	Time of recent meal (increases systolic blood pressure)

*Conditions, such as chronic kidney disease, renovascular disorders, primary aldosteronism, and coarctation of the aorta, are identifiable causes of elevated blood pressure. Chronic overtraining in athletes, use of steroids and/or nonsteroidal antiinflammatory drugs, and large increases in muscle mass can also contribute to hypertension.[23] Treatment for hypertension, dehydration, heart failure, heart attack, arrhythmias, anaphylaxis, shock (from severe infection, stroke, anaphylaxis, major trauma), and advanced diabetes can cause low blood pressure.

(From Goodman CC, Fuller K: *Pathology: implications for the physical therapist*, ed 4, Philadelphia, 2013, WB Saunders.)

BOX 3.6 Pulse Abnormalities

- Weak pulse beats alternating with strong beats
- Weak, thready pulse
- Bounding pulse (throbbing pulse followed by sudden collapse or decrease in the force of the pulse)
- Two quick beats followed by a pause (no pulse)
- Irregular rhythm (interval between beats is not equal)
- Pulse amplitude decreases with inspiration/increases with expiration
- Pulse rate too fast (>100 bpm; tachycardia)
- Pulse rate too slow (<60 bpm; bradycardia)

Blood Pressure

Blood pressure is the measurement of pressure in an artery at the peak of systole (contraction of the left ventricle) and during diastole (when the heart is at rest after closure of the aortic valve, which prevents blood from flowing back to the heart chambers). The measurement (in mm Hg) is listed as:

$$\frac{\text{Systolic (contraction phase)}}{\text{Diastolic (relaxation phase)}}$$

Blood pressure depends on many factors; the normal range differs slightly with age and varies greatly among individuals (Box 3.5). Normal systolic BP (SBP) ranges from 100 to 120 mm Hg, and diastolic BP (DBP) ranges from 60 to 80 mm Hg. Highly trained athletes may have much lower values. Target ranges for BP are listed in Table 3.2.

Assessing Blood Pressure. Blood pressure should be taken in the same arm and in the same position (supine or sitting) each time it is measured. Cuff size is important and requires the bladder width-to-length to be at least 1:2. The cuff bladder should encircle at least 80% of the arm. Blood pressure measurements are overestimated with a cuff that is too small; if a cuff is too small, go to the next size up. Keep in mind that if the cuff is too large, falsely lower BPs may be recorded.[28,29]

The PTA should not apply the BP cuff above an intravenous (IV) line where fluids are infusing or an arteriovenous (AV) shunt, on the same side where breast or axillary surgery has been performed, or when the arm or hand has been traumatized or diseased. Until research data support a change, it is recommended that clients who have undergone axillary node dissection (ALND) avoid having BP measurements taken on the affected side. Some oncology staff advise taking BP in the arm with the least amount of nodal dissection. Technique in measuring BP is a key factor in all clients, especially those with ALND.

A common mistake is to pump the BP cuff up until the systolic measurement is 200 mm Hg and then take too long to lower the pressure or to repeat the measurement a second time without waiting. Repeating the BP without a 1-minute wait time may damage the blood vessel and set up an inflammatory response. This poor technique is to be avoided, especially in clients at risk for lymphedema or who already have lymphedema.

BOX 3.7   Tips on Palpating Pulses

- Assess each pulse for strength and equality for 1 full minute; pulse rate should *not* be taken for part of a minute and then multiplied by a factor (i.e., do *not* use 15 seconds × 4, 30 seconds × 2, 6 seconds × 10).
- Expect to palpate 60 to 90 pulses per minute at all pulse sites. Begin the pulse count with zero, not "one."
- Normal pulse is 2+ and equal bilaterally (see scale in the "Pulse Rate" section).
- Apply gentle pressure; pulses are easily obliterated in some people.
- Popliteal pulse requires deeper palpation.
- Normal veins are flat; pulsations are not visible.
- Flat veins in supine that become distended in sitting may indicate heart disease.
- Pulses should be the same from side to side and should not change significantly with inspiration, expiration, or change in position.
- Pulses tend to diminish with age; distal pulses are not palpable in many older adults.
- If pulses are diminished or absent, document and report.
- Pedal pulses can be congenitally absent; the client may or may not know if absent pulse at this pulse site is normal or a change in pulse pressure.

- In the case of diminished or absent pulses, observe the client for other changes (e.g., skin temperature, texture, color, hair loss, change in toenails); ask about pain in the calf or leg with walking that goes away with rest (intermittent claudication, peripheral vascular disease).
- Carotid pulse: Assess in the seated position; have client turn the head slightly toward the side being palpated. Gently and carefully palpate along the medial edge of the sternocleidomastoid muscle. Palpate one carotid artery at a time; apply light pressure; deep palpation can stimulate carotid sinus with a sudden drop in heart rate and blood pressure. Do not poke or mash around to find the pulse; palpation must not provide a massage to the artery because of the risk of liberating a thrombus or plaque, especially in older adults.
- Femoral pulse: Femoral artery is palpable below the inguinal ligament midway between the anterior superior iliac spine and the symphysis pubis. It can be difficult to assess in the obese client. In these cases, place fingertips of both hands on either side of the pulse site; the femoral pulse should be as strong (if not stronger) than the radial pulse.
- Posterior tibial pulse: Foot must be relaxed with ankle in slight plantar flexion.

▶▶ PTA ACTION PLAN

Measuring Blood Pressure

The standard measurement technique for BP includes having the patient rest in a seated position with their back supported for 5 minutes prior to measurement.[30] The patient's feet should be flat on the floor and uncrossed. Record measurements exactly; do not round numbers up or down because this can result in inaccuracies.[31]

For clients who have had a mastectomy without ALND (i.e., prophylactic mastectomy), BP can be measured in either arm. These recommendations are to be followed for life.[32]

Until automated BP devices are improved enough to ensure valid and reliable measurements, the BP response to exercise in all clients should be taken manually with a BP cuff (sphygmomanometer) and a stethoscope.[32] It is advised to invest in the purchase of a well-made, reliable stethoscope. Older models with tubing long enough to put the earpieces in your ears and still place the bell in a lab coat pocket should be replaced. Tubing should be no more than 50 to 60 cm (12–15 inches) and 4 mm in diameter. Longer and wider tubing can distort transmitted sounds.[33]

For anyone learning to take vital signs, it may be easier to hear the BP sounds (tapping, or Korotkoff) in adults using the left arm because of the closer proximity to the left ventricle. Arm position does make a difference in BP readings; BP measurements are up to 10% higher when the elbow is at a right angle to the body with the elbow flexed at heart level. The preferred position is seated with the arms parallel and extended in a forward direction (if supine, then parallel to the body).[34]

It is more accurate to assess consecutive BP readings over time rather than using an isolated measurement for reporting BP abnormalities, but any abnormal BP measurement should be documented in the medical record and reported to the PT (or nurse). Blood pressure should also be correlated with any related diet or medication.

Before reporting abnormal BP readings, measure both sides for comparison, re-measure both sides, and have another health professional check the readings. Correlate BP measurements with other vital signs, and look for associated signs and symptoms such as pallor, fatigue, perspiration, and/or palpitations. A persistent rise or fall in BP requires medical attention and possible intervention.

Pulse Pressure. The difference between the systolic and diastolic pressure readings (SBP-DBP) is called *pulse pressure*, normally around 40 mm Hg. Pulse pressure is an index of vascular aging (i.e., loss of arterial compliance and indication of how stiff the arteries are). A widened resting pulse pressure often results from stiffening of the aorta as a result of atherosclerosis. *Resting* pulse pressure consistently greater than 60 to 80 mm Hg is a yellow (caution) flag and is a risk factor for a new onset of atrial fibrillation, especially in individuals who have type 2 diabetes.[35,36]

Widening of the pulse pressure is linked to a significantly higher risk of stroke and heart failure after the sixth decade. Some BP medications increase resting pulse pressure width by lowering DBP more than SBP, whereas others (e.g., angiotensin-converting enzyme [ACE] inhibitors) can lower pulse pressure.[37,38]

Narrowing of the resting pulse pressure (usually by a drop in SBP as the DBP rises) can suggest congestive heart failure (CHF) or a significant blood loss such as occurs in hypovolemic shock. A high pulse pressure accompanied by bradycardia is a sign of increased intracranial pressure and requires immediate evaluation.

▶▶ PTA ACTION PLAN

Reporting on Pulse Pressure

In a normal, healthy adult the pulse pressure generally increases in direct proportion to the intensity of exercise as the SBP increases and DBP stays about the same.[39] A difference of more than 80 to 100 mm Hg taken during or right after exercise should be reported. In a healthy adult, pulse pressure will return to normal within 3 to 10 minutes following moderate exercise.

The key is to watch for pulse pressures that are not accommodating during exercise. Expect to see the SBP rise slightly while the DBP stays the same. If the DBP drops while the SBP rises or if the pulse width exceeds 100 mm Hg, further assessment and evaluation are needed. Depending on all other parameters (e.g., general health of the client, past medical history, medications, concomitant associated signs and symptoms), the therapist may direct the PTA to monitor pulse pressures over a few sessions and look for a pattern (or lack of pattern) to report.

Variations in Blood Pressure. There can be some normal variation in SBP from side to side (right extremity compared with left extremity). This is usually no more than 5 to 10 mm Hg DBP or SBP (arms) and 10 to 40 mm Hg SBP (legs). A difference of 10 mm Hg or more in either systolic or diastolic measurements from one extremity to the other may be an indication of vascular problems.

? PICTURE THE PATIENT

With a change in position (supine to sitting), the normal fluctuation of BP and heart rate increases slightly (about 5 mm Hg for systolic and diastolic pressures and 5 to 10 bpm in heart rate).

In a healthy adult under conditions of minimal to moderate exercise, look for normal change (increase) in SBP of 20 mm Hg or more. Expect to see a 40 to 50 mm Hg change in SBP with intense exercise (again, this is in the healthy adult). These values are less likely with individuals taking BP medications, anyone with a significant history of heart disease, and well-conditioned athletes.

Diastolic pressure increases during upper extremity exercise or isometric exercise involving any muscle group. Activity or exercise should be monitored closely, decreased, or halted if the DBP exceeds 100 mm Hg. Diastolic measurements should be the same from side to side with less than 10 mm Hg difference observed. Diastolic pressure generally remains the same or decreases slightly during progressive exercise.[39] Systolic pressure increases with age and with exertion in a linear progression. If systolic pressure does not rise as workload increases, or if this pressure falls, it may be an indication that the functional reserve capacity of the heart has been exceeded.

The deconditioned, menopausal woman with coronary heart disease (CHD) requires careful monitoring, especially in the presence of a personal or family history of heart disease and myocardial infarct (personal or family) or sudden death in a family member.

On the other hand, females of reproductive age taking birth control pills may be at increased risk for hypertension, heart attack, or stroke. The risk of a cardiovascular event is very low with today's low-dose oral contraceptives. However, smoking, hypertension, obesity, undiagnosed cardiac anomalies, and diabetes are factors that increase a woman's risk for cardiovascular events. Any woman using oral contraceptives who presents with consistently elevated BP values should be advised by the supervising therapist to see her physician for close monitoring and follow-up.[23,40,41]

▶ PTA ACTION PLAN

Points to Ponder

Check with the supervising PT (or registered nurse) to establish a safe and accepted BP limit with activity. Always be sure that you are accurately monitoring and documenting the vital signs throughout your treatment session. Modify

the intensity and positioning of the activity to keep the patient's BP within the established limits.

This is a general (conservative) guideline when exercising a client without the benefit of cardiac testing (e.g., electrocardiogram [ECG]). This stop-point is based on the American College of Sports Medicine's guideline to stop exercise testing at 115 mm Hg DBP.[39] Other sources suggest activity should be decreased or stopped if the DBP exceeds 130 mm Hg.[41]

Other warning signs to moderate or stop exercising include the onset of angina, dyspnea, and heart palpitations. Monitor the client for other signs and symptoms such as fever, dizziness, nausea/vomiting, pallor, extreme diaphoresis, muscular cramping or weakness, and incoordination. Always honor the client's desire to slow down or stop.

Hypertension. In recent years, an unexpected increase in illness and death caused by hypertension has prompted the National Institutes of Health (NIH) to issue new guidelines for more effective BP control. According to a 2019 update by the American Heart Association, the rate of hypertension-associated mortality has increased by 23% in the US.[42]

In adults, hypertension is an SBP above 130 mm Hg or a DBP above 80 mm Hg. Consistent BP measurements between 120 and 129 (systolic) and less than 80 mm Hg diastolic are classified as prehypertensive.[43] The overall goal of treating clients with hypertension is to prevent morbidity and mortality associated with high BP. The specific objective is to achieve and maintain arterial BP below 120/80 mm Hg, if possible (Box 3.8).[33]

The older adult taking nonsteroidal antiinflammatory drugs (NSAIDs) is at risk for increased BP because these drugs are potent renal vasoconstrictors. Monitor BP carefully in these clients and look for sacral and lower extremity edema. Document and report these findings to the PT.

Always beware of *masked hypertension* (normal in the clinic but periodically high at home) and *white-coat hypertension*,

BOX 3.8 Guidelines for Hypertension and Management

The Seventh Report of the Joint National Committee on Prevention, Detection, Evaluation, and Treatment of High Blood Pressure provides a new guideline for hypertension prevention and management. The following are the report's key messages:

- In persons older than 50 years, systolic blood pressure (SBP) greater than 140 mm Hg is a much more important cardiovascular disease (CVD) risk factor than diastolic BP (DBP). Elevated SBP raises the risk of heart attacks, congestive heart failure, dementia, end-stage kidney disease, and cardiovascular mortality.
- The risk of CVD beginning at 115/75 mm Hg doubles with each increment of 20/10 mm Hg; individuals who are normotensive at age 55 have a 90% lifetime risk for developing hypertension.
- Individuals with an SBP of 120 to 139 mm Hg or a DBP of 80 to 89 mm Hg should be considered prehypertensive and require health-promoting lifestyle modifications to prevent CVD.
- If BP is more than 20/10 mm Hg above goal BP, report this to the therapist for further evaluation.

(From NHLBI: *The seventh report of the Joint National Committee on prevention, detection, evaluation, and treatment of high blood pressure. NIH publication no. 03-5233*, 2003, National Heart, Lung, and Blood Institute [NHLBI]. Available at www.nhlbi.nih.gov/.)

a clinical condition in which the client has elevated BP levels when measured in a clinic setting by a health care professional. In such cases, BP measurements are consistently normal outside of a clinical setting.

Masked hypertension may affect between 14% and 30% of adults. Patients with masked hypertension tend to demonstrate an exaggerated BP response to exercise and physical activity. White-coat hypertension occurs in 15% to 20% of adults with stage I hypertension.[44,45] These types of hypertension are more common in older adults.[46] Antihypertensive treatment for white-coat hypertension may reduce office BP but may not affect ambulatory BP. The number of adults who develop sustained high BPs is much higher among those who have masked or white-coat hypertension.[44]

At-home BP measurements can help identify adults with masked hypertension, white-coat hypertension, ambulatory hypertension, and individuals who do not experience the usual nocturnal drop in BP (decrease of 15 mm Hg), which is a risk factor for cardiovascular events.[47] Excessive morning BP surge is a predictor of stroke in older adults with known hypertension as well as a potential red-flag sign.[48,49] Documentation and communication with the supervising therapist are indicated in any of these situations.

 PTA PHYSICAL THERAPIST ASSISTANT ACTION PLAN

Follow-Up Questions

- Are you taking your medication as prescribed by your doctor?
- When was the last dose of blood pressure medication that you have taken?
- Do you monitor your blood pressure on a regular basis at home?
  - If yes, how often? What time of the day?

Points to Ponder

A more experienced PTA might be more equipped to follow up on these questions with appropriate education for the individual patient or client. The entry-level PTA will be required to report back to the PT for further guidance in educating the patient/client.

All information received should be reported to the PT if there are any medical concerns regarding the patient's compliance with medication administration at home.

Hypertension in Health Disparities and Inequalities. There is a difference in prevalence of hypertension among age group, race/ethnicity, education level, family income, foreign-born status, health insurance status, and diabetes, obesity, and disability. Additional information regarding incidence, prevalence, morbidity, and mortality beyond the scope of this text can be found through the CDC Health Disparities and Inequalities Report.[50]

Hypotension. Hypotension is a systolic pressure below 90 mm Hg or a diastolic pressure below 60 mm Hg. A BP level that is borderline low for one person may be normal for another. When the BP is too low, there is inadequate blood flow to the heart, brain, and other vital organs.

The most important factor in hypotension is how the BP changes from the normal condition. Most normal BPs are in the range of 100/60 mm Hg to 120/80 mm Hg, but a significant change, even as little as 20 mm Hg, can cause problems for some people.

Lower standing SBP (<140 mm Hg) even within the normotensive range is an independent predictor of loss of balance and falls in adults over the age of 65.[51] Diastolic BP does not appear to be related to falls. Older adult females with lower standing SBP and a history of falls are at greatest risk. The PTA has an important role in educating clients with these risk factors in preventing falls and related accidents. In older adults a decrease in BP may be an early warning sign of Alzheimer's disease.[52,53] Diastolic BP below 70 or declines in systolic pressure with hypoperfusion of the brain may raise the risk of dementia in older adults.[54,55]

▶▶ **PTA ACTION PLAN**

Points to Ponder

If the PTA has concerns regarding consistent hypotension with signs of poor activity tolerance or increased risk factors for falling, an immediate report to the PT is needed. The motivated PTA should take advantage of an important learning opportunity by discussing the clinical decision-making process the PT will use to determine the appropriate follow-up medical attention needed and modifications that will occur to the plan of care.

❓ **PICTURE THE PATIENT**

It is unclear if the steady drop in BP during the 3 years before a dementia diagnosis is a cause or effect of dementia, as reduced blood flow to the brain accelerates the development of dementia. Perhaps brain cell degeneration characteristic of dementia damages parts of the brain that regulate BP.[56]

Postural Orthostatic Hypotension. A common cause of low BP is orthostatic hypotension (OH), defined as a sudden drop in BP when changing positions, usually moving from supine to an upright position.

Physiologic responses of the sympathetic nervous system decline with aging, putting them at greater risk for OH. Older adults are prone to falls from a combination of OH and antihypertensive medications.

Postural OH is more accurately defined as a decrease in SBP of at least 20 mm Hg *or* decrease in DBP of at least 10 mm Hg *and* a 10% to 20% increase in pulse rate. Changes must be noted in *both* the BP and the pulse rate with change in position (supine to sitting, sitting to standing) (Box 3.9 and Case Example 3.1).[47]

The client should lie supine for 5 minutes prior to BP and pulse check. At least a 1-minute wait is recommended after each subsequent position change before taking the BP and pulse. Standing postural OH is measured after 3 to 5 minutes of quiet standing. Food ingestion, time of day, age, and hydration can impact this form of hypotension, as can a history of Parkinsonism, diabetes, or multiple myeloma.

Throughout the procedure, the PTA should observe and assess the client for signs and symptoms of hypotension, including dizziness, lightheadedness, pallor, diaphoresis, or syncope (or arrhythmias if using a cardiac monitor). The PTA should assist the client to a seated or supine position if any of these symptoms develop and report the results and should not test the client in the standing position if signs and symptoms of hypotension occur while sitting.

Gravitational effects on the circulatory system can cause a 10 mm Hg drop in SBP when a person changes position from supine to sitting to standing. This drop usually occurs without symptoms as the body quickly compensates to ensure there is no reduction in cardiac output.

For clients on prolonged bed rest or on antihypertensive drug therapy, there may be either no reflexive increase in heart rate or a sluggish vasomotor response. These clients may experience larger drops in BP and often experience lightheadedness.

BOX 3.9 Postural Orthostatic Hypotension (OH)

Postural OH is a medical diagnosis based on the presence of:
- Decrease of 20 mm Hg of systolic pressure and/or
- Increase of 10 mm Hg (or more) diastolic pressure and
- 10% to 20% increase in pulse rate

These changes occur with change in position (supine to upright sitting, sitting to standing). Another measurement after 1 to 5 minutes of standing may identify OH missed by earlier readings.

Monitor the client carefully since fainting is a possible risk with low blood pressure (BP), especially when combined with the dehydrating effects of diuretics. Oncology patients receiving chemotherapy who are hypotensive are also at risk for dizziness and loss of balance during the repeated BP measurement in the standing position.

This repetition is useful for older adults (65 years or older). Waiting to repeat the BP measurements reveals a client's inability to regulate BP after a change in position. The presence of low BP after a prolonged time is a red-flag finding. Be sure to check pulse rate.[24]

PICTURE THE PATIENT

Other clients at risk for postural OH include those who have just donated blood, anyone with autonomic nervous system (ANS) disease or dysfunction, and postoperative patients. Other risk factors for OH in aging adults include hypovolemia associated with dehydration and the overuse of diuretics, anticholinergic medications, antiemetics, and various over-the-counter (OTC) cough/cold preparations.[57,58]

PTA ACTION PLAN
Point to Ponder

Why does postural OH occur upon standing for the first time in a young adult who has been supine in skeletal traction for 3 weeks?

Core Body Temperature

Although the PTA does not usually assess body temperature unless directed by the PT as a precaution to activity, knowledge of normal/abnormal temperature patterns is helpful. For example, older adults (over age 65) are less likely to have a fever even in the presence of severe infection, so the predictive value of taking the body temperature is less. Because of age-related changes in the thermoregulatory system, they are also more likely to develop hypothermia than young adults. There is a tendency among the aging population to develop an increase in temperature on hospital admission or in response to any change in homeostasis. However, some persons with infectious disease remain afebrile, especially the immunocompromised and those with chronic renal disease, alcoholics, and older adults. A low-grade fever can be an early sign of life-threatening infections (most commonly pneumonia or urinary tract infection).

CASE EXAMPLE 3.1 Vital Signs

A 74-year-old retired homemaker had a total hip replacement 2 days ago. She remains an inpatient with complications related to congestive heart failure. She has a previous medical history of gallbladder removal 20 years ago, total hysterectomy 30 years ago, and surgically induced menopause with subsequent onset of hypertension.

Her medications include intravenous (IV) furosemide (Lasix), digoxin, and potassium replacement.

During the initial physical therapy intervention, the client complained of muscle cramping and headache but was able to complete the entire exercise protocol. Blood pressure was 100/76 mm Hg. Systolic measurement dropped to 90 mm Hg when the client moved from supine to standing. Pulse rate was 56 bpm with a pattern of irregular beats. Pulse rate did not change with postural change. Platelet count was 98,000 cells/mm³ when it was measured yesterday.

According to information gathered from the PT during the initial evaluation, what are the red flags that the PTA will closely monitor?

Nurses will also be monitoring the patient's signs and symptoms closely. Read the chart to stay up with what everyone else knows and/or has observed about Mrs. S. Read the physician's notes to see what, if any, medical intervention has been ordered based on laboratory values (e.g., platelet levels) or vital signs (e.g., changes in medication). If there is a new order or change in status, the PT must be notified prior to the PTA working with this patient.

Do not hesitate to discuss concerns and observations with the nursing staff. This helps them know you are aware of the medical side of care, but it also gives you some perspective from the nursing side. What do they see as significant? What requires immediate medical attention?

Be sure to report anything observed but not already recorded in the chart, such as muscle cramping, headache, irregular heartbeat with bradycardia, low pulse, and orthostatic hypotension.

In this case, report to the registered nurse and physical therapist and document:
1. Irregular heartbeat with bradycardia (a possible sign of digoxin/digitalis toxicity)
2. Muscle cramping (possible side effects of furosemide) and headache (possible side effect of digoxin)
3. Vital signs; her blood pressure was not too unusual and pulse rate did not change with position change (probably because of medications) so she does not have medically defined orthostatic hypotension.

The response of vital signs to exercise must be monitored carefully and charted; monitor vital signs throughout intervention. Record the time it takes for the client's vital signs to return to normal after exercise or treatment. This can be used as a means of documenting measurable outcomes. Mrs. S. may not ambulate any further or faster in the afternoon compared with the morning, but her vital signs may reflect closer to normal values and a faster return to homeostasis as a measurable outcome.

Postoperative fever is common and may be from an infectious or noninfectious cause. Medical evaluation is needed to make this determination. In the home health setting, wound infection, abscess formation, or peritonitis may appear as a hectic fever pattern 3 to 4 days postoperatively with increases and declines of body temperature but no return to baseline (normal). Such a situation would warrant telephone consultation with the physician's office nurse.

Any client who reports constitutional symptoms (see Box 1.3) should be discussed with the therapist. The PTA can ask about the presence of any of these symptoms in a patient or client who reports a fever or elevated temperature. The PTA may also ask about other signs and symptoms of infection (e.g., redness of skin, red streaks in skin, swelling, heat, fatigue, headache, chills). Any one sign or symptom is important, but a group or constellation of clinical signs and/or symptoms may be very significant and must be observed closely.

>> PTA ACTION PLAN

Points to Ponder

The PTA should not exercise a client who has a suspected or documented fever without consulting with the PT first. Exercise with a fever stresses the cardiopulmonary system, which may be further complicated by dehydration. Severe dehydration can occur from vomiting, diarrhea, medications (e.g., diuretics), or heat exhaustion.

? PICTURE THE PATIENT

Clinical signs and symptoms of dehydration can include the following:

Mild
- Thirst
- Dry mouth, dry lips

Moderate
- Very dry mouth, cracked lips
- Sunken eyes, sunken fontanel (infants)
- Poor skin turgor
- Postural hypotension
- Headache

Severe
- All signs of moderate dehydration
- Rapid, weak pulse (>100 bpm at rest)
- Rapid breathing
- Confusion, lethargy, irritability
- Cold hands and feet
- Inability to cry or urinate

Clients at greatest risk of dehydration include postoperative patients, aging adults, and athletes. Severe fluid volume deficit can cause vascular collapse and shock. Clients at risk of shock include burn or trauma patients, clients in anaphylactic shock or diabetic ketoacidosis, and individuals experiencing severe blood loss.[57]

>> PTA ACTION PLAN

Summary on Documenting and Reporting Vital Signs

The following findings should always be documented and reported to the PT:
- Any of the yellow caution signs presented in Box 3.10.
- Individuals who report consistent ambulatory hypertension using out-of-office or at-home readings, adults who do not show a drop in BP at night (15 mm Hg lower than daytime measures), and older adults with diagnosed hypertension who have an excessive surge in morning BP measurements.
- African Americans with elevated BP; they should be evaluated by a medical doctor
- Pulse amplitude that fades with inspiration and strengthens with expiration
- Irregular pulse and/or irregular pulse combined with symptoms of dizziness or shortness of breath (SOB); tachycardia or bradycardia.
- Pulse increase over 20 bpm lasting more than 3 minutes after rest or changing position.
- Persistent low-grade (or higher) fever, especially associated with constitutional symptoms—most commonly sweats but also unintended weight loss, malaise, nausea, and vomiting.
- Any unexplained fever without other systemic symptoms, especially in the person taking corticosteroids or otherwise immunosuppressed.
- Weak and rapid pulse accompanied by fall in BP (pneumothorax).
- Clients who are neurologically unstable as a result of a recent CVA, head trauma, spinal cord injury, or other central nervous system (CNS) insult often exhibit new arrhythmias during the period of instability; when the client's pulse is monitored, any new arrhythmias noted should also be reported immediately to the nursing staff or physician.
- Always take BP in any client with neck pain, upper quadrant symptoms, or thoracic outlet syndrome.

WALKING SPEED: THE SIXTH VITAL SIGN

Walking speed is used by some as a general indicator of function, including health status, motor control, muscle strength, and endurance.[59] The test can be a reliable and valid measure of functional ability with predictive values to assess future health status, functional decline, potential for hospitalization, and even mortality.[60]

RECOGNIZING AND REPORTING NEUROLOGIC RED FLAGS

Acute insult or injury to the neurologic system may cause changes in neurologic status, requiring ongoing observation, especially in the older adult. Systemic disease can produce nerve damage; careful assessment can help the PTA recognize red-flag findings. A family history of neurologic disorders or a personal history of diabetes, hypertension, high cholesterol, cancer, seizures, or heart disease may be significant.

Major Areas to Observe

Major areas to observe include the following:
- Mental and emotional status
- Cranial nerve function (e.g., eye movement, vision, hearing, taste, facial movements and sensation, voice, swallowing, tongue movement, sense of smell, speech)

BOX 3.10 Guidelines for Blood Pressure

Consider the following as yellow (caution) flags that require closer monitoring and possible medical referral:

- SBP greater than 120 mm Hg and/or DBP greater than 80 mm Hg, especially in the presence of significant risk factors (age, medications, personal or family history)
- Decrease in DBP below 70 mm Hg in adults age 75 or older (risk factor for Alzheimer's)
- Persistent rise or fall in BP over time (at least three consecutive readings over 2 weeks), especially in a client taking NSAIDs (check for edema) or any woman taking birth control pills (should be closely monitored by physician)
- Steady fall in BP over several years in adults over 75 (risk factor for Alzheimer's)
- Lower standing SBP (<140 mm Hg) in adults over age 65 with a history of falls (increased risk for falls)
- A difference in pulse pressure greater than 40 mm Hg
- More than 10 mm Hg difference (SBP or DBP) from side to side (upper extremities)
- Approaching or more than 40 mm Hg difference (SBP or DBP) from side to side (lower extremities)
- BP in lower extremities is lower than in the upper extremities
- DBP increases more than 10 mm Hg during activity or exercise
- SBP does not rise as workload increases; SBP falls as workload increases
- SBP exceeds 200 mm Hg during exercise or physical activity; DBP exceeds 100 mm Hg during exercise or physical activity; these values represent the upper limits and may be too high for the client's age, general health, and overall condition.
- BP changes in the presence of other warning signs, such as first-time onset or unstable angina, dizziness, nausea, pallor, or extreme diaphoresis
- Sudden fall in BP (>10–15 mm Hg SBP) or more than 10 mm Hg DBP with concomitant rise (10%–20% increase) in pulse (orthostatic hypotension); watch for postural hypotension in hypertensive clients, especially anyone taking diuretics (decreased fluid volume/dehydration)
- Use a manual sphygmomanometer to measure BP during exercise; most standard automatic units are not designed for this purpose

BP, Blood pressure; *DBP*, diastolic blood pressure; *NSAIDs*, nonsteroidal antiinflammatory drugs; *SBP*, systolic blood pressure.

- Motor function (gross motor and fine motor; coordination, gait, balance)
- Sensory function (light touch, vibration, pain, pressure, and temperature)
- Reflexes
- Neural tension
- Vision

The PTA should report headaches, confusion (increased confusion), dizziness, seizures, or other neurologic signs and symptoms, and should note the presence of any incoordination, tremors, weakness, or abnormal speech patterns.

Neurologic symptoms with no apparent cause, such as paresthesias, dizziness, and weakness, may actually be symptoms of depression. This is particularly true if the neurologic symptoms are symmetric or not anatomic.[61,62] Any of these findings should be documented and reported to the PT.

? PICTURE THE PATIENT

Clinical signs and symptoms of neurologic impairment include the following:
- Confusion/increased confusion
- Depression
- Irritability
- Drowsiness/lethargy
- Dizziness/lightheadedness
- Loss of consciousness
- Blurred vision or other change in vision
- Slurred speech or change in speech pattern
- Headache
- Balance/coordination problems
- Falls (or near falls)
- Significant change in upright posture
- Weakness
- Change in memory
- Change in muscle tone for an individual with previously diagnosed neurologic condition
- Seizure activity
- Loss of sensation, presence of numbness, and/or tingling anywhere in the body
- Nerve palsy; transient paralysis
- Change in one or more reflexes (increased or decreased reflex responses)

Reflexes

Deep tendon reflexes (DTRs) often tested by the PT include the following:
- Jaw (cranial nerve V)
- Biceps (C5–6)
- Brachioradialis (C5–6)
- Triceps (C7–8)
- Patella (L3–4)
- Achilles (S1–2)

These reflexes are assessed for symmetry and briskness using the following scale[25]:

0	No response, absent
+1	Low normal, decreased; slight muscle contraction
+2	Normal, visible muscle twitch producing movement of arm/leg
+3	More brisk than normal, increased or exaggerated; may not indicate disease
+4	Hyperactive; very brisk, clonus; spinal cord disorder suspected

A change in one or more DTRs is a yellow (caution) flag. Some individuals have very brisk reflexes normally, whereas others are much more hyporeflexive. Whenever encountering increased or decreased reflexes (hyperreflexes and hyporeflexes, respectively), the therapist may ask the PTA to routinely follow several guidelines:

- Test reflexes above and below and from side to side in order to gauge overall reflexive response. A "normal" hyperreflexive response will be present in most, if not all, reflexes. The same is true for generalized hyporeflexive responses.
- Offer the client distraction while testing through conversation or by asking such silly questions as, "What color is your toothbrush?" "What day of the week were you born?" or "Count out loud backwards by three starting at 89."
- Retest unusual reflexes later in the day or on another day.
- Have another clinician test the individual.

The isolated DTR that does not fit the client's physiologic pattern must be considered a red flag. One red flag by itself does not require immediate medical follow-up. But a hyporesponsive patellar tendon reflex that is reproducible and is accompanied by back, hip, or thigh pain in the presence of a past history of prostate cancer offers a different picture altogether.

A diminished reflex may be interpreted as the sign of a possible "space-occupying lesion"—most often, a disc protruding from the disc space and either pressing on a spinal nerve root or irritating the spinal nerve root (i.e., chemicals released by the herniation in contact with the nerve root can cause nerve root irritation).

Tumors (whether benign or malignant) can also press on the spinal nerve root, mimicking a disc problem. A small lesion can put just enough pressure to irritate the nerve root, resulting in a hyperreflexive DTR. A large tumor can obliterate the reflex arc, resulting in diminished or absent reflexes. Either way, changes in DTRs must be considered a yellow (caution) or red (warning) flag sign to be documented, reported, and further investigated.

Neural Tension

Excessive nerve tightness or adhesion can cause adverse neural tension in the peripheral nervous system. When the nerve cannot slide or glide in its protective sheath, neural extensibility and mobility are impaired. The clinical result can be numbness, tingling, and pain. This could be caused by disc protrusion, scar tissue, or space-occupying lesions, including cysts, bone spurs, tumors, and cancer metastases.[63,64]

PTs utilize neural tension tests to assess the effects of stress on underlying tissues. The most common neural tension tests include the straight leg raise test, the seated slump test, and the upper limb neural tension test.[65]

A positive neural tension test does not reveal the underlying problem, only that the peripheral nerve is involved. History and physical examination are still very important in assessing the clinical presentation.

Someone with full ROM accompanied by negative articular signs but with impaired neural extensibility and mobility raises a yellow (caution) flag. A second look at the history and a more thorough neurologic exam may be warranted.

Reducing symptoms with neural mobilization performed by the PT does not rule out the possibility of cancer. A red flag is raised with any client who responds well to neural mobilization but experiences a recurrence of symptoms. This could be a sign that the tumor has grown larger or cancer metastases have progressed, once again interfering with neural mobility.

▶▶ PTA ACTION PLAN

Points to Ponder

If there are no observed changes of the nervous system (e.g., reflexes, muscle tone assessment, gross manual muscle testing, sensation), from what was further recorded in the baseline evaluation, evaluation by the PT may not be required. For example, sensory function is not assessed if motor function is intact, and there are no client reports of specific sensory problems or changes.

Keep in mind that fatigue and side effects of medications can affect the neurologic system. Should the PTA observe any of the impairments listed, he or she should take the time needed to make specific observations during any follow-up treatment sessions.

Falls and Fall Prevention

Around the world, falls are the leading cause of traumatic brain injury and death among persons aged 65 or older.[66-68] Older adults who fall often sustain more severe head injuries than their younger counterparts. Falls are a major cause of intracranial lesion among older persons because of their greater susceptibility to subdural hematoma.[67]

By assessing risk factors (prediction) and offering preventive and protective strategies, the PTA can make a significant difference in the number of fall-related injuries and fractures. There are many ways to look at fall assessment. For the purpose of a general survey, there are four main categories:

- Well adult (no falling pattern)
- Just starting to fall
- Falls frequently (more than once every 6 months)
- Fear of falling

Healthy older adults who have no falling patterns may have a fear of falling in specific instances (e.g., getting out of the bath or shower; walking on ice, curbs, or uneven terrain). Fear of falling can be considered a mobility impairment or functional limitation. It restricts the client's ability to perform specific actions, thereby preventing the client from doing the things he or she wants to do. Functionally, this may appear as an inability to take a tub bath, walk on grass unassisted, or even attempt household tasks such as getting up on a sturdy step stool to change a light bulb (Case Example 3.2).

Risk Factors for Falls. If all other senses and reflexes are intact and muscular strength and coordination are normal, the affected individual can regain balance without falling. Many times, this does not happen. All health care professionals must work together to make early identification of adults at increased risk for falls.

With careful questioning, any potential problems with balance may come to light. The PTA can then alert the therapist of these findings. The therapist will determine the need for testing static and dynamic balance and look for potential risk factors and systemic or medical causes of falls (Table 3.3).

All of the variables and risk factors listed in Table 3.3 for falls are important. Older adults may have impaired balance, slower reaction times, and decreased strength, leading to more frequent falls. Sleep deprivation can lead to slowing in motor reaction time, thus increasing the risk of falls.[69-71] Medications, especially polypharmacy, can contribute to falls.[72-75] There are some key areas the PTA can pay attention to that contribute to falls among the aging adult population[76,77]:

- Vision/hearing impairments
- Balance impairments; dizziness
- Environmental factors
- Blood pressure regulation
- Medications/substances
- Elder assault

As we age, cervical spinal motion declines, as does peripheral vision. These two factors alone contribute to changes in our vestibular system and the balance mechanism.[78,79] Macular degeneration, glaucoma, cataracts, or any other visual problems can result in loss of depth perception and even greater loss of visual acuity.

CASE EXAMPLE 3.2 Fracture After a Fall

A 67-year-old female fell and sustained a complete transverse fracture of the left fibula and an incomplete fracture of the tibia. The client reported she lost her footing while walking down four steps at the entrance of her home.

She was immobilized in a plaster cast for 9 weeks. Extended immobilization was required after the fracture because of a slow rate of healing resulting from osteopenia/osteoporosis. She was non–weight-bearing and ambulated with crutches while her foot was immobilized. Initially, this client was referred to physical therapy for range of motion (ROM), strengthening, and gait training.

The client is married and lives with her husband in a single-story home. Her goals were to ambulate independently with a normal gait.

Past Medical History: Type 2 diabetes, hypertension, osteopenia, and history of alcohol use. Client used tobacco ($1^1/_2$ packs a day for 35 years) but has not smoked for the past 20 years. Client described herself as a "weekend alcoholic," meaning she did not drink during the week but drank six or more beers a day on weekends.

Current medications include tolbutamide, enalapril, hydrochlorothiazide, alendronate (Fosamax), supplemental calcium, and multivitamin.

Intervention by PT/PTA team: The client was seen six times before a scheduled surgery interrupted the plan of care. Progress was noted as increased ROM and increased strength through the left lower extremity, except dorsiflexion.

Seven weeks later, the client returned to the previous PT for strengthening and gait training resulting from a "limp" on the left side. She reported that she noticed the limping had increased since she had both her big toenails removed. She also noted increased toe dragging, stumbling, and leg cramps (especially at night). She reported that she had decreased her use of alcohol since she fractured her leg because of the pain medications and recently because of fear of falling.

Minimal progress was noted in improving balance or strength in the lower extremity. The client felt that her loss of strength could be attributed to inactivity following the foot surgery, even though she reported doing her home exercise program.

As a result of the thoroughness of the observations and communication by the PTA, a neurologic screening exam was repeated by the PT, with hyperreflexia observed in the lower extremities, bilaterally. There was a positive Babinski reflex on the left. The findings were reported to the primary care physician, who requested that physical therapy continue.

During the next week and a half, the client reported that she fell twice. She also reported that she was "having some twitching in her [left] leg muscles." The client also reported "coughing a lot while [she] was eating; food going down the wrong pipe."

Outcome: The client presented with a referral for weakness and gait abnormality thought to be related to the left fibular fracture and fall that did not respond as expected and, in fact, resulted in further loss of function.

The physician was notified of the client's need for a cane, no improvement in strength, fasciculations in the left lower extremity, and the changes in her neurologic status. The client returned to her primary care provider, who then referred her to a neurologist.

Results: Upon examination by the neurologist, the client was diagnosed with amyotrophic lateral sclerosis. A new physical therapy plan of care was developed based on the new diagnosis.

Small Group Activity

- Make a list of physical impairments with which this patient is presenting.
- Make a list of functional limitations that the PT would consider when developing goals with the patient.
- Discuss the red-flag observations that the PTA should have noticed while working with the patient.

(From Chanoski C: *Adapted from case report presented in partial fulfillment of DPT 910, principles of differential diagnosis*, Chester, 2005, Institute for Physical Therapy Education, Widener University, used with permission.)

TABLE 3.3 Risk Factors for Falls

Age Changes	Environmental/ Living Conditions	Pathologic Conditions	Medications	Others
Muscle weakness; loss of joint motion (especially lower extremities)	Poor lighting	Vestibular disorders; episodes of dizziness or vertigo from any cause	Antianxiety; benzodiazepines	History of falls
	Throw rugs, loose carpet, complex carpet designs	Orthostatic hypotension (especially before breakfast)	Anticonvulsants	Female sex; postmenopausal status
Abnormal gait	Cluster of electric wires or cords	Chronic pain condition	Antidepressants	Living alone
Impaired or abnormal balance	Stairs without handrails	Neuropathies	Antihypertensives	Elder abuse/assault
Impaired proprioception or sensation	Bathroom without grab bars	Cervical myelopathy	Antipsychotics	Nonambulatory status (requiring transfers)
Delayed muscle response/ increased reaction time	Slippery floors (water, urine, floor surface, ice); icy sidewalks, stairs, or streets	Osteoarthritis; rheumatoid arthritis	Diuretics	Gait changes (decreased stride length or speed)
		Visual or hearing impairment; multifocal eyeglasses; change in perception of color; loss of depth perception; decreased contrast sensitivity	Narcotics	Postural instability; reduced postural control
↓ Systolic blood pressure (<140 mm Hg in adults over 65 years old)	Restraints	Cardiovascular disease	Sedative-hypnotics	Fear of falling; history of falls
	Use of alcohol or other drugs	Urinary incontinence	Phenothiazines	Dehydration from any cause
		Central nervous system disorders (e.g., stroke, Parkinson's disease, multiple sclerosis)	Use of more than four medications (polypharmacy/ hyperpharmacotherapy)	Recent surgery (general anesthesia, epidural)
Stooped or forward-bent posture	Footwear, especially slippers	Motor disturbance		Sleep disorder/disturbance; sleep deprivation; daytime drowsiness; brief disorientation after waking up from a nap*
		Osteopenia, osteoporosis		
		Pathologic fractures		
		Any mobility impairments (e.g., amputation, neuropathy, deformity)		
		Cognitive impairment; dementia; depression		

*From Stone KL: Self-reported sleep and nap habits and risk of mortality in a large cohort of older women, *J Am Geriatr Soc* 57(4):604–611, 2009.

The ANS's ability to regulate blood pressure is also affected by age. A sudden drop in blood pressure can precipitate a fall. Coronary heart disease, peripheral vascular disease, diabetes mellitus, and blood pressure medications are just a few of the factors that can put additional stress on the regulating function of the ANS.

Lower standing balance, even within normotensive ranges, is an independent predictor of falls in community-dwelling older adults. Older females (65 years old or older) with a history of falls and with lower SBP should pay more attention to the prevention of falls and related accidents.[48]

The subject of balance impairment and falls as it relates to medical conditions and medications is very important. Chronic diseases and multiple pathologies are more important predictors of falling than even polypharmacy (the use of four or more medications during the same period).[80–82] The presence of chronic musculoskeletal pain is associated with a 1.5-fold increased risk of falling for adults ages 70 and up.[82]

Multiple comorbidities often mean the use of multiple drugs (polypharmacy). These two variables together increase the risk of falls in older adults. Some medications (especially psychotropics such as tranquilizers and antidepressants, including amitriptyline, doxepin, sertraline [Zoloft], fluoxetine [Prozac], paroxetine [Paxil], mirtazapine [Remeron], citalopram [Celexa], and bupropion [Wellbutrin]) are red-flag risk factors for loss of balance and injuries from falls.

PTA ACTION PLAN
What to Watch for

The PTA should watch for clients with chronic conditions who are taking any of these drugs. Anyone with fibromyalgia, depression, cluster migraine headaches, chronic pain, obsessive-compulsive disorders (OCDs), panic disorder, and anxiety who is on a psychotropic medication must be monitored carefully for dizziness, drowsiness, and postural orthostatic hypotension (a sudden drop in BP with an increase in pudisorders and can occur withlse rate). In addition, alcohol can interact with many medications, increasing the risk of falling.

It is not uncommon for clients on hypertensive medication (diuretics) to become dehydrated, dizzy, and lose their balance. Postural OH can (and often does) occur in the aging adult—even in someone taking BP-regulating medications.

Orthostatic hypotension as a risk factor for falls may occur as a result of volume depletion (e.g., diabetes mellitus, sodium or potassium depletion), venous pooling (e.g., pregnancy, varicosities of the legs, immobility following a motor vehicle or cerebrovascular accident), side effects of medications such as antihypertensives, starvation associated with anorexia or cachexia, and sluggish normal regulatory mechanisms associated with anatomic variations or as a result of other conditions such as metabolic disorders or diseases of the CNS.[57,58]

PICTURE THE PATIENT

Falling is a primary symptom of Parkinson's disease. Any time a client reports episodes of dizziness, loss of balance, or a history of falls, further screening and possible medical referral are needed. This is especially true in the presence of other neurologic signs and symptoms such as headache, confusion, depression, irritability, visual changes, weakness, memory loss, and drowsiness or lethargy.

PTA ACTION PLAN
Follow-Up Questions

Some potential screening questions may include the following:
- Do you have any episodes of dizziness?
If yes, does turning over in bed cause (or increase) dizziness?
- Do you have trouble getting in or out of bed without losing your balance?
- Can/Do you get in and out of your tub or shower?
- Do you avoid walking on grass or curbs to avoid falling?
- Do you avoid negotiating stairs in your home to avoid falling?
- Have you started taking any new medications, drugs, or pills of any kind?
- Has there been any change in the dosage of your regular medications?
- Have you changed your level of activity or stopped doing leisure activities to avoid falling?

RECOGNIZING AND REPORTING RED-FLAG CLINICAL PRESENTATIONS

The Integumentary System: Skin and Nail Beds

The first thing every PTA encounters with each client or patient is what can be observed on the outside, primarily the skin and nail beds. Changes in the skin and nail beds may be the first sign of inflammatory, infectious, and immunologic disorders and can occur with involvement of a variety of organs.

For example, dermatitis can occur 6 to 8 weeks before primary signs and symptoms of pulmonary malignancy develop. Clubbing of the fingers can occur quickly in various acute illnesses and conditions. Skin, hair, and nail bed changes are common with endocrine disorders. Renal disease, rheumatic disorders, and autoimmune diseases are all accompanied by skin and nail bed changes in many physical therapy clients.

PTA ACTION PLAN
Observing Skin Conditions

The supervising therapist should be notified of any new skin lesions, especially in children (Fig. 3.1). Many conditions in adults and children can be treated effectively; some, but not all, can be cured. When assessing skin conditions of any kind, even benign lesions such as psoriasis (Fig. 3.2) or eczema, the PTA should always use standard precautions because any disruption of the skin increases the risk of infection. The presence of skin lesions may point to a problem with the integumentary system or may be an integumentary response to a systemic problem that must be further evaluated by the therapist.

For example, pruritus is the most common manifestation of dermatologic disease but is also a symptom of underlying systemic disease in up to 50% of individuals with generalized itching.[83] In both situations, skin rash is a common accompanying sign. The most common visceral system causing pruritus is the hepatic system.[84] Look for other associated signs and symptoms of liver or gallbladder impairment, such as nails of Terry (Fig. 3.3), carpal tunnel syndrome, liver palms (palmar erythema; Fig. 3.4), liver flap (asterixis; Fig. 3.5), and spider angiomas (Figs. 3.6 and 3.7).

At the same time, be aware that pruritus, or itch, is very common among aging adults. The natural attrition of glands that

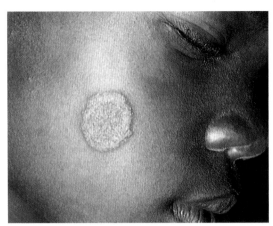

FIG. 3.1 Tinea corporis or ringworm of the body presents anywhere on the body in adults or children but more commonly on the chest, abdomen, back of arms, face, and dorsum of the feet. The circular lesions with clear centers can form singly or in clusters and represent a fungal infection that is both contagious and treatable. Tinea pedis (not shown), also known as ringworm of the feet or "athlete's foot" occurs most often between the toes but also along the sides of the feet and the soles (easily spread and treatable). (From Hurwitz S: *Clinical pediatric dermatology: a textbook of skin disorders of childhood and adolescence*, ed 2, Philadelphia, 1993, WB Saunders.)

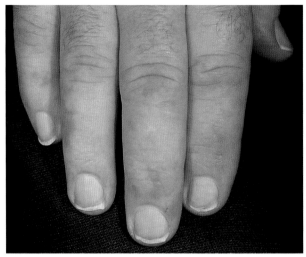

FIG. 3.3 Nails of Terry. Opaque white nails of Terry in a patient with cirrhosis. Various forms of nail disease have been described in patients with cirrhosis. This is an example of the classic white nails of Terry characterized by an opaque nail plate with a narrow line of pink at the distal end instead of the more normal pink nail plate in the White persons. Nails of Terry can also present as a result of malnutrition, diabetes mellitus, hyperthyroidism, trauma, and sometimes for unknown reasons (idiopathic). (From Callen JP, Jorizzo JL, editors: *Dermatological signs of internal disease*, ed 4, Philadelphia, 2009, WB Saunders.)

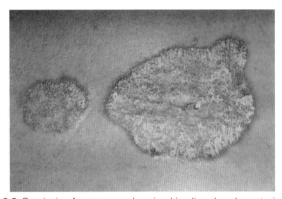

FIG. 3.2 Psoriasis. A common chronic skin disorder characterized by red patches covered by thick, dry silvery scales that are the result of excessive build-up of epithelial cells. Lesions often come and go and can be anywhere on the body but are most common on extensor surfaces, bony prominences, scalp, ears, and genitals. Arthritis of the small joints of the hands often accompanies the skin disease (psoriatic arthritis). (From Lookingbill DP, Marks JG: *Principles of dermatology*, ed 3, Philadelphia, 2000, WB Saunders.)

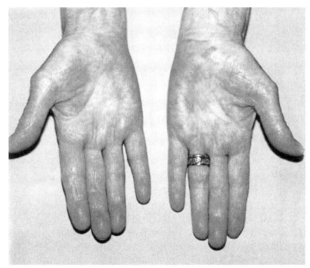

FIG. 3.4 Palmar erythema, caused by liver impairment, presents as a warm redness of the skin over the palms and soles of the feet in the White population. Darker skin tones may change from tan to gray. Look for other signs of liver disease such as nail bed changes, spider angiomas, liver flap, and bilateral carpal or tarsal tunnel syndrome. Palmar erythema can occur in healthy individuals and in association with nonhepatic diseases. (From Barrison I, editor: *Gastroenterology in practice*, St. Louis, 1992, Mosby.)

moisturize the skin combined with the effects of sun exposure, medications, excessive bathing, and harsh soaps can result in dry, irritable skin.[85,86]

The PTA may see scratch marks or even broken skin where the sufferer has scratched violently. Open, red (often bleeding) sores appear most commonly on the face and arms but can be anywhere on the body. These lesions can become inflamed, swollen, and pus filled in the presence of a *Staphylococcus* infection. Left untreated, pathogens can enter the bloodstream, causing dangerous sepsis or deeper abscess. There is no cure, but medical evaluation is needed; the PT should be notified immediately.

? PICTURE THE PATIENT

Some clients may describe formication, also referred to as a tactile hallucination (e.g., the sensation of ants crawling on the skin), is sometimes described as an itching, prickling, or crawling feeling.[87] The most common cause is menopause, but chronic drug or alcohol use can also cause formication. Some schizophrenics also experience formication.[88] As one of the many side effects of crystal methamphetamine addiction, formication is also referred to as speed bumps, meth sores, and crank bugs.

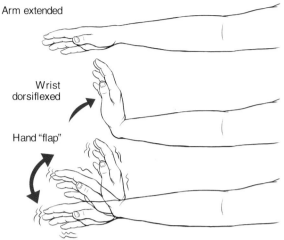

FIG. 3.5 To test for asterixis or liver flap, have the client extend the arms, spread the fingers, extend the wrist, and observe for the abnormal "flapping" tremor at the wrist. If a tremor is not readily apparent, ask the client to keep the arms straight while gently hyperextending the client's wrist. An alternative method of testing for this phenomenon involves having the client relax the legs in the supine position with the knees bent. The feet are flat on the table. As the legs fall to the sides, watch for a flapping or tremoring of the legs at the hip. The knees appear to come back toward the midline repeatedly.

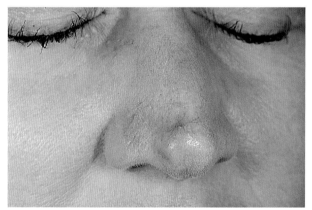

FIG. 3.6 Spider angioma. Permanently enlarged and dilated capillaries visible on the surface of the skin caused by vascular dilation are called spider angiomas. These capillary radiations can be flat or raised in the center. They present on the upper half of the body, primarily on the face, neck, chest, or abdomen and occur as a normal development or in association with pregnancy, chronic liver disease, or estrogen therapy. They do not go away when the underlying condition is treated; laser therapy is available to remove them for cosmetic reasons. (From Swartz MH: *Textbook of physical diagnosis: history and examination*, ed 6, Philadelphia, 2009, Saunders.)

Responding to Skin Lesions

▶▶ PTA ACTION PLAN

Skin Lesions: What to Report

Clients often point out skin lesions or ask the PTA about lumps and bumps. Good lighting and good exposure are essential for inspection. Always compare one side to the other, and assess for abnormalities in all of the following:

Texture	Tenderness
Size	Shape, contour, symmetry

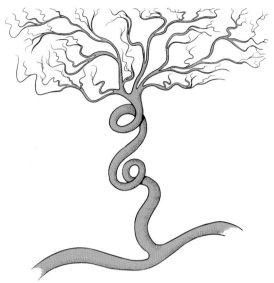

FIG. 3.7 Arterial spider. Schematic diagram of an arterial spider formed by a coiled arteriole that spirals up to a central point and then branches out into thin-walled vessels that merge with normal capillaries, resembling a spider in appearance. Exposure to heat (e.g., hot tubs, warm shower) will cause temporary vasodilation. The skin lesion will appear larger until vasoconstriction occurs.

Position, alignment	Mobility or movement
Color	Location

The hands, arms, feet, and legs can be observed throughout the treatment session for changes in texture, color, temperature, clubbing, circulation, including capillary filling, and edema. Abnormal texture changes include shiny, stiff, coarse, dry, or scaly skin.

Skin mobility and turgor are affected by the fluid status of the client. Dehydration and aging reduce skin turgor, and edema decreases skin mobility. Chronically ill or hospitalized patients should be examined frequently for signs of skin breakdown. Check all pressure points, including the ears, sacrum, scapulae, shoulders, area over the greater trochanters, heels, malleoli, and the back of the head.

▶▶ PTA ACTION PLAN

Coordinating Clinical Observations

As directed by the PT, the PTA may coordinate with nursing staff to remove prostheses, restraints, and dressings to look beneath them. Anyone with an IV line, catheter, or other insertion sites must be examined for signs of infiltration (e.g., pus, erythema), phlebitis, and tape burns.

Observe for signs of edema. Edema is an accumulation of fluid in the interstitial spaces. Pitting edema, in which pressing a finger into the skin leaves an indentation, often indicates a chronic condition (e.g., chronic kidney failure, liver failure, CHF) but can occur acutely as well (e.g., face) (Fig. 3.8). The location of edema helps the therapist identify the potential cause. Bilateral edema of the legs may be seen in clients with heart failure or with chronic venous insufficiency.

Abdominal and leg edema can be seen in clients with heart disease, cirrhosis of the liver (or other liver impairment), and protein malnutrition. Edema may also be noted in dependent areas, such as the sacrum, when a person is confined to bed. Localized edema in one extremity may be the result of venous obstruction (thrombosis) or lymphatic blockage of the extremity (lymphedema).

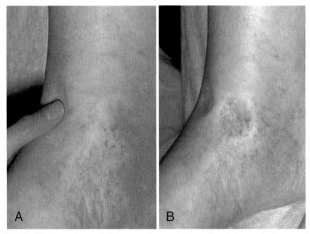

FIG. 3.8 Pitting edema (A) in a patient with cardiac failure. A depression (B) ("pit") remains in the edema for some minutes after firm fingertip pressure is applied. (From Forbes CD, Jackson WD: *Color atlas and text of clinical medicine*, ed 3, London, 2003, Mosby.)

Points to Ponder
The PTA notifies the PT of any new findings or changes (e.g., size, depth, shape, color, drainage) in previously observed and recorded skin lesions. If the PTA is conducting an accurate assessment during observation and inspection of the skin, it is likely he or she will recognize changes in staging of any skin lesions (e.g., worsening dehydration, advancing pressure ulcers). Any progression or worsening of the clinical presentation requires consultation with the PT.

If the PT instructs the PTA in proper technique of assessing for dehydration, the PTA is allowed to follow up with continued assessment. It is acceptable for the PTA to inquire about further assessment techniques in this (or any other) area of the general survey.

Palpation

Palpation is used to discriminate among textures, dimensions, consistencies, and temperature. It is used to define things that are inspected and to reveal things that cannot be inspected. Textures are best detected using the fingertips, whereas dimensions or contours are detected using several fingers, the entire hand, or both hands, depending on the area being examined.

Inspection and palpation are often performed at the same time; be sure and look at the client and not at your hands. Muscle tension interferes with palpation, so the client must be positioned and draped appropriately in a room with adequate lighting and temperature.

Assess skin temperature with both hands at the same time. The back of the PTA's hands senses temperature best because of the thin layer of skin. Use the palm or heel of the hand to assess for vibration. The finger pads are best to assess texture, size, shape, position, pulsation, consistency, and turgor. Heavy or continued pressure dulls the examiner's palpatory skill and sensation.

Light palpation is used first, looking for areas of tenderness followed by deep palpation to elicit deep pain. Light palpation (skin is depressed up to 1/4 to 1/2 inch) is also used to assess texture, temperature, moisture, pulsations, vibrations, and superficial lesions. During deep palpation, enough pressure is

used to depress the skin up to 1 inch; applying too much pressure decreases sensation.

Tender or painful areas are assessed last while carefully observing the client's face for signs of discomfort.

Change in Skin Temperature

Skin temperature can be an indication of vascular supply. If directed by the PT, the PTA can use a handheld, noninvasive, infrared thermometer to measure skin surface temperature. The most common use of this device is for temperature observation and comparison of both feet in individuals with diabetes for the purpose of identifying increased skin temperatures, intended as an early warning of inflammation, impending infection, and possible foot ulceration.

? PICTURE THE PATIENT

Temperature differences of four or more degrees between the right and left foot are predictive for foot ulcers and must be reported to the PT (or nursing staff, as appropriate); self-monitoring has been shown to reduce the risk of ulceration in high-risk individuals.[88–90] Other signs and symptoms of vascular changes of an affected extremity may include paresthesia, muscle fatigue and discomfort, or cyanosis with numbness, pain, and loss of hair from a reduced blood supply (Box 3.11).

≫ PTA ACTION PLAN
Points to Ponder

The PT is required to oversee the education that the PTA is providing to the patient regarding the patient's plan of care. This will involve detailed communication between the PTA and PT on a regular basis. The PTA should be sure that the self-monitoring technique for skin inspection that he or she is teaching the patient is consistent with that of the interdisciplinary team's approach.

The information collected from observations made of the peripheral vascular system (according to Box 3.11) should be documented in the medical record and immediately reported to the supervising PT or registered nurse if abnormal changes are found.

Change in Skin Color

Capillary filling of the fingers and toes is an indicator of peripheral circulation. A capillary refill test is performed by pressing down on the nail bed and releasing. Observe first for blanching (whitening), followed by return of color within 3 seconds after release of pressure (normal response).[34]

Skin color changes can occur with a variety of illnesses and systemic conditions. Clients may notice a change in their skin color before anyone else does, so be sure and ask about it. Look for pallor; increased or decreased pigmentation; yellow, green, or red skin color; and cyanosis.

The first signs of vascular occlusive disease are often skin changes (see Box 3.11). The PTA must keep in mind common risk factors, including bed rest or prolonged immobility, use of IV catheters, obesity, MI, heart failure, pregnancy, recent surgery, and any problems with coagulation.

BOX 3.11 Observation of the Peripheral Vascular System

Inspection

Compare extremities side to side:
  Size
  Symmetry
  Skin
  Nail beds
  Color
  Hair growth
  Sensation
Capillary refill time (fingers and toes)
Rubor (redness) on dependency (feet dangling down)

Palpation
*Pulses**

Upper quadrant	Lower quadrant
Carotid	Femoral
Brachial	Popliteal
Radial	Dorsalis pedis
Ulnar	Posterior tibial

Characteristics of Pulses
Rate
Rhythm
Strength (amplitude)
  +4 = bounding
  +3 = full, increased
  +2 = normal
  +1 = diminished, weak
  0 + absent

Check for symmetry (compare right to left)
Compare upper extremity to lower extremity

Arterial Insufficiency of Extremities

Pulses	Decreased or absent
Color	Pale on elevation
	Dusky rubor on dependency
Temperature	Cool/cold
Edema	None
Skin	Shiny, thin pale skin; thick nails; hair loss
	Ulcers on toes
Sensation	Pain: increased with exercise (claudication) or leg elevation; relieved by dependent dangling position
	Paresthesias

Venous Insufficiency of Extremities

Pulses	Normal arterial pulses
Color	Pink to cyanotic
	Brown pigment at ankles
Temperature	Warm
Edema	Present
Skin	Discolored, scaly (eczema or stasis dermatitis)
	Ulcers on ankles, toes, fingers
	Varicose veins
Sensation	Pain: increased with standing or sitting; relieved with elevation or support hose

* Pulses may be palpated by the PTA if indicated by the PT as a precaution for activity.

❓ PICTURE THE PATIENT

Skin changes associated with impairment of the hepatic system include jaundice, pallor, and orange or green skin. In some situations, jaundice may be the first and only manifestation of hepatic disease. It is first noticeable in the sclera of the eye as a yellow hue when bilirubin level reaches 2 to 3 mg/dL. Dark-skinned persons may have a normal yellow color to the outer sclera. Jaundice involves the whole sclera up to the iris.

When the bilirubin level reaches 5 to 6 mg/dL, the skin becomes yellow. Other skin and nail bed changes associated with liver disease include nails of Terry (see Fig. 3.3), palmar erythema (see Fig. 3.4), and spider angioma (see Figs. 3.6 and 3.7).

A bluish cast to skin color can occur with cyanosis when O_2 levels are reduced in the arterial blood (central cyanosis) or when blood is oxygenated normally but blood flow is decreased and slow (peripheral cyanosis). Cyanosis is first observed in the hands and feet, lips, and nose as a pale blue change in color. The client may report numbness or tingling in these areas.

Central cyanosis is caused by advanced lung disease, congestive heart disease, and abnormal SaO₂. Peripheral cyanosis occurs with CHF (decreased blood flow), venous obstruction, anxiety, and cold environment.[91]

Peripheral vascular disease (PVD), both arterial and venous conditions, is a common problem observed in the extremities of older adults, especially those with a history of heart disease. Rubor (dusky redness) is a common finding in PVD as a result of arterial insufficiency.

⏩ PTA ACTION PLAN

Observing for PVD

When the legs are raised above the level of the heart, pallor of the feet and lower legs develops quickly (usually within 1 minute). When the same client sits up and dangles the feet down, the skin returns to a pink color quickly (usually in about 10 to 15 seconds). A minute later, the pallor is replaced by rubor, usually accompanied by pain and diminished pulses. Skin is cool to the touch, and trophic changes may be seen (e.g., hair loss over the foot and toes, thick nails, thin skin).

Rubor on dependency is another test used to observe the adequacy of arterial circulation.[25] Place the client in the supine position and observe the color of the soles of the feet. Normal feet should be pink or flesh colored in Whites and tan or brown in clients with dark skin tones. The feet of clients with impaired circulation are often chalky white (Whites) or gray or white in clients with darker skin.

Elevate the legs to 45 degrees (above the heart level). For clients with a compromise of the arterial blood supply, any color present will quickly disappear in this position; in other words, the elevated foot develops increased pallor. No change (or little change) is observed in the normal individual. Bring the individual to a sitting position with the legs dangling. Venous filling is delayed following foot elevation. Color change in the lower leg and foot may take 30 seconds or more and will be a very bright red (dependent rubor).[91]

Diffuse hyperpigmentation can occur with Addison disease, sarcoidosis, pregnancy, leukemia, hemochromatosis, celiac sprue (malabsorption syndrome), scleroderma, and chronic renal failure.[92]

Diffuse hyperpigmentation can occur with Addison disease, sarcoidosis, pregnancy, leukemia, scleroderma, and chronic renal failure. The pigmentation presents as patchy tan to brown spots most often but may occur as yellow-brown or yellow to tan with scleroderma and renal failure. Any area of the body can be affected, although pigmentation changes in pregnancy tend to affect just the face (melasma or the mask of pregnancy).

Assessing Dark Skin. Clients with dark skin may require a slightly different approach to skin assessment than the White population. Color changes are often observed first in the fingernails, lips, mucous membranes, conjunctiva of the eye, and palms and soles of dark-skinned people.

Pallor may present as yellow or ashen gray as a result of an absence of the normally present underlying red tones in the skin. The palms and the soles show changes more clearly than the skin. Skin rashes may present as a change in skin texture, so palpating for changes is important. Edema can be palpated as "tightness," and darker skin may appear lighter. Inflammation may be perceived as a change in skin temperature instead of redness or erythema of the skin.

Jaundice may appear first in the sclera but can be confused for the normal yellow pigmentation of dark-skinned clients. Be aware that the normal oral mucosa (gums, borders of the tongue, and lining of the cheeks) of dark-skinned individuals may appear freckled.

Petechiae are easier to see when present over areas of skin with lighter pigmentation, such as the abdomen, gluteal area, and volar aspect of the forearm. Petechiae and ecchymosis (bruising) can be differentiated from erythema by applying pressure over the involved area. Pressure will cause erythema to blanch, whereas the skin will not change in the presence of petechiae or ecchymosis.

▶ PTA ACTION PLAN

What to Watch for

Observe for any obvious changes in any of the areas mentioned above. Observation of the hands should be done at the level of the client's heart. In addition, the anemic client's hands should be warm; if they are cold, the paleness is due to vasoconstriction.

Red Flags for Skin Cancer

When examining a skin lesion or mass of any kind, all health care professionals are encouraged to follow the American Cancer Society (ACS) and the Skin Cancer Foundation method of using the following ABCDEs to assess skin lesions for cancer detection (Fig. 3.9):

A—Asymmetry
B—Border
C—Color
D—Diameter
E—Evolving

The ABCDE criteria have been verified in multiple studies, documenting the effectiveness and diagnostic accuracy of this

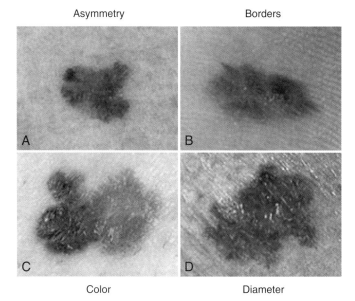

Asymmetry   Borders

Color   Diameter

FIG. 3.9 Common characteristics associated with early melanomas are described and shown in this photo. (A) Asymmetry: a line drawn through the middle does not produce matching halves. (B) Borders are uneven, fuzzy, or have notched or scalloped edges. (C) Color changes occur with shades of brown, black, tan, or other colors being present at the same time. (D) Diameter is greater than the width of a pencil eraser. The Evolving stage (not shown) indicates any change in size, shape, color, elevation, or another trait, or any new symptom, such as bleeding, itching, or crusting, requires evaluation. (Used with permission from Dermik Laboratories http://dermnetnz.org/.)

screening technique. Their efficacy has been confirmed with digital image analysis; sensitivity ranges from 57% to 90% and specificity from 59% to 90%.[93]

Round, symmetric skin lesions such as common moles, freckles, and birthmarks are considered "normal." If an existing mole or other skin lesion starts to change and a line drawn down the middle shows two different halves, medical evaluation is needed. The PTA should notify the PT immediately of any unusual or suspicious observations.

Common moles and other "normal" skin changes usually have smooth, even borders or edges. Malignant melanomas, the most deadly form of skin cancer, have uneven, notched borders.

Benign moles, freckles, "liver spots," and other benign skin changes are usually a single color (most often a single shade of brown or tan) (Fig. 3.10). A single lesion with more than one shade of black, brown, or blue may be a sign of malignant melanoma.

Even though some of us have moles we think are embarrassingly large, the average mole is really less than one-fourth of an inch (about the size of a pencil eraser). Anything larger than this should be inspected carefully.

The Skin Cancer Foundation (www.skincancer.org) has many public education materials available to help the PTA recognize and accurately report suspicious skin lesions to the PT. In addition to their website, they have posters, brochures, videos, and other materials available for use in the clinic. It is highly recommended that these types of education materials be available in waiting rooms as part of a nationwide primary prevention program.

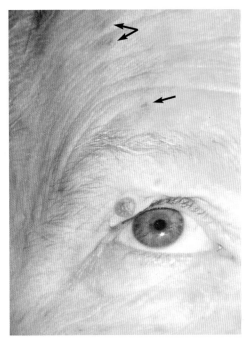

FIG. 3.10 Seborrheic keratosis, a benign well-circumscribed, raised, tan-to-black lesion often presents on the face, neck, chest, or upper back. This lesion represents a build-up of keratin, which is the primary component of the epidermis. There is a family tendency to develop these lesions. The more serious lesions are the red patches located on this client's forehead *(arrows)*: precancerous lesions called *actinic ker atosis*, the result of chronic sun exposure. These lesions have a "sandpaper" feel when palpated. Medical treatment is needed for this premalignant lesion. (Courtesy Catherine C. Goodman, 2005.)

BOX 3.12 Risk Factor Assessment for Skin Cancer

- Advancing age
- Personal or family history of skin cancer (particularly melanoma)
- Moles with any of the ABCDE features, or moles that are changing in any way
- Complexion that is fair or light with green, blue, or gray eyes
- Skin that sunburns easily; skin that never tans
- History of painful sunburns with blistering during childhood or the adolescent years
- Use of tanning beds or lamps
- Short, intense episodes of sun exposure: the indoor worker who spends the weekend out in the sun without skin protection (or any sporadic exposure to strong sunshine of normally covered skin)
- Transplant recipient

(Data from Skin Cancer Foundation, http://www.skincancer.org/skin-cancer-information/skin-cancer-facts. Accessed March 8, 2014.)

Other websites (such as www.skincheck.org [Melanoma Education Foundation] and http://sydney.edu.au/medicine/melanoma-foundation/about-melanoma/index.php [The Melanoma Foundation of the University of Sydney Australia]) provide a dditional photos of suspicious lesions with more screening guidelines. The client's risk is much higher if any of the risk factors listed in Box 3.12 are present.

PTA ACTION PLAN
Information to Collect for the Therapist

For all lesions, masses, or aberrant tissue, observe or palpate for heat, induration, scarring, or discharge. Make note of how long the client has had the lesion, if it has changed in the last 6 weeks to 6 months, and whether it has been evaluated by the PT. Always ask appropriate follow-up questions with this assessment.

Follow-Up Questions
- Does it itch, hurt, feel sore, or burn?
- Does anyone else in your household have anything like this?
- Have you taken any new medications (prescribed or OTC) in the last 6 weeks?
- Have you traveled somewhere new in the last month?
- Have you been exposed to anything in the last month that could cause this? (Consider exposure as a result of occupational, environmental, and hobby interests.)
- Do you have any other skin changes anywhere else on your body?
- Have you had a fever or sweats in the last 2 weeks?
- Are you having any trouble breathing or swallowing?
- Have you had any other symptoms of any kind anywhere else in your body?

Points to Ponder
How you ask is just as important as what you say. Do not frighten people by first telling them you always screen for skin cancer. It may be better to introduce the subject by saying that as health care professionals, therapists are trained to observe many body parts, including the skin, joints, posture, and so on. You notice the client has an unusual mole (or rash, or whatever you have observed), and you wonder if this is something that has been there for years. Has it changed in the last 6 weeks to 6 months? Has the client ever shown it to the doctor?

Observing Surgical Scars

It is always a good idea to look at surgical scars (Fig. 3.11), especially sites of local cancer removal. Any suspicious scab or tissue granulation, redness, or discoloration must be noted (or photographed if possible).

Start by asking the client if he or she has noticed any changes in the scar. Continue by asking the following:

PTA ACTION PLAN
Follow-Up Questions

- Would you have any objections if I looked at (or examined) the scar tissue?
  If the client declines or refuses, be sure to follow up with counsel to perform self-inspection and report any changes to the physician.
  In Fig. 3.12, the small scab and granular tissue forming above the scar represent red flags of suspicious local recurrence. Even if the client suggests this is from "picking" at the scar, a medical evaluation is well advised.
  The PTA has a responsibility to report these findings to the PT; all health care professionals are encouraged to make every effort to ensure client/patient compliance with follow-up.

Common Skin Lesions

Vitiligo. A lack of pigmentation from melanocyte destruction (vitiligo) (Fig. 3.13) can be hereditary and have no significance, or it can be caused by conditions such as hyperthyroidism,

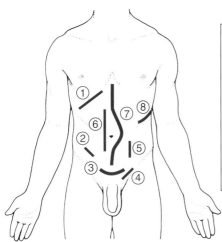

1. Cholecystectomy; a subcostal incision, when made on the right, provides exposure of the gallbladder and common bile duct; used on the left for splenectomy
2. Appendectomy, sometimes called McBurney's or Gridiron incision
3. Transverse suprapubic incision for hysterectomy and other pelvic surgeries
4. Inguinal hernia repair (herniorrhaphy or hernioplasty)
5. Anterior rectal resection (left paramedian incision)
6. Incision through the right flank (right paramedian); called laparotomy or celiotomy; sometimes used to biopsy the liver
7. Midline laparotomy
8. Nephrectomy (removal of the kidney) or other renal surgery

FIG. 3.11 Abdominal surgical scars. Not shown: puncture sites for laparoscopy, usually close to the umbilicus and one or two other sites.

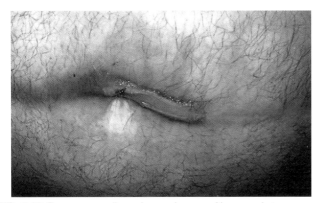

FIG. 3.12 Squamous cell carcinoma in scar. Always ask to see and examine scars from previous surgeries, especially when there has been a history of any kind of cancer, including skin cancer. Even this black and white photo shows many skin changes to suggest the need for medical evaluation. At the far right of the raised scar tissue is a normal, smooth scar. This is what the entire scar should look like. There is a horizontal line of granulation along the upper edge of the scar, as well as a scabbed-over area in the middle of the raised scar. There is also a change in skin color on either side of the scar. (From Swartz MH: *Textbook of physical diagnosis*, ed 4, Philadelphia, 2001, WB Saunders.)

stomach cancer, pernicious anemia, diabetes mellitus, or autoimmune diseases.[83]

Lesions can occur anywhere on the body but tend to develop in sun-exposed areas, body folds, and around body openings. Intraarticular steroid injections can cause a temporary loss of pigmentation at the injection site. Anyone with any kind of skin type and skin color can be affected by vitiligo.

Café Au Lait. Café au lait ("coffee with milk") spots describe the light-brown macules (flat lesion, different in color) on the skin as shown in Fig. 3.14. This benign skin condition may be associated with Albright's syndrome or a hereditary disorder called *neurofibromatosis*. The diagnosis is considered when a child presents with five or more of these skin lesions or if any single patch is greater than 1.5 cm in diameter.

Skin Rash. Many possible causes of skin rash exist, including viruses (e.g., chickenpox, measles, Fifth disease, shingles),

systemic conditions (e.g., meningitis, lupus, hives), parasites (e.g., lice, scabies), and reactions to chemicals.

A common cause of skin rash seen in a physical therapy practice is medications, especially antibiotics (Fig. 3.15). The reaction may occur immediately or there may be a delayed reaction of hours up to 6 to 8 weeks after the drug is stopped.

Skin rash can also occur before visceral malignancy of many kinds. Watch for skin rash or hives in someone who has never had hives before, especially if there has been no contact with medications, new foods, new detergents, new perfumes, or travel.

Hemorrhagic Rash. Hemorrhagic rash requires documentation and an immediate report to the PT. A hemorrhagic rash occurs when small capillaries under the skin start to bleed, forming tiny blood spots under the skin (petechiae). The petechiae increase over time as bleeding continues.

Dermatitis. Dermatitis (sometimes referred to as eczema) is characterized by skin that is red, brown, or gray; sore; itchy; and sometimes swollen. The skin can develop blisters and weeping sores. Skin changes, especially in the presence of open lesions, put the client at increased risk of infection. In chronic dermatitis, the skin can become thick and leathery.

Different types of dermatitis are diagnosed on the basis of medical history, etiology (if known), and presenting signs and symptoms. Contributing factors include stress, allergies, genetics, infections, and environmental irritants. For example, contact dermatitis occurs when the skin reacts to something it has come into contact with, such as soap, perfume, metals in jewelry, and plants (e.g., poison ivy or oak).

Dyshidrotic dermatitis can affect skin that gets wet frequently. It presents as small, itchy bumps on the sides of the fingers or toes and progresses to a rash. Atopic dermatitis often accompanies asthma or hay fever. It appears to affect genetically predisposed clients who are hypersensitive to environmental allergens. This type of dermatitis can affect any part of the body but often involves the skin inside the elbow and on the back of the knees.

Rosacea. Rosacea is a chronic facial skin disorder seen most often in adults between the ages of 30 and 60 years. It can cause a

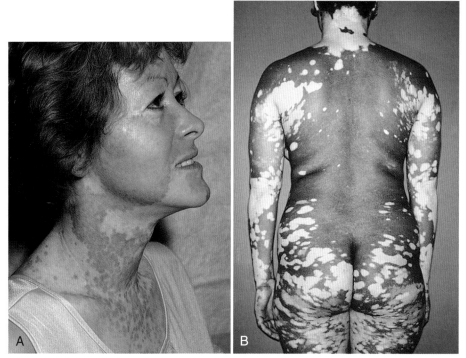

FIG. 3.13 *Vitiligo* is a term derived from the Greek word for "calf" used to describe patches of light skin caused by loss of epidermal melanocytes. (A) Note the patchy loss of pigment on the face, neck and chest. (B) This condition can affect any part of the face, hands, or body and can be very disfiguring, especially in dark-skinned individuals. This skin change may be a sign of hyperthyroidism. (From Swartz MH: *Textbook of physical diagnosis*, ed 5, Philadelphia, 2006, WB Saunders.)

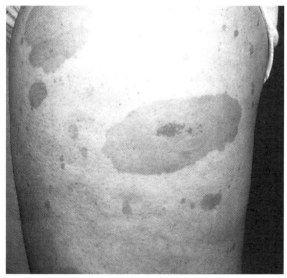

FIG. 3.14 Café-au-lait patches of varying sizes in a client with neuro-fibromatosis. Occasional (fewer than five) tan macules are not significant and can occur normally. Patches 1.5 cm or larger in diameter raise the suspicion of underlying pathology, even if there is only one present. (From Epstein O, Perkin GD, deBono DP, et al.: *Clinical examination*, London, 1992, Gower Medical Publishing, used with permission, Elsevier Science.)

facial rash easily mistaken for the butterfly rash associated with lupus. Features include erythema, flushing, telangiectasia, papules, and pustules affecting the cheeks and nose of the face. An enlarged nose is often present, and the condition progressively gets worse (Fig. 3.16).[92]

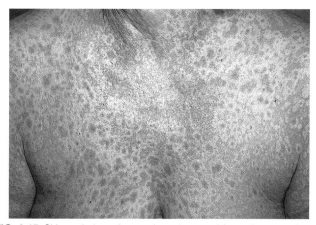

FIG. 3.15 Skin rash (reactive erythema) caused by a drug reaction to phenobarbital. Hypersensitivity reactions to drugs are most common with antibiotics (especially penicillin), sulfonamides ("sulfa drugs," anti-infectives), and phenobarbital, as shown here. (From Callen JP, Paller AS, Greer KE, et al.: *Color atlas of dermatology*, ed 2, Philadelphia, 2000, WB Saunders.)

Rosacea can be controlled with dermatologic or other medical treatment in some cases. There may be a link between rosacea and GI disease caused by the *H. pylori* bacteria.[94,95] Such cases may respond favorably to antibiotics. The PT will refer the client when medical referral is needed.

Thrombocytopenia. Decrease in platelet levels can result in thrombocytopenia, a bleeding disorder characterized by petechiae (tiny purple or red spots), multiple bruises, and

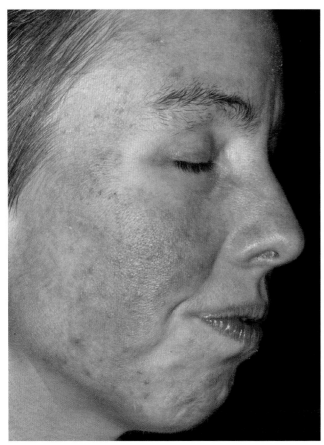

FIG. 3.16 Rosacea, a form of adult acne, may be associated with *Helicobacter pylori;* medical evaluation and treatment are needed to rule out this possibility. (From Habif T: *Clinical dermatology: a color guide to diagnosis and therapy,* ed 5, Philadelphia, 2010, Mosby.)

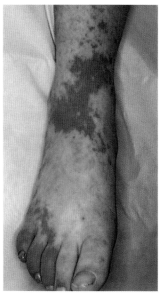

FIG. 3.17 Purpura. Petechiae and ecchymoses are seen in this flat macular hemorrhage from thrombocytopenia (platelet level < 100,000 mm³). This condition also occurs in older adults as blood leaks from capillaries in response to minor trauma. It can occur in fair-skinned people with skin damage from a lifetime of exposure to ultraviolet (UV) radiation. Exposure to UVB and UVA rays can cause permanent damage to the structural collagen that supports the walls of the skin's blood vessels. Combined with thinning of the skin that occurs with aging, radiation-impaired blood vessels are more likely to rupture with minor trauma. (From Hurwitz S: *Clinical pediatric dermatology: a textbook of skin disorders of childhood and adolescence,* ed 2, Philadelphia, 1993, WB Saunders.)

hemorrhage into the tissues (Fig. 3.17). Joint bleeds, nose and gum bleeds, excessive menstruation, and melena (dark, tarry, sticky stools from oxidized blood in the GI tract) can occur with thrombocytopenia.[95]

There are many causes of thrombocytopenia. In a physical therapy practice, the most common causes seen are bone marrow failure from radiation treatment, leukemia, or metastatic cancer; cytotoxic agents used in chemotherapy; and drug-induced platelet reduction, especially among adults with rheumatoid arthritis treated with gold or inflammatory conditions treated with aspirin or other NSAIDs.

Postoperative thrombocytopenia can be heparin-induced for patients receiving IV heparin.[96] The PTA should watch for limb ischemia, cyanosis of fingers or toes, and signs and symptoms of a stroke, heart attack, or pulmonary embolus.

Xanthomas. Xanthomas are benign fatty fibrous yellow plaques, nodules, or tumors that develop in the subcutaneous layer of skin (Fig. 3.18), often around tendons. The lesion is characterized by the intracellular accumulation of cholesterol and cholesterol esters.[83] These are most often associated with disorders of lipid metabolism, primary biliary cirrhosis, and uncontrolled diabetes (Fig. 3.19).[97] They may have no pathologic significance but can occur in association with malignancy such as leukemia, lymphoma, or myeloma.[83,98] Xanthomas require a

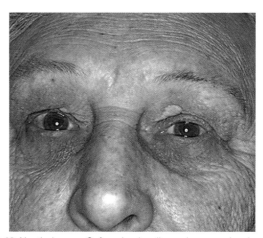

FIG. 3.18 Xanthelasma. Soft, raised yellow plaques, also known as *xanthomas,* commonly occur with aging and may be a sign of high cholesterol levels. As shown here on the eyelid, these benign lesions also occur on the extensor surfaces of tendons, especially in the hands, elbows, and knees. They may have no pathologic significance, but they often appear in association with disorders of lipid metabolism. (From Albert DM, Jakobeic FA: *Principles and practice of ophthalmology,* vol 3, Philadelphia, 1994, WB Saunders.)

medical referral if they have not been evaluated by a physician. When associated with diabetes, these nodules will resolve with adequate glucose control.[83,92]

Education and prescriptive exercise are important features of treatment for the client with xanthomas from poorly controlled

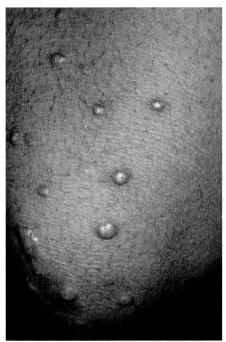

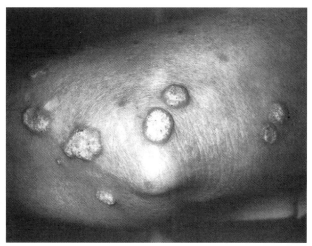

FIG. 3.20 Skin lesions associated with discoid lupus erythematosus. These disk-shaped lesions look like warts or squamous cell carcinoma. A medical examination is needed to make the definitive differential diagnosis. (From Callen JP, Jorizzo J, Greer KE, et al.: *Dermatological signs of internal disease*, Philadelphia, 1988, WB Saunders.)

FIG. 3.19 A slightly different presentation of xanthomas, this time associated with poorly controlled diabetes mellitus. Although the lesion is considered "benign," the presence of these skin lesions in anyone with diabetes signals the need for immediate medical attention. Together, the therapist and the PTA play a key role in client education and the development of an appropriate exercise program to bring blood glucose levels under adequate control. (From Callen JP, Jorizzo J, Greer KE, et al.: *Dermatological signs of internal disease*, Philadelphia, 1988, WB Saunders.)

BOX 3.13 Rheumatic Diseases Accompanied by Skin Lesions

- Acute rheumatic fever
- Discoid lupus erythematosus
- Dermatomyositis
- Gonococcal arthritis
- Lyme disease
- Psoriatic arthritis
- Reactive arthritis
- Rubella
- Scleroderma
- Systemic lupus erythematosus
- Vasculitis

---

diabetes. Gaining control of glucose levels using the three keys of intervention (diet, exercise, and insulin or oral hypoglycemic medication) is essential and requires a team management approach.

Rheumatologic Diseases. Skin lesions are often the first sign of an underlying rheumatic disease (Box 3.13). In fact, the skin has been called a "map" to rheumatic diseases. The butterfly rash over the nose and cheeks associated with lupus erythematosus can be seen in the acute (systemic) phase, whereas discoid lesions are more common with chronic integumentary form of lupus (Fig. 3.20).[99]

Individuals with dermatomyositis often have a heliotrope rash and/or Gottron's papules. Scleroderma is accompanied by many skin changes; pitting of the nails is common with psoriatic arthritis. Skin and nail bed changes are common with some sexually transmitted diseases that also have a rheumatologic component (see Fig. 3.20).[100]

Steroid Skin and Steroid Rosacea. Steroid skin is the name given when bruising or ecchymosis occurs as a result of the chronic use of topical or systemic corticosteroids (Fig. 3.21). In the case of topical steroid creams, this is a red flag that pain is not under control and medical attention for an underlying (probably inflammatory) condition is needed. If the therapist has not documented this condition in the medical record, the PTA is advised to bring the presence of this skin lesion to the PT's attention.

The use of topical corticosteroids for more than 2 weeks to treat chronic skin conditions affecting the face can cause a condition characterized by rosacea-like eruptions known as *steroid rosacea*.[98] Attempts to stop using the medication may result in severe redness and burning called *steroid addiction syndrome* (Fig. 3.22).[101,102]

Erythema Chronicum Migrans. One or more erythema migrans rash may occur with Lyme disease. There is no one prominent rash. The rash varies in size and shape and may have purple, red, or bruised-looking rings. The rash may appear as a solid red, expanding rash or blotch or as a central red spot surrounded by clear skin that is ringed by an expanding red rash. It may be smooth or bumpy to the touch, and it may itch or ooze. The Centers for Disease Control and Prevention website provides a photo gallery of possible rashes associated with Lyme disease.[100]

This rash, which develops in most people with Lyme disease, appears most often 1 to 2 weeks after the disease is transmitted (via tick bite) and may persist for 3 to 5 weeks. It usually is not painful or itchy but may be warm to the touch. The bull's-eye rash may be more difficult to see on darker-skinned people. A dark, bruise-like appearance is more common in those cases.

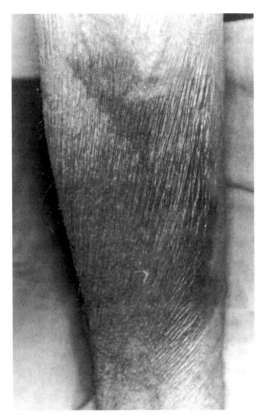

FIG. 3.21 Ecchymosis as a result of steroid application Also note the cutaneous atrophy produced by topical steroids. This skin condition is referred to as "steroid skin" when associated with chronic oral or topical steroid use. Medical referral may be needed for better pain control. (From Callen JP, Jorizzo J, Greer KE, et al.: *Dermatological signs of internal disease*, Philadelphia, 1988, WB Saunders.)

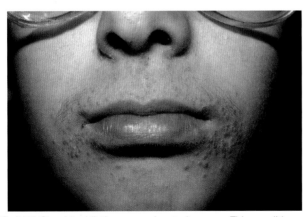

FIG. 3.22 Steroid addiction appearing to be acne. This condition was caused by long-term application of a moderate-potency steroid and mycostatin combined. (From Weston WL: *Weston color textbook of pediatric dermatology*, ed 4, St. Louis, 2007, Mosby.)

Effects of Radiation. Radiation for the treatment of some cancers has some specific effects on the skin. Pigment-producing cells can be affected by either low-dose radiation causing hyperpigmentation or by high-dose radiation resulting in depigmentation (vitiligo). Pigmentation changes can be localized or generalized.[103]

Radiation recall reaction can occur months later as a postirradiation effect. The physiologic response is much like overexposure to the sun with erythema of the skin in the same pattern as the radiation exposure without evidence of disease progression at that site. It is usually precipitated by some external stimuli or event, such as exposure to the sun, infection, or stress.

Radiation recall is also more likely to occur when an individual receives certain chemotherapies (e.g., cyclophosphamide, paclitaxel, doxorubicin, gemcitabine) after radiation.[104,105] The chemotherapy causes the previously radiated area to become inflamed and irritated.

Radiation dermatitis and *x-ray keratosis*, separate from radiation recall, are terms used to describe acute (expected) skin irritation caused by radiation at the time of radiation.

Skin changes can also occur as a long-term effect of radiation exposure. Radiation levels administered to oncology patients even 10 years ago were much higher than today's current treatment regimes. Long-term effects may be visible at previous radiation sites.

Sexually Transmitted Diseases/Infections. Sexually transmitted diseases (STDs) are a variety of clinical syndromes caused by pathogens that can be acquired and transmitted through sexual activity.[106] STDs, also known as sexually transmitted infections (STIs), are often accompanied by skin and/or nail bed lesions and joint pain. Being able to recognize STIs is helpful in the clinic. Someone presenting with joint pain of "unknown cause" and also demonstrating signs of an STI may help bring the correct diagnosis to light sooner than later.

Around the world, STIs pose a major health problem. In 1970, there were two major STIs; today, there are 25. The prevalence of STIs is rapidly increasing to epidemic proportions in the United States. In 2012 more than 51% of all STIs occurred in people 25 years of age or younger.[107]

STIs have been positively identified as a risk factor for cancer. Not all STIs are linked with cancer, but studies have confirmed that human papilloma virus (HPV) is the primary cause of cervical cancer. HPV is the leading viral STI in the United States. More than 70 types of HPV have been identified: 23 infect the cervix and 13 types are associated with cancer in males and females. Infection with one of these viruses does not predict cancer, but the risk of cancer is increased.[106]

Syphilis is on the rise again with the number of cases increasing by 36% between 2017 and 2021 among gay and bisexual males, suggesting an erosion of safe sex practices.[108] It is highly contagious, spread from person to person by direct contact with a syphilis sore on the body of an infected person. Sores occur at the site of infection, mainly on the external genitals, vagina, anus, or rectum. Sores can also occur on the lips and in the mouth.

Transmission occurs during vaginal, anal, or oral sex. An infected pregnant woman can also pass the disease to her unborn child. Syphilis cannot be spread by contact with toilet seats, doorknobs, swimming pools, hot tubs, bathtubs, shared clothing, or eating utensils.

In the first stage of syphilis, a syphilis chancre may appear (Fig. 3.23) at the site of inoculation (usually the genitals, anus, or mouth). The chancre occurs 4 weeks after initial infection

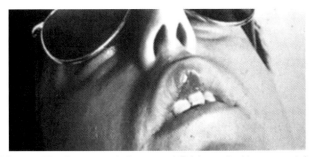

FIG. 3.23 The first stage (primary syphilis) is marked by a very infectious sore called a *chancre*. The chancre is usually small, firm, round with well-demarcated edges, and painless. It appears at the spot where the bacteria entered the body. Chancres last 1 to 5 weeks and heal on their own. (From *A close look at venereal disease*, Public service slide presentation. Courtesy Pfizer Laboratories, Pfizer Inc., New York. Permission granted, 2004.)

and is often not noticed in females when present in the genitalia. The chancre is often accompanied by lymphadenopathy.

Without treatment the spread of the bacteria through the blood causes the second stage (secondary syphilis). Therapists may see lesions associated with secondary syphilis (Fig. 3.24). Neurologic (untreated) infection may present as cranial nerve dysfunction, meningitis, stroke, acute or chronic altered mental status, loss of vibration sense, and auditory or ophthalmic abnormalities.[106]

The client may report or present with a characteristic rash that can appear all over the body, most often on the palms and soles. The appearance of these skin lesions occurs after the primary chancre disappears. During this time, the risk of human immunodeficiency virus (HIV) transmission from unsafe sexual practices is increased two- to fivefold.

Syphilis can be tested for with a blood test and treated successfully with antibiotics. Left untreated, tertiary (late-stage) syphilis can cause paralysis, blindness, personality changes or dementia, and damage to internal organs and joints. The PTA can facilitate early detection and treatment through immediate documentation and communication with the PT.

Herpes Virus. Several herpes viruses are accompanied by characteristic skin lesions. HSV-1 and HSV-2 are the most common. Most people have been exposed at an early age and already have immunity. In fact, four out of five Americans harbor HSV-1. Because of the universal distribution of these viruses, most individuals have developed immunity by the ages of 1 to 2 years.

The HSV-1 and HSV-2 viruses are virtually identical, sharing approximately 50% of their DNA. Both types infect the body's mucosal surfaces, usually the mouth or genitals, and then establish latency in the nervous system.[109] Both can cause skin and nail bed changes.

Cold sores caused by HSV-1 (also known as recurrent herpes labialis, or "fever blister") are found on the lip or the skin near the mouth. HSV-1 usually establishes latency in the trigeminal ganglion, a collection of nerve cells near the ear. HSV-1 generally only infects areas above the waistline and occurs when oral secretions or mucous membranes infected with HSV come in contact with a break in the skin (e.g., torn cuticle, skin abrasion).

HSV-1 can be transmitted to the genital area during oral sex. In fact, HSV-1 can be transmitted oral-to-oral, oral-to-genital, anal-to-genital, and oral-to-anal. HSV-1 actually predominates for oral transmission, whereas a second herpesvirus (genital herpes; HSV-2) is more often transmitted sexually.

HSV-2, also known as "genital herpes," can cause cold sores but usually does not; rather, it is more likely to infect body tissues below the waistline as it resides in the sacral ganglion at the base of the spine.

Most HSV-1 and HSV-2 infections are not a major health threat in most people, but slowing the spread of genital herpes is important. The virus is more of a social problem than a medical one. The exception is that genital lesions from herpes can make it easier for a person to become infected with other viruses,

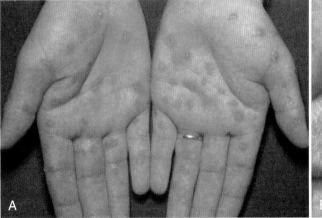
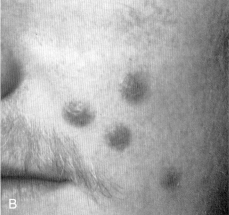

FIG. 3.24 Maculopapular rash associated with secondary syphilis appears as a pink, dusky, brownish-red or coppery, indurated, oval or round lesion with a raised border. These are referred to as "copper penny" spots. The lesions do not bleed and are usually painless. They usually appear scattered on the palms (A) or the bottom of the feet (not shown) but may also present on the face (B). The second stage begins 2 weeks to 6 months after the initial chancre disappears. The client may report joint pain with general flu-like symptoms (e.g., headache, sore throat, swollen glands, muscle aches, fatigue). Patchy hair loss may be described or observed. (From Mir MA: *Atlas of clinical diagnosis*, London, 1995, WB Saunders, p 198.)

including HIV, which increases the risk of developing acquired immunodeficiency syndrome (AIDS).

Nonmedical treatment with OTC products is now available for cold sores. Outbreaks of genital herpes can be effectively treated with medications, but these do not "cure" the virus. HSV-1 is also the cause of herpes whitlow, an infection of the finger, and "wrestler's herpes," a herpes infection on the chest or face.

Herpetic Whitlow. Herpetic whitlow, an intense painful infection of the terminal phalanx of the fingers, is caused by Herpes simplex virus (HSV)-1 (60%) and HSV-2 (40%). The thumb and index fingers are most commonly involved. There may be a history of fever or malaise several days before symptoms occur in the fingers.[110]

Common initial symptoms of infection include tingling pain or tenderness of the affected digit, followed by throbbing pain, swelling, and redness. Fluid-filled vesicles form and eventually crust over, ending the contagious period. The client with red streaks down the arm and lymphadenopathy may have a secondary infection. Take the client's vital signs (especially body temperature) and report all findings to the physician.

As in other herpes infections, viral inoculation of the host occurs through exposure to infected body fluids via a break in the skin such as a paper cut or a torn cuticle. Autoinoculation can occur in anyone with other herpes infections such as genital herpes. It is an occupational risk among health care workers exposed to infected oropharyngeal secretions of clients, which is easily prevented by using standard precautions.[111]

Herpes Zoster. Varicella-zoster virus (VZV) (or herpes zoster or "shingles") is another herpes virus with skin lesions characteristic of the condition. VZV is caused by the same virus that causes chickenpox. After an attack of chickenpox, the virus lies dormant in the nerve tissue, usually the dorsal root ganglion. If the virus is reactivated, the virus can reappear in the form of shingles.

Shingles is an outbreak of a rash or blisters (vesicles with an erythematosus base) on the skin that may be associated with severe pain (Fig. 3.25). The pain is associated with the involved nerve root and associated dermatome and generally presents on one side of the body or face in a pattern characteristic for the involved site (Fig. 3.26). Early signs of shingles include burning or shooting pain and tingling or itching. The rash or blisters are present between 1 and 14 days.

Complications of shingles involving cranial nerves include hearing and vision loss. Postherpetic neuralgia (PHN), a condition in which the pain from shingles persists for months and sometimes years, after the shingles rash has healed, can also occur. Postherpetic neuralgia can be very debilitating. Early intervention within the first 72 hours of onset with antiretroviral medications may diminish or eliminate PHN. Early identification and intervention are very important to outcomes.

Adults with shingles are infectious to anyone who has not had chickenpox. Anyone who has had chickenpox can develop shingles when immunocompromised. Other risk factors for VZV include age (young or old) and immunocompromise from HIV infection, chemotherapy or radiation treatment, transplants, aging, and stress.

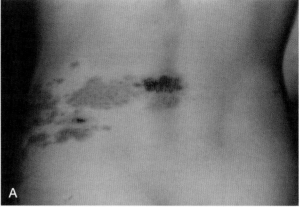
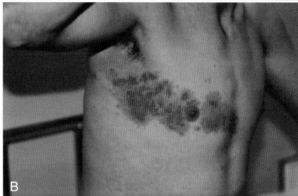

FIG. 3.25 Herpes zoster (shingles). (A) Lesions appear unilaterally along the path of a spinal nerve. (B) Eruptions involving the T4 dermatome. (A, From Callen J, Greer K, Hood H, et al.: *Color atlas of dermatology*, Philadelphia, 1993, WB Saunders; B, From Marx J, Hockberger R, Walls R: *Rosen's emergency medicine: concepts and clinical practice*, ed 6, St. Louis, 2006, Mosby.)

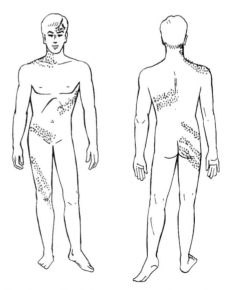

FIG. 3.26 Symptoms of shingles appear on only one side of the body, usually on the torso or face. Most often, the lesions are visible externally. In unusual cases, clients report the same symptoms internally along the dermatome but without a corresponding external skin lesion. (From Malasanos L, Barkauskas V, Stoltenberg-Allen K: *Health assessment*, ed 4, St. Louis, 1990, Mosby.)

Cutaneous Manifestations of Abuse

Signs of child abuse or domestic violence in adults may be seen as skin lesions. Cigarette burns leave a punched-out ulceration with dry, purple crusts (see www.dermatlas.org). Splash marks or scald lines from thermal (hot water) burns occur most often on the buttocks and distal extremities.[112] Bruising from squeezing and shaking involving the mid-portion of the upper arms is a suspicious sign.

Accidental bruising in young children is common; the PTA should watch for nonaccidental bruising found in atypical areas, such as the buttocks, hands, and trunk, or in a child who is not yet walking upright up or cruising (walking along furniture or holding an object while taking steps). To make an accurate assessment, it is important to differentiate between inflicted cutaneous injuries and mimickers of physical abuse. For example, infants with bruising may be demonstrating early signs of bleeding disorders.[112] Mongolian spots can also be mistaken for bruising from child abuse (see the next section).

Mongolian Spots. Discoloration of the skin in newborn infants called Mongolian spots (Fig. 3.27) can be mistaken for signs of child abuse. The Mongolian spot is a congenital, developmental condition exclusively involving the skin and is very common in children of Asian, African, Indian, Native American, Eskimo, Polynesian, or Hispanic origins.[113]

These benign pigmentation changes appear as flat dark blue or black areas and come in a variety of sizes, shapes, and colors. The skin changes result from entrapment of melanocytes (skin cells containing melanin, the normal pigment of the skin) during their migration from the neural crest into the epidermis.

If the PTA observes any suspicious skin bruising and it has not been identified and documented, it is appropriate to bring it to the therapist's attention.

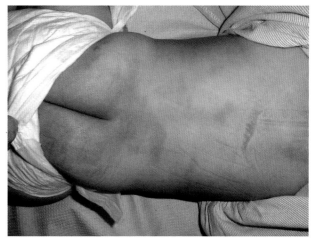

FIG. 3.27 Mongolian spots (congenital dermal melanocytosis). Mongolian spots are common among people of Asian, East Indian, Native American, Inuit, African, and Latino or Hispanic heritage. They are also present in about 1 in 10 fair-skinned infants. The spots—bluish gray to deep brown to black skin markings—often appear on the base of the spine, on the buttocks and back, and even sometimes on the shoulders, ankles, or wrists. Mongolian spots may cover a large area of the back. When the melanocytes are close to the surface, they look deep brown. The deeper they are in the skin, the more bluish they look, and are often mistaken for signs of child abuse. These spots "fade" with age as the child grows and usually disappear by age 5. (Courtesy Dr. Dubin Pavel, 2004.)

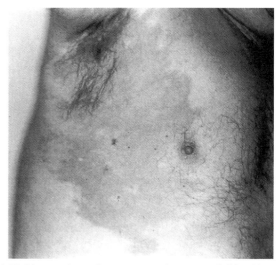

FIG. 3.28 Metastatic carcinoma presenting as a cellulitic skin rash on the anterior chest wall as a result of carcinoma of the lung. This rash can be red, tan, or brown with a flat or raised appearance. When associated with a paraneoplastic syndrome, it may appear far from the site of the primary cancer. (From Callen JP, Jorizzo J, Greer KE, et al.: *Dermatological signs of internal disease*, Philadelphia, 1988, WB Saunders.)

Cancer-Related Skin Lesions

When observing any skin lesions, keep in mind that there are cancer-related skin lesions to monitor. For example, skin rash can present as an early sign of a condition called a *paraneoplastic syndrome* before other manifestations of cancer or cancer recurrence (Fig. 3.28).

Pinch purpura, a purplish, brown, or red discoloration of the skin, can be mistaken by the therapist for a birthmark or port wine stain (Fig. 3.29). The question "How long have you had this?" can help differentiate between something the person has had his or her entire life and a suspicious skin lesion or recent change in the integument.

When purpura causes a raised and palpable skin lesion, it is called *palpable purpura*. The palpable hemorrhages are caused by red blood cells extravasated (escaped) from damaged vessels into the dermis. This type of purpura can be associated with cutaneous vasculitis, pulmonary-renal syndrome, or drug reaction. The lower are affected most often.

Many older adults assume this is a "normal" sign of aging, and in fact, purpura does occur more often in aging adults; see Fig. 3.17; they do not see a physician when it first appears. Early detection and referral are always the keys to a better prognosis. In asking the three important questions, the PTA plays an instrumental part in recognizing and reporting unusual skin lesions.

A client with a past medical history of cancer now presenting with a suspicious skin lesion (Fig. 3.30) that has not been evaluated by the physician must be advised to have this evaluated as soon as possible. The PTA must be aware of how to present this recommendation to the client. There is a need to avoid frightening the client while conveying the importance of early diagnosis of any unusual skin lesions.

Kaposi Sarcoma. Kaposi sarcoma is a form of skin cancer common in older Jewish males of Mediterranean descent that presents with a wide range of appearances. It is not contagious to touch and does not usually cause death or disfigurement.

More recently, Kaposi sarcoma has presented as an opportunistic disease in adults with HIV/AIDS. With the more successful treatment of AIDS with antiretroviral agents, opportunistic diseases, such as Kaposi sarcoma, are on the decline.

Even though this skin lesion will not transmit skin cancer or HIV, all health care workers are always advised to use standard precautions with anyone who has skin lesions of any type.

Lymphomas. Round patches of reddish-brown skin with hair loss over the area are lymphomas, a type of neoplasm of lymphoid tissue (Fig. 3.31). The most common forms of lymphoma are Hodgkin disease and non-Hodgkin lymphoma.

Typically, the appearance of a painless, enlarged lymph node or skin lesion of this type is followed by weakness, fever, and weight loss. A history of chronic immunosuppression (e.g., antirejection drugs for organ transplants, chronic use of immunosuppressant drugs for inflammatory or autoimmune diseases, cancer treatment) in the presence of this clinical presentation is a major red flag.

▶▶ PTA ACTION PLAN

Three Simple Questions Reviewed

As previously pointed out, the PTA can use three simple questions to assess the need for further evaluation of any previously undocumented lesions or lesions that appear to have changed in any way from the initial report:
- How long have you had this?
- Has it changed in any way over the last 3 to 6 weeks?
- Has the physical therapist (or your doctor) seen it?

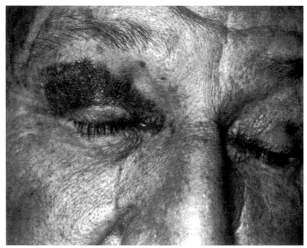

FIG. 3.29 Pinch purpura in an individual with multiple myeloma caused by amyloidosis of the skin. The purpura shown here is a recent skin change for this client. (From Callen JP, Jorizzo J, Greer KE, et al.: *Dermatological signs of internal disease*, ed 2, Philadelphia, 1995, WB Saunders.)

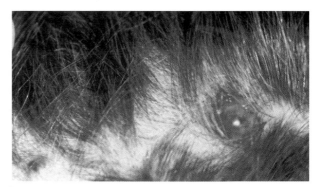

FIG. 3.30 Metastatic renal carcinoma presenting as a nodule in the scalp. Observing any skin lesions, no matter what part of the body the PTA is examining, must be followed by these three assessment questions: (1) How long have you had this? (2) Has it changed in any way over the last 3 to 6 weeks? and (3) Has the physical therapist (or your doctor) seen it? (From Callen JP, Jorizzo J, Greer KE, et al.: *Dermatological signs of internal disease*, Philadelphia, 1988, WB Saunders.)

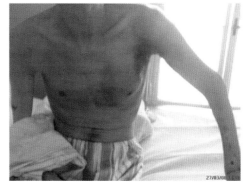

FIG. 3.31 Lymphomas seen on the chest of an adult male arise in individuals who are chronically immunosuppressed for any reason. (From Czepiel J, Kluba-Wojewoda U, Biesiada G, et al. The case of a diffuse large B-cell lymphoma (DLBCL) in a course of HIV. *HIV AIDS Rev* 9 (1): 25, 2010.)

BOX 3.14   Hand and Nail Bed Assessment

Observe the Hands for the Following
- Palmar erythema (see Fig. 3.4)
- Tremor (e.g., liver flap or asterixis; see Fig. 3.5)
- Pallor of palmar creases (anemia, gastrointestinal [GI] malabsorption)
- Palmar xanthomas (lipid deposits on palms of hands; hyperlipidemia, diabetes)
- Turgor (lift skin on back of hands; hydration status)
- Edema

Observe the Fingers and Toenails for the Following
- Color (capillary refill time, nails of Terry: see Fig. 3.3)
- Shape and curvature
- Clubbing:
  - **C**rohn or **C**ardiac/cyanosis
  - **L**ung (cancer, hypoxia, cystic fibrosis)
  - **U**lcerative colitis
  - **B**iliary cirrhosis
  - Present at **b**irth (harmless)
  - **N**eoplasm
  - **GI** involvement
- Nicotine stains
- Splinter hemorrhages (see Fig. 3.36)
- Leukonychia (whitening of nail plate with bands, lines, or white spots; inherited or acquired from malnutrition from eating disorders, alcoholism, or cancer treatment; myocardial infarction [MI], renal failure, poison, anxiety)
- Koilonychia ("spoon nails"; see Fig. 3.34); congenital or hereditary, iron-deficiency anemia, thyroid problem, syphilis, rheumatic fever
- Beau's lines (see Fig. 3.35); decreased production of the nail by the matrix caused by acute illness or systemic insult such as chemotherapy for cancer; recent MI, chronic alcohol abuse, or eating disorders. This can also occur in isolated nail beds from local trauma.
- Adhesion to the nail bed. Look for onycholysis (loosening of nail plate from distal edge inward; Graves' disease, psoriasis, reactive arthritis, obsessive-compulsive behavior: "nail pickers")
- Pitting (psoriasis, eczema, alopecia areata)
- Thinning/thickening

Observing the Nail Beds

As with assessment of the skin, nail beds (fingers and toes) should be evaluated observed for color, shape, thickness, texture, and the presence of lesions (Box 3.14). Systemic changes affect both fingernails and toenails, but the signs are typically more prominent in the faster-growing fingernails.[114]

The normal nail consists of three parts: the nail bed, the nail plate, and the cuticle (Fig. 3.32). The nail bed is highly vascularized and gives the nail its pink color. The hard nail is formed at the proximal end (the matrix). About one-fourth of the nail is covered by skin (the proximal nail fold). The cuticle seals and protects the space between the proximal fold and the nail plate.

Many individual variations in color, texture, and grooming of the nails are influenced by factors unrelated to disease, such as occupation, chronic use of nail polish or acrylics, or exposure to chemical dyes and detergents. Longitudinal lines of darker color (pigment) may be seen in the normal nails of clients with darker skin.

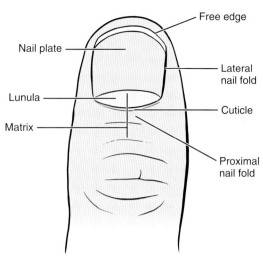

FIG. 3.32 Normal nail structure. The nail matrix forms the nail plate and begins about 5–8 mm beneath the proximal nail fold and extends distally to the edge of the lunula (half-moon), where the nail bed begins. The lunula is the exposed part of the nail matrix, distal to the proximal nail fold; it is not always visible.

❓ PICTURE THE PATIENT

In the older adult, minor variations associated with the aging process may be observed (e.g., gradual thickening of the nail plate, appearance of longitudinal ridges, yellowish-gray discoloration).

In the normal individual, pressing or blanching the nail bed of a finger or toe produces a whitening effect; when pressure is released, a return of color should occur within 3 seconds. If the capillary refill time exceeds 3 seconds, the lack of circulation may be due to arterial insufficiency from atherosclerosis or spasm.

Nail Bed Changes

Some of the more common nail bed changes seen in a physical therapy practice are included in this chapter. With any nail or skin condition, the PTA should ask if the nails have always been like this or if any changes have occurred in the last 6 weeks to 6 months. Documentation and reporting may not be needed if the PT is aware of the new onset of nail bed changes.

Again, as with visual inspection of the skin, this section of the text is only a cursory look at the most common nail bed changes; many more are not included here. A well-rounded library should include at least one text with color plates and photos of various nail bed changes.[87,115–117] This is to provide the PTA with background information, which can be used during the observation and assessment portion of the PTA's visit with the client.

Onycholysis. Onycholysis, a painless loosening of the nail plate, occurs from the distal edge inward (Fig. 3.33). Fingers and toes may both be affected as a consequence of dermatologic conditions such as dermatitis, fungal disease, lichen planus, and psoriasis. Systemic diseases associated with onycholysis include myeloma, neoplasia, Graves' disease, anemia, and reactive arthritis.[118]

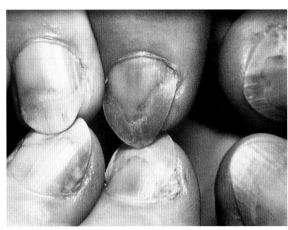

FIG. 3.33 Onycholysis. Loosening of the nail plate, usually from the tip of the nail, progressing inward and from the edge of the nail moving inward. Possible causes include Graves' disease, psoriasis, reactive arthritis, and obsessive-compulsive behaviors (nail pickers). (From Arndt KA, Wintroub BU, Robinson JK, et al.: *Primary care dermatology*, Philadelphia, 1997, WB Saunders.)

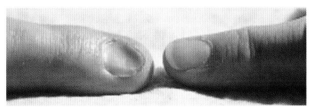

FIG. 3.34 Koilonychia (spoon nails). In this side-by-side view, the affected nail bed is on the left and the normal nail on the right. With a spoon nail, the rounded indentation would hold a drop or several drops of water, hence the name. (From Swartz MH: *Textbook of physical diagnosis*, ed 6, Philadelphia, 2009, WB Saunders.)

Medications, such as tetracycline, fluoroquinolones (antibiotics), anticancer drugs, NSAIDs, psoralens, retinoids, zidovudine, and quinine, can cause photo-onycholysis (toes must be exposed to the sun for the condition to occur).[118]

Local causes from chemical, physical, cosmetic, or traumatic sources can bring on this condition. In the case of trauma, a limited number of nails are affected. For example, in clients with onycholysis as a result of nervous or obsessive-compulsive behaviors, only one or two nails are targeted. The individual picks around the edges until the nail is raised and separated from the nail bed. When there is an underlying systemic disorder, it is more common to see all the nail plates affected.

Koilonychia. Koilonychia or "spoon nails" may be a congenital or hereditary trait and, as such, is considered "normal" for that individual. These are thin, depressed nails with lateral edges tilted upward, forming a concave profile (Fig. 3.34).

Koilonychia can occur as a result of hypochromic anemia, iron deficiency (with or without anemia), poorly controlled diabetes of more than 15 years' duration, chemical irritants, local injury, developmental abnormality, or psoriasis. It can also be an outward sign of thyroid problems, syphilis, and rheumatic fever.[87,115]

Beau's Lines. Beau's lines are transverse grooves or ridges across the nail plate as a result of a decreased or interrupted production of the nail by the matrix (Fig. 3.35). The cause is usually an acute illness or systemic insult such as chemotherapy for cancer. Other common conditions associated with Beau's lines are poor peripheral circulation, eating disorders, cirrhosis associated with chronic alcohol use, and recent myocardial infarction (MI).[57]

Since the nails grow at an approximate rate of 3 mm each month, the date of the initial onset of illness or disease can be estimated by the location of the line. The dent appears first at the cuticle and moves forward as the nail grows. Measure the distance (in millimeters) from the dent to the cuticle, and add 3 to account for the distance from the cuticle to the matrix. This is the number of weeks ago the person first had the problem.

Beau's lines are temporary until the impaired nail formation is corrected (if and when the individual returns to normal health). These lines can also occur as a result of local trauma to the hand or fingers.

In the case of an injury, the dent may be permanent. Hand therapists see this condition most often. If it is not the result of a recent injury, the client may be able to remember sustaining an injury years ago.

Splinter Hemorrhages. Splinter hemorrhages may be the sign of a silent MI or the client may have a known history of MI. These red-brown linear streaks (Fig. 3.36) can also signal other systemic conditions, such as bacterial endocarditis, vasculitis, or renal failure.

In a hospital setting, they are not uncommon in the cardiac care unit (CCU) or other ICU. In such a case, the therapist may simply take note of the nail bed changes and correlate them with

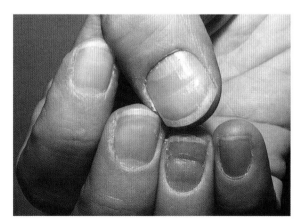

FIG. 3.35 Beau's lines or grooves across the nail plate. A depression across the nail extends down to the nail bed. This occurs with shock, illness, malnutrition, or trauma severe enough to impair nail formation, such as acute illness, prolonged fever, or chemotherapy. A dent appears first at the cuticle and moves forward as the nail grows. All nails can be involved, but with local trauma, only the involved nail will be affected. This photo shows a client after insult, following full recovery. At the time of the illness, nail loss is obvious, often with change in nail bed color, as occurs with chemotherapy. (From Callen JP, Greer KE, Hood AF, et al.: *Color atlas of dermatology*, Philadelphia, 1994, WB Saunders.)

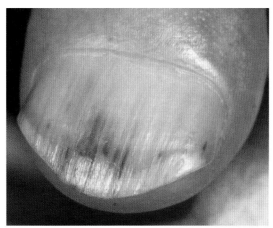

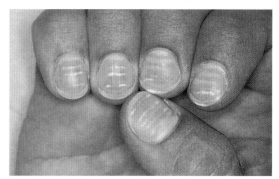

FIG. 3.37 Leukonychia punctata. Transverse white bands result from repeated minor trauma to the full nail matrix. (From Baran, Dawber, *and Levene, 1991.*)

FIG. 3.36 Splinter hemorrhages. These red-brown streaks, or embolic lesions, occur with subacute bacterial endocarditis, sepsis, rheumatoid arthritis, vitamin C deficiency, or hematologic neoplasm. They can occur from local trauma, in which case only the injured nail beds will have the telltale streak. Splinter hemorrhages may also be a nonspecific sign. (From Hordinsky MK, Sawaya ME, Scher RK: *Atlas of hair and nails*, Philadelphia, 2000, Churchill Livingstone.)

the pathologic insult, probably already a part of the medical record. If the condition is not documented by other medical staff, the PTA should bring this to the attention of the PT for further evaluation.

When present in only one or two nail beds, local trauma may be linked to the nail bed changes. Asking the client about recent trauma or injury to the hand or fingers may bring this to light.

Leukonychia. Leukonychia, or white nail syndrome, is characterized by dots or lines of white that progress to the free edge of the nail as the nail grows (Fig. 3.37). White nails can be congenital, but more often, they are acquired in association with hypocalcemia, severe hypochromic anemia, Hodgkin disease, renal failure, malnutrition from eating disorders, MI, leprosy, hepatic cirrhosis, and arsenic poisoning.[57]

Acquired leukonychia is caused by a disturbance to the nail matrix. Repeated trauma, such as keyboard punching, is a potential acquired cause of this condition.[119] When the entire nail plate is white, the condition is called *leukonychiatotalis* (Case Example 3.3).

Paronychia. Paronychia is an infection of the fold of skin at the margin of a nail bed. There is an obvious red, swollen site of inflammation that is tender or painful. This may be acute as with a bacterial infection, or chronic, in association with an occupationally induced fungal infection referred to as "wet work" from having the hands submerged in water for long periods.

The client may also have a history of finger exposure to chemical irritants, acrylic nails or nail glue, or sculpted nails. Paronychia of one or more fingers is not uncommon in people who pick, bite, or suck their nails. Health care professionals with these nervous habits working in a clinical setting (especially hospitals) are at increased risk for paronychia from infection with bacteria such as *Streptococcus* or *Staphylococcus*. Green coloration of the nail may indicate *Pseudomonas* infection.

Paronychia infections may spread to the pulp space of the finger, developing a painful felon (an infection with localized abscess). Untreated infection can spread to the deep spaces of the hand and beyond.

It is especially important to recognize any nail bed irregularity because it may be a clue to malignancy. Likewise, anyone with diabetes mellitus, immunocompromise, or a history of steroids and retroviral use is at increased risk for paronychia formation. Early identification and reporting are imperative to avoid more serious consequences.

Clubbing. Thickening and widening of the terminal phalanges of the fingers and toes result in a painless club-like appearance recognized by the loss of the angle between the nail and the nail bed (see Figs. 3.33 and 3.34).

Clubbing of the fingers Fig. 3.38) and toes usually results from chronic oxygen deprivation in these tissue beds. It is most often observed in clients with cystic fibrosis, advanced COPD, congenital heart defects, and cor pulmonale, but they can occur within 10 days in someone with an acute systemic condition such as a pulmonary abscess, malignancy, or polycythemia. Clubbing may be the first sign of a paraneoplastic syndrome associated with cancer.[120,121]

Most of the time, clubbing is due to pulmonary disease and resultant hypoxia (diminished availability of blood to the body tissues), but clubbing can be a sign of heart disease, peripheral vascular disease, and disorders of the liver and GI tract.

Clubbing can be assessed by the Schamroth method (see Fig. 3.39). Any positive findings in the nail beds should be viewed in light of the entire clinical presentation. For example, a positive Schamroth test without observable clinical changes in skin color, capillary refill time, or shape of the fingertips may not signify systemic disease but rather a normal anatomic variation of nail curvature.[34]

PRECAUTIONS/CONTRAINDICATIONS TO THERAPY

The following parameters are listed as precautions/contraindications rather than one or the other because these signs and

CASE EXAMPLE 3.3 Leukonychia

A 24-year-old White male was seen in physical therapy for a work-related back injury.

During a routine therapy session one day, the client showed the PTA his nails and asked what could be the cause of the white discoloration in all the nail beds.

He reported that the nails seemed to grow out from time to time. There was tenderness along the sides of the nails and at the distal edge of the nails. It was obvious the nails were bitten and that several nails were red and swollen. The client admitted to picking at his nails when he was nervous. He was observed tapping his nails on the table repeatedly during the exam. No changes of any kind were observed in the feet.

The PTA referred back to the initial evaluation documentation for information regarding the past medical history. The client's history was found to be negative for any significant health problems. He was not taking any medications, over-the-counter drugs, or recreational drugs. He did not smoke and denied the use of alcohol. His job as a supervisor in a machine shop did not require the mechanical use of his hands. He was not exposed to any unusual chemicals or solvents at work.

Result: When asked, "How long have you had this?" The client reported for 2 years. When asked, "Have your nails changed in the last 6 weeks to 6 months?" The answer was, "Yes, the condition seems to come and go." When asked, "Has your doctor seen these changes?" the client did not think so.

The PTA did not know what was causing the nail bed changes and suggested the client ask his physician about the condition at his next appointment. The PTA then informed the client that she would discuss their conversation with the supervising PT for follow-up as well.

The physician also observed the client repeatedly tapping his nails and performed a screening exam for anxiety.

The nail bed condition was diagnosed as leukonychia from repeated microtrauma to the nail matrix. The patient was referred to psychiatry to manage the observed anxiety symptoms. The nails returned to normal in about 3 months (90–100 days) after the client stopped tapping, restoring normal growth to the nail matrix.

Critical Thinking Activity

In a small group, discuss the following questions:
- Is it beyond the scope of the PTA to even address the concerns of the client regarding the fingernails during this treatment session?
- Did the PTA ask appropriate questions to gain enough information for follow-up with the PT?
- Is the PTA required to document the discussion that occurred with the client today?

*Unexplained or poorly tolerated by client.
(From Maino K, Stashower ME: Traumatic transverse leukonychia, *SKINmed* 3(1):53–55, 2004. From WebMD. Accessed online at http://www.medscape.com/viewarticle/467074.)

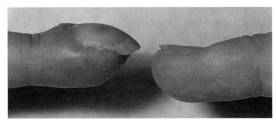

FIG. 3.38 Rapid development of digital clubbing (fingers as shown on the left or toes [not shown]) over the course of a 10- to 14-day period requires immediate medical evaluation. Clubbing can be assessed using the Schamroth method shown in Fig. 3.39. (From Swartz MH: *Textbook of physical diagnosis*, ed 6, Philadelphia, 2009, WB Saunders.)

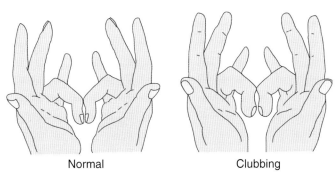

Normal   Clubbing

FIG. 3.39 Schamroth method. Assessment of clubbing. The client places the fingernails of opposite fingers together and holds them up to a light. If the examiner can see a diamond shape between the nails, there is no clubbing. Clubbing is identified by the absence of the diamond shape. It occurs first in the thumb and index finger. (From Ignatavicius DD, Bayne MV: Assessment of the cardiovascular system. In Ignatavicius DD, Bayne MV, editors: *Medical-surgical nursing*, Philadelphia, 1993, WB Saunders.)

symptoms may have different significance depending on the client's overall health, age, medications taken, and other factors. What may be a precaution for one client may be a clear contraindication for another and vice versa. The presence of any of these signs or symptoms requires documentation and discussion with the PT.

- Resting heart rate: 120 to 130 bpm*
- Resting systolic pressure: 180 to 200 mm Hg*
- Resting diastolic pressure: 105 to 110 mm Hg*
- Marked dyspnea
- Loss of palpable pulse or irregular pulse with symptoms of dizziness, nausea, or SOB

Anemic individuals may demonstrate an increased normal resting pulse rate that should be monitored during exercise. Anyone with unstable BP may require initial standing with a tilt table or monitoring of the BP before, during, and after treatment. Again, it is recommended that the PTA seek guidance from the PT when determining safe BP parameters.

GUIDELINES FOR IMMEDIATE COMMUNICATION WITH THE PHYSICAL THERAPIST

- Anyone with diabetes mellitus, who is immunocompromised, or who has a history of steroid and retroviral use now presenting with red, inflamed, swollen nail bed(s) or any skin lesion involving the feet must be referred for medical evaluation immediately.
- Recurrent cancer can appear as a single lump, a pale or red nodule just below the skin surface, a swelling, a dimpling of

the skin, or a red rash. Report any of these changes to a physician immediately.

- Immediate medical referral is advised for any client reporting a new onset of SOB who is tachypneic, diaphoretic, or cyanotic; any suspicion of anaphylaxis is also an emergency situation.
- Cough with sputum production that is yellow, green, or rust colored.
- Abrupt change in mental status, confusion or increasing confusion, and new onset of delirium requires medical attention.
- Outbreak of vesicular rash associated with herpes zoster. Medical referral within 72 hours of the initial appearance of skin lesions is needed; client will begin a course of antiretroviral medication to manage symptoms and help prevent postherpetic neuropathy.

▶▶ PTA ACTION PLAN

Some Final Points to Ponder

- Under the direct supervision of the PT, the PTA carries out certain portions of the physical assessment with every client by observing general health and nutrition, mental status, mood or affect, skin and body contours, mobility, and function on a daily basis.
- Measuring vital signs is a key component of the screening assessment. Vital signs, observations, and reported associated signs and symptoms are among the best screening tools available to the PTA. These same parameters can be useful to the PT to plan and progress safe and effective exercise programs for clients who have true neuromuscular or musculoskeletal problems and also have other health concerns or comorbidities.
- Documentation of physical findings is important. From a legal point of view, if it is not documented, it is not assessed. Record important normal and abnormal findings.
- The PTA should make general skin and nail bed observations on a regular basis. Changes in the skin and nail beds may be the first sign of inflammatory, infectious, and immunologic disorders and can occur with the involvement of a variety of organs.
- Even the experienced PTA should be aware to avoid expressing premature concern to the client when observing yellow- or red-flag situations. Prompt and professional collaboration and communication with the appropriate medical personnel is a key responsibility of the PTA.

REFERENCES

1. Wainner RS, Whitman JM, Cleland JA, Flynn TW: Regional interdependence: a musculoskeletal examination model whose time has come, *J Orthop Sports Phys Ther* 37(11):658–660, 2007.
2. Sieber FE: Sedation depth during spinal anesthesia and the development of postoperative delirium in elderly patients undergoing hip fracture repair, *Mayo Clin Proc* 85(1):18–26, 2010.
3. Talmo CT, Aghazadeh M, Bono JV: Perioperative complications following total joint replacement, *Clin Geriatr Med* 28(3):471–487, 2012.
4. Flink BJ, Rivelli SK, Cox EA, et al: Obstructive sleep apnea and incidence of postoperative delirium after elective knee replacement in the nondemented elderly, *Anesthesiology* 116(4):788–796, 2012.
5. Krenk L, Rasmussen LS, Hansen TB, et al: Delirium after fast-track hip and knee arthroplasty, *Br J Anaesth* 108(4):607–611, 2012.
6. Jain FA, Brooks JO 3rd, Larsen KA, et al: Individual risk profiles for postoperative delirium after joint replacement surgery, *Psychosomatics* 52(5):410–416, 2011.
7. Lee KH, Ha YC, Lee YK, et al: Frequency, risk factors, and prognosis of prolonged delirium in elderly patients after hip fracture surgery, *Clin Orthop Relat Res* 469(9):2612–2620, 2011.
8. Bjorklund KB, Hommel A, Thorngren KG, et al: Reducing delirium in elderly patients with hip fracture: a multi-factorial intervention study, *Acta Anaesthesiol Scand* 54(6):678–688, 2010.
9. Alfonso DT, Toussaint RJ, Alfonso BD, et al: Nonsurgical complications after total hip and total knee arthroplasty, *Am J Orthop* 35(11):503–510, 2006.
10. Silverstein JH, Deiner SG: Perioperative delirium and its relationship to dementia, *Prog Neuropsychopharmacol Biol Psychiatry* 43:108–115, 2013.
11. Lundström M, Stenvall M, Olofsson B: Symptom profile of postoperative delirium in patients with and without dementia, *J Geriatr Psychiatry Neurol* 25(3):162–169, 2012.
12. National Institutes of Health: *Calculate your body mass index.* http://www.nhlbi.nih.gov/guidelines/obesity/BMI/bmicalc.htm. Accessed February 1, 2014.
13. Dr. Steven B: *Hall's Body Mass Index seeker.* http://www.halls.md/body-mass-index/bmi.htm. Accessed December 11, 2012.
14. National Center for Chronic Disease Prevention and Health Promotion: *Body mass index for children and teens.* http://www.cdc.gov/nccdphp/dnpa/bmi/bmi-for-age.htm. Accessed December 11, 2012.
15. Severin R, Sabbahi A, Albarrati A, Phillips SA, Arena S: Blood pressure screening by outpatient physical therapists: a call to action and clinical recommendations, *Phys Ther* 100(6):1008–1019, 2020.
16. Frese EM, Fick A, Sadowsky HS: Blood pressure measurement guidelines for physical therapists, *Cardiopulm Phys Ther J* 22(2):5–12, 2011.
17. Severin R, Wang E, Wielechowski A, Phillips SA: Outpatient physical therapist attitudes toward and behaviors in cardiovascular disease screening: a national survey, *Phys Ther* 99:833–848, 2019.
18. Billek-Sawhney B, Sawhney R: Cardiovascular considerations in outpatient physical therapy, *J Orthop Sports Phys Ther* 27:57, 1998.
19. Gonzalez Della Valle A, Chiu YL, Ma Y, et al: The metabolic syndrome in patients undergoing knee and hip arthroplasty: trends and in-hospital outcomes in the United States, *J Arthroplasty* 27(10):1743–1749, 2012.
20. APTA Guide to Physical Therapist Practice 4.0. American Physical Therapy Association; 2023.
21. American College of Sports Medicine (ACSM): *Guidelines for exercise testing and prescription*, ed 8, Philadelphia, 2009, Lippincott, Williams & Wilkins.
22. Fritz S, Lusardi M: White paper: "Walking speed: the sixth vital sign," *J Geriatric Phys Ther* 32(2):2–5, 2009.

23. Hussain SF: Progestogen-only pills and high blood pressure: is there an association? A literature review, *Contraception* 69(2):89–97, 2004.

24. Shaw DK: What's so vital about vital signs? *Q Rev* 44(4):1–5, 2009.

25. Marshall GL, Little JW: Deep tendon reflexes: a study of quantitative methods, *J Spinal Cord Med* 25(2):94–99, 2002. Summer

26. Philips Medical Systems: *Understanding pulse oximetry SpO₂ concepts*, 2002. http://incenter.medical.philips.com/doclib/enc/fetch/586262/586457/Understanding_Pulse_Oximetry.pdf%3Fnodeid%3D586458%26vernum%3D2. Accessed December 18, 2012.

27. Hardwick KD: Insightful options, *Rehab Magazine* 15(7):30–33, 2002.

28. Ostchega Y, Prineas RJ, Paulose-Ram R, et al: National health and nutrition examination survey 1999-2000: effect of observer training and protocol standardization on reducing blood pressure measurement error, *J Clin Epidemiol* 56:768–774, 2003.

29. Liu Y: National Health and Nutrition Examination Survey 1999-2000: effect of observer training and protocol standardization on reducing blood pressure measurement error, *J Clin Epidemiol* 57(6):651, 2004 (author reply 652).

30. Muntner P, Shimbo D, Carey RM, et al: Measurement of blood pressure in humans: a scientific statement from the American Heart Association, *Hypertension* 73:e35–e66, 2019.

31. Nelson MR, Quinn S, Bowers-Ingram L, et al: Cluster-randomized controlled trial of oscillometric vs. manual sphygmomanometer for blood pressure management in primary care (CRAB), *Am J Hypertens* 22(6):598–603, 2009.

32. Levin DK: Measuring blood pressure in legs, *Medscape Int Med* 6(1), 2004. Available at: http://www.medscape.com/viewarticle/471829. Accessed November 25, 2012

33. Chobanian A.V., Bakris G.L., Black H.R., et al: The seventh report of the Joint National Committee on Prevention, Detection, Evaluation, and Treatment of High Blood Pressure. Hypertension. 2003;42:1206–1252.

34. Jarvis C: *Physical examination and health assessment*, ed 6, Philadelphia, 2011, WB Saunders.

35. Mitchell GF: Pulse pressure and risk of new onset atrial fibrillation, *JAMA* 297(7):709–715, 2007.

36. Valbusa F, Bonapace S, Bertolini L, et al: Increased pulse pressure independently predicts incident atrial fibrillation in patients with type 2 diabetes, *Diabetes Care* 35(11):2337–2339, 2012.

37. Franklin SS: Pulse pressure as a risk factor, *Clin Exp Hypertens* 26(7-8):645–652, 2004.

38. Bernstein KE, Ong FS, Blackwell WL, et al: A modern understanding of the traditional and nontraditional biological functions of Angiotensin-converting enzyme, *Pharmacol Rev* 65(1):1–46, 2012.

39. American College of Sports Medicine: *ACSM guidelines for exercise testing and prescription*, ed 9, Philadelphia, 2013, Lippincott, Williams & Wilkins.

40. Burkman R, Schlesselman JJ, Zieman M: Safety concerns and health benefits associated with oral contraception, *Am J Obstet Gynecol* 190(4 Suppl):S5–S22, 2004.

41. Hillegass EA: *Essentials of cardiopulmonary physical therapy*, ed 3, Philadelphia, 2010, Saunders.

42. Benjamin Ej, Muntner P, Alonso A, et al: Heart disease and stroke statistics – 2019 update: a report from the American Heart Association, *Circulation.* 139(10):00659, 2019.

43. Whelton PK, Carey RM, Aronow WS, et al: 2017 ACC/AHA/AAPA/ABC/ACPM/AGS/APhA/ASH/ASPC/NMA/PCNA guideline for the prevention, detection, evaluation, and management of high blood pressure in adults: executive summary: a report of the American College of Cardiology/American Heart Association Task Force on clinical practice guidelines, *Hypertension* 71(6):1269–1324, 2018.

44. Mancia G: Long-term risk of sustained hypertension in white-coat or masked hypertension, *Hypertension* 54(2):226–232, 2009.

45. Peacock J, Diaz KM, Viera AJ, Schwartz JE, Shimbo D: Unmasking masked hypertension: prevalence, clinical implications, diagnosis, correlates and future directions, *J Hum Hypertens* 28:521–528, 2014.

46. Bulpitt CJ, Beckett N, Peters R, et al: Does white coat hypertension require treatment over age 80? Results of the hypertension in the very elderly trial ambulatory blood pressure side project, *Hypertension* 61(1):89–94, 2013.

47. Mancia G, Verdecchia P: Hypertension compendium: clinical value of ambulatory blood pressure, evidence and limtes, *Circ Res* 116:1034–1045, 2015.

48. Kario K: Morning surge in blood pressure and cardiovascular risk, *Hypertension* 56:765–773, 2010.

49. Yano Y, Kario K: Nocturnal blood pressure, morning blood pressure surge, and cerebrovascular events, *Curr Hypertens Rep* 14(3):219–227, 2012.

50. Centers for Disease Control and Prevention: CDC Health Disparities and Inequalities Report, *MMWR* 62(Suppl 3):1–189, 2013.

51. Kario K, Tobin JN, Wolfson LI, et al: Lower standing systolic blood pressure as a predictor of falls in the elderly: a community-based prospective study, *J Am Coll Cardiol* 38(1):246–252, 2001.

52. Sierra C: Hypertension and mild cognitive impairment, *Curr Hypertens Rep* 14(6):548–555, 2012.

53. Feldstein CA: Association between chronic blood pressure changes and development of Alzheimer's disease, *J Alzheimers Dis* 32(3):753–763, 2012.

54. de la Torre JC: Cardiovascular risk factors promote brain hypoperfusion leading to cognitive decline and dementia, *Cardiovasc Psychiatry Neurol*:367516, 2012.

55. Scuteri A, Cunha PG: Decreasing arterial aging by controlling blood pressure levels and hypertension: a step forward, *Curr Vasc Pharmacol* 10(6):702–704, 2012.

56. Qui C, von Strauss E, Winblad B, et al: Decline in blood pressure over time and risk of dementia: a longitudinal study from the Kungsholmen project, *Stroke* 35(8):1810–1815, 2004.

57. Goldman L, Schafer AI: *Goldman's Cecil medicine*, ed 24, Philadelphia, 2012, Saunders.

58. Fillit HM: *Brocklehurst's textbook of geriatric medicine*, ed 7, Philadelphia, 2010, Saunders.

59. Montero-Odasso M, Schapira M, Soriano ER, et al: Gait velocity as a single predictor of adverse events in healthy seniors aged 75 years and older, *J Gerontol A Biol Sci Med Sci* 60A:1304–1309, 2005.

60. Middleton A, Fritz S, Lusardi M: Walking speed: the functional vital sign, *J Aging Phys Act* 23(2):314–322, 2015.

61. Singla S, Jhamb S, Singh KD, Kumar A: Depression affects autonomic system of the body? Yes, it does!, *J Educ Health Promot* 9:217, 2020.

62. Dros J, Maarsingh OR, Beem L, et al: Functional prognosis of dizziness in older adults in primary care: a prospective cohort study, *J Am Geriatr Soc* 60(12):2263–2269, 2012.

63. Dutton M: *Dutton's orthopaedic examination evaluation and intervention*, ed 3, New York, 2012, McGraw-Hill Medical.

64. Butler DS: *Mobilisation of the nervous system*, Philadelphia, 1991, Churchill Livingstone.

65. Davis DS, Anderson IB, Carson MG, Elkins CL, Stuckey LB: Upper Limb Neural Tension and Seated Slump Tests: The False Positive Rate among Healthy Young Adults without Cervical or Lumbar Symptoms, *J Man Manip Ther* 16(3):136–141, 2008.

66. GBD 2016 Traumatic Brain Injury and Spinal Cord Injury Collaborators: Global, regional, and national burden of traumatic brain injury and spinal cord injury, 1990-2016: a systematic analysis for the global burden of disease study 2016, *Lancet Neurol* 18:56–87, 2019.

67. Harvey LA, Close JC: Traumatic brain injury in older adults: characteristics, causes and consequences, *Injury* 43(11):1821–1826, 2012.

68. Gaetani P, Revay M, Sciacca S, et al: Traumatic brain injury in the elderly: considerations in a series of 103 patients older than 70, *J Neurosurg Sci* 56(3):231–237, 2012.

69. Stone KL: Actigraphy-measured sleep characteristics and risk of falls in older women, *Arch Intern Med* 168(16):1768–1775, 2008.

70. Grundstrom AC, Guse CE, Layde PM: Risk factors for falls and fall-related injuries in adults 85 years of age and older, *Arch Gerontol Geriatr* 54(3):421–428, 2012.

71. Mesas AE, López-García E, Rodríguez-Artalejo F: Self-reported sleep duration and falls in older adults, *J Sleep Res* 20(1 Pt 1):21–27, 2011.

72. Ming Y, Zecevic A: Medications & polypharmacy influence on recurrent fallers in community: a systematic review, *Can Geriatr J* 21(1):14–25, 2018.

73. Olazarán J, Valle D, Serra JA, et al: Psychotropic medications and falls in nursing homes: a cross-sectional study, *J Am Med Dir Assoc* 14(3):213–217, 2013.

74. Lamis RL, Kramer JS, Hale LS, et al: Fall risk associated with inpatient medications, *Am J Health Syst Pharm* 69(21):1888–1894, 2012.

75. Kojima T, Akishita M, Nakamura T, et al: Polypharmacy as a risk for fall occurrence in geriatric outpatients, *Geriatr Gerontol Int* 12(3):425–430, 2012.

76. Santos SS, da Silva ME, de Pinho LB, et al: Risk of falls in the elderly: an integrative review based on the North American nursing diagnosis association, *Rev Esc Enferm USP* 46(5):1227–1236, 2012.

77. Olsson Möller U, Midlöv P, Kristensson J, et al: Prevalence and predictors of falls and dizziness in people younger and older than 80 years of age: a longitudinal cohort study, *Arch Gerontol Geriatr* 56(1):160–168, 2013.

78. Patino CM, McKean-Cowdin R, Azen SP, et al: Central and peripheral visual impairment and the risk of falls and falls with injury, *Ophthalmology* 117(2):199–206, 2010.

79. Jacobson GP, McCaslin DL, Grantham SL, Piker EG: Significant vestibular system impairment is common in a cohort of elderly patients referred for assessment of falls risk, *J Am Acad Audiol* 19(10):799–807, 2008.

80. Lawlor DA, Patel R, Ebrahim S: Association between falls in elderly women and chronic diseases and drug use: cross sectional study, *BMJ* 327(7417):712–717, 2003.

81. Gnjidic D, Hilmer SN, Blyth FM, et al: Polypharmacy cutoff and outcomes: five or more medicines were used to identify community-dwelling older men at risk of different adverse outcomes, *J Clin Epidemiol* 65(9):989–995, 2012.

82. Leveille S: Chronic musculoskeletal pain and the occurrence of falls in an older population, *JAMA* 302(20):2214–2221, 2009.

83. Habif TP: *Skin disease: diagnosis and treatment*, ed 3, Philadelphia, 2011, Saunders.

84. Feldman M: *Sleisenger and Fordtran's gastrointestinal and liver disease*, ed 9, Philadelphia, 2010, Saunders.

85. Webster GF: Common skin disorders in the elderly, *Clin Cornerstone* 4(1):39–44, 2001.

86. James WD: *Andrews' diseases of the skin: clinical dermatology*, Philadelphia, 2011, Saunders.

87. Lavery LA, Higgins KR, Lanctot DR, et al: Preventing diabetic foot ulcer recurrence in high-risk patients: use oftemperature monitoring as a self-assessment tool, *Diabetes Care* 30(1):14–20, 2007.

88. Armstrong DG: Skin temperature monitoring reduces the risk for diabetic foot ulceration in high-risk patients, *Am J Med* 120(12):1042–1046, 2007.

89. Armstrong DG: Does dermal thermometry predict clinical outcome in diabetic foot infection? Analysis of data from the SIDESTEP* trial, *Wound J* 3(4):302–307, 2006.

90. Farid KJ, Winkelman C, Rizkala A, Jones K: Using temperature of pressure-related intact discolored areas of skin to detect deep tissue injury: an observational, retrospective, correlational study, *Ostomy Wound Manage* 58(8):20–31, 2012.

91. McGee S: *Evidence-based physical diagnosis*, ed 3, Philadelphia, 2012, Saunders.

92. Bolognia JL: *Dermatology*, ed 3, Philadelphia, 2012, Saunders.

93. Rigel DS: The evolution of melanoma diagnosis: 25 years beyond the ABCDs, *Ca J Clin* 60(5):301–316, 2010.

94. Tüzün Y, Keskin S, Kote E: The role of *Helicobacter pylori* infection in skin diseases: facts and controversies, *Clin Dermatol* 28(5):478–482, 2010.

95. Rakel D: *Integrative medicine*, ed 3, Philadelphia, 2012, Saunders.

96. Hoffman R: *Hematology: basic principles and practice*, ed 6, Philadelphia, 2012, Saunders.

97. Kuo CC: Diabetic eruptive xanthoma, *Acta Clin Belg* 66(4):321–322, 2011.

98. Habif TP: *Clinical dermatology: a color guide to diagnosis and therapy*, ed 5, St. Louis, 2010, Mosby.

99. Yazici Y, Erkan D, Scott R, et al: The skin: a map to rheumatic diseases, *J Musculoskel Med* 18(1):43–53, 2001.

100. CDC: *Lyme disease signs and symptoms*. https://www.cdc.gov/lyme/signs_symptoms/rashes.html Accessed July 16, 2023.

101. Weston WL: *Color textbook of pediatric dermatology*, St. Louis, 2007, Mosby.

102. Fitzpatrick JE: *Dermatology secrets plus*, ed 4, St. Louis, 2010, Mosby.

103. Guillot B, Bessis D, Dereure O: Mucocutaneous side effects of antineoplastic chemotherapy, *Expert Opin Drug Saf* 3(6):579–587, 2004.

104. Borroni G, Vassallo C, Brazzelli V, et al: Radiation recall dermatitis, panniculitis, and myositis following cyclophosphamide therapy: histopathologic findings of a patient affected by multiple myeloma, *Am J Dermatopathol* 26(3):213–216, 2004.

105. Friedlander PA, Bansal R, Schwartz L, et al: Gemcitabine-related radiation recall preferentially involves internal tissues and organs, *Cancer* 100(9):1793–1799, 2004.

106. Workowski KA, Berman S: Sexually transmitted diseases treatment guidelines, 2010, *MMWR* 59(RR-12):1–110, 2010.

107. Centers for Disease Control and Prevention: *CDC fact sheet: STD trends in the United States. 2011 National Data*. https://www.cdc.gov/nchhstp/newsroom/fact-sheets/std/std-us-2021.html Accessed July 16, 2023.

108. CDC: *Use same CDC website reference as in comment CM19.* https://www.cdc.gov/nchhstp/newsroom/fact-sheets/std/std-us-2021.html

109. World Health Organization: *Herpes simplex virus.*https://www.who.int/en/news-room/fact-sheets/detail/herpes-simplex-virus Accessed July 16, 2023.

110. Wolfe SW: *Green's operative hand surgery*, ed 6, Philadelphia, 2011, Churchill Livingstone.

111. Bennett JV, Jarvis WR, Brachman PS: *Hospital infections*, ed 5, Philadelphia, 2014, Lippincott Williams & Wilkins, pp 50.

112. Mudd SS, Findlay JS: The cutaneous manifestations and common mimickers of physical child abuse, *J Pediatr Health Care* 18(3):123–129, 2004.

113. Kliegman RM: *Nelson textbook of pediatrics*, ed 19, Philadelphia, 2011, Saunders.

114. Stanley WJ: Nailing a key assessment: learn the significance of certain nail anomalies, *Nursing* 33(8):50–51, 2003.

115. Callen J, Jorizzo J, Bolognia J, et al: *Dermatological signs of internal disease*, ed 4, Philadelphia, 2009, Saunders.

116. Hordinsky MK, Sawaya ME, Scher RK, et al: *Atlas of hair and nails*, Philadelphia, 2000, Churchill Livingstone.

117. Schalock PC: *Lippincott's primary care dermatology*, Baltimore, 2010, Lippincott, Williams & Wilkins.

118. Zaias N, Escovar SX, Zaiac MN: Finger and toenail onycholysis, *J Eur Acad Dermatol Venereol* 29(5), 2015. 848-538

119. Maino K, Stashower ME: Traumatic transverse leukonychia, *SKINmed* 3(1):53–55, 2004. Available at: http://www.medscape.com/viewarticle/467074 (posted 01/25/2004). Accessed January 2, 2013

120. Mason RJ: *Murray and Nadel's Textbook of Respiratory Medicine*, ed 5, Philadelphia, 2010, Saunders.

121. Leslie KO, Wick MR: *Leslie & Wick: Practical Pulmonary Pathology*, ed 2, Philadelphia, 2011, Saunders.

Review of Systems for the Physical Therapist Assistant

After conducting a follow-up interview and reassessment of pain type/pain patterns, the physical therapist assistant (PTA) may recognize one or more red-flag characteristics of systemic disease in the patient/client's report or observed as part of the clinical presentation.

Anytime there is an apparent pattern or cluster of associated signs and symptoms as shown in Box 4.1, the PTA is encouraged to record and report such findings to the physical therapist (PT). This type of review helps bring to the therapist's attention any signs or symptoms the client has not recognized, has forgotten, or thought unimportant to mention. After compiling a list of the client's signs and symptoms, compare those to the list in Box 4.1. Are there any identifying clusters to document and report? See Case Example 4.1.

For example, cutaneous (skin) manifestations and joint pain may occur as a result of systemic diseases, such as Crohn's disease (regional enteritis) or psoriatic arthritis, or as a delayed reaction to medications. Likewise, hair and nail changes, temperature intolerance, and unexplained excessive fatigue are cluster signs and symptoms associated with the endocrine system.

Changes in urinary frequency, flow of urine, or color of urine point to urologic involvement. The PTA can watch for other groupings of signs and symptoms associated with each system. In this way the PTA assists the PT by reporting any questionable signs and symptoms of a systemic nature that may point to a problem outside the scope of physical therapy practice. Early identification and intervention for many medical conditions can result in improved outcomes, including decreased morbidity and mortality.

RECOGNIZING AND REPORTING HEMATOLOGIC RED FLAGS

Hematologic considerations in the orthopedic population fall into two main categories: bleeding and clotting. People with known abnormalities of hemostasis (either hypocoagulation or hypercoagulation problems) will require close observation.[1] All surgical patients and neurologically compromised or immobilized individuals must also be observed carefully for any signs or symptoms of venous thromboembolism.

The hematologic system is composed of the blood, blood vessels, and the organs that produce the blood. Blood contains erythrocytes (red blood cells or RBCs), leukocytes (white blood cells), and platelets (thrombocytes) suspended in plasma, a pale yellow fluid. Blood is the circulating tissue of the body; plasma and its formed elements circulate through the heart, arteries, capillaries, and veins. The erythrocytes carry oxygen to and remove carbon dioxide from the tissues. Leukocytes act in the inflammatory and immune response. The plasma carries antibodies and nutrients to tissues and removes wastes from tissues. Platelets, together with coagulation factors in plasma, control the clotting of blood.

Many red-flag signs and symptoms can be associated with hematologic disorders. Some of the most important indicators of dysfunction in this system include problems associated with exertion (often minimal exertion) such as dyspnea, chest pain, palpitations, severe weakness, and fatigue. Neurologic symptoms, such as headache, drowsiness, dizziness, apathy, depression, syncope, or polyneuropathy, can also indicate a variety of possible problems in this system.[2,3]

Significant skin and fingernail-bed changes that can occur with hematologic problems might include pallor of the face, hands, nail beds, and lips; cyanosis or clubbing of the fingernail beds; and wounds or easy bruising or bleeding in skin, gums, or mucous membranes, often with no reported trauma to the area. The presence of blood in the stool or vomit or severe pain and swelling in joints and muscles can sometimes be a critical indicator of bleeding disorders that can be life threatening.[2,3]

Many hematologic-induced signs and symptoms seen in the physical therapy practice occur as a result of medications. For example, chronic or long-term use of steroids and nonsteroidal antiinflammatory drugs (NSAIDs) can lead to gastritis and peptic ulcer with gastrointestinal (GI) bleeding and subsequent iron deficiency anemia.[4] Leukopenia, a common problem occurring during chemotherapy, or as a symptom of certain types of cancer, can produce symptoms of infections such as fever, chills, tissue inflammation; severe mouth, throat, and esophageal pain; and mucous membrane ulcerations.[5]

Thrombocytopenia (decreased platelets) associated with easy bruising and spontaneous bleeding is a result of the pharmacologic treatment of common conditions seen in a physical therapy practice, such as rheumatoid arthritis and cancer.

Platelet Disorders

Platelets (thrombocytes) function primarily in hemostasis (stopping bleeding) and in maintaining capillary integrity. They function in the coagulation (blood clotting) mechanism by forming hemostatic plugs in small ruptured blood vessels or by adhering to any injured lining of larger blood vessels.

BOX 4.1 Review of Systems

When conducting a general review of systems, ask the client about the presence of any other problems anywhere else in the body. Depending on the client's answer, you may want to prompt him or her about any of the following common signs and symptoms* associated with each system:

General Questions
___Fever, chills, sweating (constitutional symptoms)
___Appetite loss, nausea, vomiting (constitutional symptoms)
___Fatigue, malaise, weakness (constitutional symptoms)
___Excessive, unexplained weight gain or loss
___Vital signs: blood pressure, temperature, pulse, respirations
___Insomnia
___Irritability
___Hoarseness or change in voice; frequent or prolonged sore throat
___Dizziness, falls

Integumentary (Include Skin, Hair, and Nails)
___Recent rashes, nodules, or other skin changes
___Unusual hair loss or breakage
___Increased hair growth (hirsutism)
___Nail-bed changes
___Itching (pruritus)

Musculoskeletal/Neurologic
___Joint pain, redness, warmth, swelling, stiffness, deformity
___Frequent or severe headaches
___Vision or hearing changes
___Vertigo
___Paresthesias (numbness, tingling, "pins and needles" sensation)
___Change in muscle tone
___Weakness; atrophy
___Abnormal deep tendon (or other) reflexes
___Problems with coordination or balance; falling
___Involuntary movements; tremors
___Radicular pain
___Seizures or loss of consciousness
___Memory loss
___Paralysis
___Mood swings; hallucinations

Rheumatologic
___Presence/location of joint swelling
___Muscle pain, weakness
___Skin rashes
___Reaction to sunlight
___Raynaud phenomenon
___Nail-bed changes

Cardiovascular
___Chest pain or sense of heaviness or discomfort
___Palpitations
___Limb pain during activity (claudication; cramps, limping)
___Discolored or painful feet; swelling of hands and feet
___Pulsating or throbbing pain anywhere, but especially in the back or abdomen
___Peripheral edema; nocturia
___Sudden weight gain; unable to fasten waistband or belt, unable to wear regular shoes
___Persistent cough
___Fatigue, dyspnea, orthopnea, syncope
___High or low blood pressure, unusual pulses

___Differences in blood pressure from side to side with position change (10 mm Hg or more; 20 mm Hg increase or decrease/diastolic or systolic; associated symptoms: dizziness, headache, nausea, vomiting, diaphoresis, heart palpitations, increased primary pain or symptoms)
___Positive findings on auscultation

Pulmonary
___Cough, hoarseness
___Sputum, hemoptysis
___Shortness of breath (dyspnea, orthopnea); altered breathing (e.g., wheezing, pursed-lip breathing)
___Night sweats; sweats anytime
___Pleural pain
___Cyanosis, clubbing
___Positive findings on auscultation (e.g., friction rub, unexpected breath sounds)
___Pulmonary embolism and deep vein thrombosis

Psychological
___Sleep disturbance
___Stress levels
___Fatigue, psychomotor agitation
___Changes in personal habits, appetite
___Depression, confusion, anxiety
___Irritability, mood changes

Gastrointestinal
___Abdominal pain
___Indigestion; heartburn
___Difficulty in swallowing
___Nausea/vomiting; loss of appetite
___Diarrhea or constipation
___Change in stools; change in bowel habits
___Fecal incontinence
___Rectal bleeding; blood in stool or vomit
___Skin rash followed by joint pain (Crohn's disease)

Hepatic/Biliary
___Change in taste/smell
___Anorexia
___Feeling of abdominal fullness, ascites
___Asterixis (muscle tremors)
___Change in urine color (dark, cola colored)
___Light-colored stools
___Change in skin color (yellow, green)
___Skin changes (rash, itching, purpura, spider angiomas, palmar erythema)

Hematologic
___Skin color or nail-bed changes
___Bleeding: nose, gums, easy bruising, melena
___Hemarthrosis, muscle hemorrhage, hematoma
___Fatigue, dyspnea, weakness
___Rapid pulse, palpitations
___Confusion, irritability
___Headache

Genitourinary
___Reduced stream, decreased output
___Burning or bleeding during urination; change in urine color
___Urinary incontinence, dribbling

BOX 4.1 Review of Systems—cont'd

___Impotence, pain with intercourse
___Hesitation, urgency
___Nocturia, frequency
___Dysuria (painful or difficult urination)
___Testicular pain or swelling
___Genital lesions
___Penile or vaginal discharge
___Impotence (males) or other sexual difficulty (males or females)
___Infertility (males or females)
___Flank pain

Gynecologic
___Irregular menses, amenorrhea, menopause
___Pain with menses or intercourse
___Vaginal discharge, vaginal itching
___Surgical procedures
___Pregnancy, birth, miscarriage, and abortion histories
___Spotting or bleeding, especially for the postmenopausal female 12 months after last period (without hormone replacement therapy)

Endocrine
___Hair and nail changes
___Change in appetite, unexplained weight change
___Fruity breath odor
___Temperature intolerance, hot flashes, diaphoresis (unexplained perspiration)
___Heart palpitations, tachycardia
___Headaches
___Low urine output, absence of perspiration
___Cramps
___Edema, polyuria, polydipsia, polyphagia
___Unexplained weakness, fatigue, paresthesia

___Carpal/tarsal tunnel syndrome
___Periarthritis, adhesive capsulitis
___Joint or muscle pain (arthralgia, myalgia), trigger points
___Prolonged deep tendon reflexes
___Sleep disturbance

Cancer
___Constant, intense pain, especially bone pain at night
___Unexplained weight loss (10% of body weight in 10–14 days); most clients in pain are inactive and gain weight
___Loss of appetite
___Excessive fatigue
___Unusual lump(s), thickening, change in a lump or mole, sore that does not heal; other unusual skin lesions or rash
___Unusual or prolonged bleeding or discharge anywhere
___Change in bowel or bladder habits
___Chronic cough or hoarseness; change in voice
___Rapid onset of digital clubbing (10–14 days)
___Proximal muscle weakness, especially when accompanied by change in one or more deep tendon reflexes

Immunologic
___Skin or nail-bed changes
___Fever or other constitutional symptoms (especially recurrent or cyclical symptoms)
___Lymph node changes (tenderness, enlargement)
___Anaphylactic reaction
___Symptoms of muscle or joint involvement (pain, swelling, stiffness, weakness)
___Sleep disturbance

* Cluster of three to four or more lasting longer than 1 month.

CASE EXAMPLE 4.1 Recognizing and Reporting the Correct Observations

A 47-year-old male with low back pain of unknown cause has come to his physical therapy session at an outpatient clinic. After gathering your daily subjective information from the client, you ask him:
• Are there any other symptoms of any kind anywhere else in your body?

The client tells you he does break out into an unexpected sweat from time to time but does not think he has a temperature when this happens. He has increased back pain when he passes gas or has a bowel movement, but then the pain goes back to the "regular" pain level (reported as 5 on a scale from 0 to 10).

Other reported symptoms include the following:
• Heartburn and indigestion
• Abdominal bloating after meals
• Chronic bronchitis from smoking (3 packs/day)
• Alternating diarrhea and constipation

Critical Thinking Activity
• Do these symptoms fall into any one category? See Box 4.1.
• What is the next step for the physical therapist assistant (PTA)?

It appears that many of the symptoms are gastrointestinal in nature. Since the client has mentioned unexplained sweating, but no known fevers, you take the time to measure all vital signs, especially body temperature.

These follow-up questions are appropriate for the PTA to ask:
• Have you ever been treated for an ulcer or internal bleeding while taking any over-the-counter pain relievers?
• Have you experienced any unexpected weight loss in the last few weeks?

• Have you traveled outside the United States in the last year?
• What is the effect of eating or drinking on your abdominal pain? Back pain?
• Do you have a sense of urgency so that you have to find a bathroom for a bowel movement or diarrhea right away without waiting?
• Have the client pay attention to his symptoms over the next 24 to 48 hours:
  • Immediately after eating
  • Within 30 minutes of eating
  • One to two hours later

Your decision to have the physical therapist (PT) see this patient depends on your findings from the client's responses to your clinical questions. This does not appear to be an emergency since the client is not in acute distress. An elevated temperature or other unusual vital signs would be examples of the need for an immediate examination by the PT. Documentation of observations is important, and the PT should be notified appropriately (by phone and/or report).

Small Group Activity
• Develop a list of possible responses to the follow-up questions that would appropriately direct the PTA to immediately report to the PT for examination of the patient.
• Develop a list of possible responses to the follow-up questions that would appropriately direct the PTA to continue with treatment plans for today; document responses and observations and discuss with the PT at a later time, but *before* the patient's next appointment.

Thrombocytosis refers to a condition in which the number of platelets is abnormally high (usually a temporary situation), whereas *thrombocytopenia* refers to a condition in which the number of platelets is abnormally low. The most common red-flag signs and symptoms are listed in Box 4.2.

Platelets are affected most often by anticoagulant drugs, including aspirin, heparin, warfarin (Coumadin), and other antithrombotic drugs now appearing on the market (e.g., fondaparinux [Arixtra]). In a physical therapy practice the most common causes seen with thrombocytopenia are bone marrow failure from radiation treatment, leukemia, or metastatic cancer; cytotoxic agents used in chemotherapy[6]; and drug-induced platelet reduction, especially among adults with rheumatoid arthritis treated with gold or inflammatory conditions treated with aspirin or other NSAIDs.

? PICTURE THE PATIENT

The PTA must be alert for obvious skin, joint, or mucous membrane symptoms of thrombocytopenia, which include severe bruising, external hematomas, joint swelling, and the presence of multiple petechiae observed on the skin or gums. These symptoms usually indicate a platelet count well below 100,000/mm³.

BOX 4.2 Common Signs and Symptoms of Platelet Disorders

Thrombocytosis
Thrombosis
Splenomegaly (enlarged spleen)
Easy bruising

Thrombocytopenia
Bleeding after minor trauma
Spontaneous bleeding
- Petechiae (small red dots)
- Ecchymoses (bruises)
- Purpura spots (bleeding under the skin)
- Epistaxis (nosebleed)
Menorrhagia (excessive menstruation)
Gingival bleeding
Melena (black, tarry stools)

≫ PTA ACTION PLAN
Precautions During Exercise

Strenuous exercise or any exercise that involves straining or bearing down could precipitate a hemorrhage, particularly of the eyes or brain. Blood pressure (BP) cuffs, safety/gait belts, and resistance exercise equipment (e.g., TheraBand) must be used with caution. Any mechanical compression or soft tissue mobilization is contraindicated without the PT's approval.

ANEMIA

Anemia is a reduction in the oxygen-carrying capacity of the blood as a result of an abnormality in the quantity or quality of erythrocytes. Anemia is not a disease but is a symptom of any number of different blood disorders. The most common causes of anemia include excessive blood loss, increased destruction of erythrocytes, and decreased production of erythrocytes. Decreased capacity of the blood to carry oxygen may result in disturbances in the function of many organs and tissues, and these symptoms can be different with each person. Rapid onset of anemia after a surgery could result in dyspnea, palpitations, weakness, and fatigue.

≫ PTA ACTION PLAN
Communication With the Physical Therapist

Any clinical sign or symptom that has already been pointed out by the PT and/or discussed with the therapist or nursing staff need only be documented and reported when there has been a significant change in size, intensity, new associated symptoms, or other warning signs. The PT should alert the PTA as to the most important findings to look for and report.

Diminished exercise tolerance is expected in individuals with anemia. Exercise testing and prescribed exercise(s) in clients with anemia must be instituted with extreme caution. The PTA should proceed very gradually with physical activity and exercise to tolerance and/or perceived exertion levels.[7–9] In addition, any major change in exercise parameters (frequency, intensity, duration, or mode/type of exercise) for any anemic client should be approved first by the PT (Case Example 4.2).

CASE EXAMPLE 4.2 Anemia

A 72-year-old female, status post hip fracture, was treated surgically with nails (used for the fixation of the ends of fractured bones) and was referred to physical therapy for follow-up treatment before hospital discharge. The initial evaluation and examination of physical therapists (PTs) were unremarkable for physical therapy precautions or contraindications.

When the physical therapist assistant (PTA) met with the client for the first time, she had already been ambulating alone in her room from the bed to the bathroom and back using a hospital wheeled walker. She was wearing thigh-length support hose, hospital gown, and open-heeled slippers from home. Although the nursing report indicated she was oriented to time and place, she seemed confused and required multiple verbal cues to follow the PTA's directions.

After ambulating a distance of approximately 50 feet using her wheeled walker and standby assistance from the PTA, the client reported that she could not "catch her breath" and asked to sit down. She placed her hand over her heart and commented that her heart was "fluttering." Blood pressure and pulse measurements were taken and recorded as 145/72 mm Hg and 90 bpm, respectively.

The PTA consulted with nursing staff immediately regarding this episode and was given the "go-ahead" to complete the therapy session. The PTA documented the episode in the medical record and left a note for the physician, briefly describing the incident and ending with the question: "Are there any medical contraindications to continuing progressive therapy?" The PTA then verbally followed up with the supervising PT to notify of the patient's current condition and of the note left for the physician.

Result: A significant fall in hemoglobin often occurs after hip fracture and surgical intervention resulting from the blood loss caused by the fracture and surgery.

In this case, although the physician did not offer a direct reply to the PT, the physician's notes indicated a suspected diagnosis of anemia. Follow-up blood work was ordered and the diagnosis was confirmed. Nursing staff conferred with the physician, and the physical therapy staff was advised to work within the patient's tolerance using perceived exertion as a guide while monitoring pulse and blood pressure.

RECOGNIZING AND REPORTING CARDIOVASCULAR RED FLAGS

The cardiovascular system consists of the heart, capillaries, veins, and lymphatics and functions in coordination with the pulmonary system to circulate oxygenated blood through the arterial system to all cells. This system then collects deoxygenated blood from the venous system and delivers it to the lungs for reoxygenation.

Cardinal symptoms of cardiac disease usually include chest, neck, and/or arm pain or discomfort, palpitation, dyspnea, syncope (fainting), fatigue, cough, diaphoresis, and cyanosis. Edema and leg pain (claudication) are the most common symptoms of the vascular component of a cardiovascular pathologic condition. Symptoms of cardiovascular involvement should also be reviewed by system (Table 4.1).

Chest Pain or Discomfort

Chest pain or discomfort is a common presenting symptom of cardiovascular disease and must be documented and reported. Chest pain may be cardiac or noncardiac in origin and may radiate to the neck, jaw, upper trapezius muscle, upper back, shoulder, or arms (most commonly the left arm).

TABLE 4.1 Cardiovascular Signs and Symptoms by System

System	Symptoms
General	Weakness Fatigue Weight change Poor exercise tolerance Peripheral edema
Integumentary	Pressure ulcers Loss of body hair Cyanosis (lips and nail beds)
Central nervous system	Headaches Impaired vision Dizziness or syncope
Pulmonary	Labored breathing, dyspnea Productive cough
Genitourinary	Urinary frequency Nocturia Concentrated urine Decreased urinary output
Musculoskeletal	Chest, shoulder, back, neck, jaw, or arm pain Myalgias Muscular fatigue Muscle atrophy Edema Claudication
Gastrointestinal	Nausea and vomiting Ascites (abdominal distention)

Modified from Goodman CC, Fuller K: *Pathology: implications for the physical therapist*, ed 3, Philadelphia, 2009, WB Saunders.

Radiating pain down the arm follows the pattern of ulnar nerve distribution. Pain of cardiac origin can be experienced in the somatic areas because the heart is supplied by the C3–T4 spinal segments, referring visceral pain to the corresponding somatic area. For example, the heart and the diaphragm, supplied by the C5–C6 spinal segment, can refer pain to the shoulder (see Figs. 2.4 and 2.5).

Cardiac-related chest pain may arise as a result of angina, myocardial infarction, pericarditis, endocarditis, mitral valve prolapse, or dissecting aortic aneurysm. Location and description (frequency, intensity, and duration) vary according to the underlying pathologic condition.

Cardiac chest pain is often accompanied by associated signs and symptoms such as nausea, vomiting, diaphoresis, dyspnea, fatigue, pallor, or syncope. These associated signs and symptoms help differentiate true musculoskeletal symptoms from those associated with a systemic problem.

▶ PTA ACTION PLAN

Change in Anginal Pattern

Changes in the pattern of angina, such as increased intensity, decreased threshold of stimulus, or longer duration of pain, require immediate intervention by the physician. Clients in treatment within the hospital setting should be returned to the care of the nursing staff immediately. In the case of outpatients, clients should be encouraged to contact their physician by telephone for further instructions before leaving the physical therapy department.

Palpitation

Palpitation, the presence of an irregular heartbeat, may also be referred to as arrhythmia or dysrhythmia, which may be caused by a relatively benign condition (e.g., mitral valve prolapse, "athlete's heart," caffeine, anxiety, exercise, menopause) or a severe condition (e.g., coronary artery disease, cardiomyopathy, complete heart block, ventricular aneurysm, atrioventricular valve disease, mitral or aortic stenosis).[10]

The sensation of palpitations has been described as a bump, pound, jump, flop, flutter, or racing sensation of the heart. Associated symptoms may include lightheadedness or syncope. Palpated pulse may feel rapid or irregular, as if the heart "skipped" a beat.

Occasionally, a client will report "fluttering" sensations in the neck. Generally, unless accompanied by other symptoms, these sensations in the neck are caused by anxiety, random muscle fasciculation, or minor muscle strain or overuse.

Palpitations can be considered physiologic (i.e., when fewer than six per minute occur, this may be considered within normal function of the heart). However, palpitation lasting for hours or occurring in association with pain, shortness of breath (SOB), fainting, or severe lightheadedness requires medical evaluation. Palpitation in any person with a history of unexplained sudden death in the family requires medical referral.[11]

Dyspnea

Dyspnea, also referred to as breathlessness or SOB, can be cardiovascular in origin, but it may also occur as a result of a pulmonary pathologic condition, fever, certain medications, allergies, poor physical conditioning, or obesity. Early onset of dyspnea may be described as having to breathe too much or as an uncomfortable feeling during breathing after exercise or exertion. With severe compromise of the cardiovascular or pulmonary systems, dyspnea may occur at rest.

The severity of dyspnea is determined by the extent of disease. Thus the more severe the heart disease is, the easier it is to bring on dyspnea. Extreme dyspnea includes paroxysmal nocturnal dyspnea (PND) and orthopnea (breathlessness that is relieved by sitting upright with pillows used to prop the trunk and head).

Dyspnea relieved by specific breathing patterns (e.g., pursed-lip breathing) or by specific body position (e.g., leaning forward on the arms to lock the shoulder girdle) is more likely to be pulmonary than cardiac in origin. Because breathlessness can be a terrifying experience for many persons, any activity that provokes the sensation is avoided, thus quickly reducing functional activities.

▶ PTA ACTION PLAN
What to Watch for and Report

The PTA should watch for individuals who do not report SOB because they no longer do the things that bring on difficulty breathing. Anyone who cannot climb a single flight of stairs without feeling moderately to severely winded or who awakens at night or experiences SOB when lying down should be brought to the therapist's attention. The PTA should also notify the therapist if anyone with known cardiac involvement develops progressively worse dyspnea.

Cardiac Syncope

Cardiac syncope (fainting) or more mild lightheadedness can be caused by reduced oxygen delivery to the brain. Lightheadedness that results from orthostatic hypotension (sudden drop in BP) may occur with any quick change in a prolonged position (e.g., going from a supine position to an upright posture or standing up from a sitting position) or physical exertion involving increased abdominal pressure (e.g., straining with a bowel movement, lifting, getting up out of a chair or on and off a bedpan or the toilet).[12]

Noncardiac conditions, such as anxiety and emotional stress, can cause hyperventilation and subsequent lightheadedness (vasovagal syncope). Side effects, such as orthostatic hypotension, may also occur during the period of initiation and regulation of cardiac medications (e.g., vasodilators). Syncope that occurs without any warning period of lightheadedness, dizziness, or nausea may be a sign of heart valve or arrhythmia problems and should be reported immediately.[10]

Fatigue

Fatigue provoked by minimal exertion indicates a lack of energy, which may be cardiac in origin (e.g., coronary artery disease, aortic valve dysfunction, cardiomyopathy, or myocarditis) or may occur as a result of a neurologic, muscular, metabolic, or pulmonary pathologic condition. Often, fatigue of a cardiac nature is accompanied by associated symptoms such as dyspnea, chest pain, palpitations, or headache.

▶ PTA ACTION PLAN
Monitoring Fatigue

Fatigue that goes beyond expectations during or after exercise, especially in a client with a known cardiac condition, must be closely monitored. It should be remembered that beta blockers prescribed for cardiac problems can also cause unusual fatigue symptoms.

For the client experiencing fatigue without a prior diagnosis of heart disease, monitoring vital signs may indicate a failure of the BP to rise with increasing workloads. Such a situation may indicate cardiac output that is inadequate in meeting the demands of exercise. However, poor exercise tolerance is often the result of deconditioning, especially in the older adult population. The therapist may want to consider further testing (e.g., exercise treadmill test) to determine whether fatigue is cardiac induced.

Cough

Cough is usually associated with pulmonary conditions, but it may occur as a pulmonary complication of a cardiovascular pathologic complex. Left ventricular dysfunction, including mitral valve dysfunction resulting from pulmonary edema or left ventricular congestive heart failure (CHF), may result in a cough when aggravated by exercise, metabolic stress, supine position, or PND. The cough is often hacking and may produce large amounts of frothy, blood-tinged sputum. In the case of CHF, cough develops because a large amount of fluid is trapped in the pulmonary tree, irritating the lung mucosa.[13] Any of these findings must be reported and documented.

Cyanosis

Cyanosis is a bluish discoloration of the lips and nail beds of the fingers and toes that accompanies inadequate blood oxygen levels (reduced amounts of hemoglobin). Although cyanosis can accompany hematologic or central nervous system (CNS) disorders, most often, visible cyanosis accompanies cardiac and pulmonary problems and is a red-flag observation.

Edema

Edema in the form of a 3-lb or greater weight gain or a gradual, continuous gain over several days, which results in swelling of the ankles, legs, abdomen, and hands, combined with SOB, fatigue, and dizziness, may be red-flag symptoms of CHF.[11]

Noncardiac causes of edema may include pulmonary hypertension, kidney dysfunction, cirrhosis, burns, infection, lymphatic obstruction, use of NSAIDs, or allergic reaction. Right upper quadrant pain described as a constant aching or sharp pain may occur when there is edema associated with liver impairment (e.g., cirrhosis).

When edema and other accompanying symptoms persist despite rest or intervention as prescribed, reevaluation by the therapist is required.

Claudication

Claudication or leg pain occurs with peripheral vascular disease (arterial or venous), often occurring simultaneously with coronary artery disease. Claudication can be more functionally debilitating than other associated symptoms, such as angina or dyspnea, and may occur in addition to these other symptoms. The presence of pitting edema along with leg pain is usually associated with vascular disease.[11]

Vascular claudication may occur in the absence of physical findings but is usually accompanied by skin discoloration and trophic changes (e.g., thin, dry, hairless skin) in the presence of vascular disease. The PTA may assess core temperature, peripheral pulses, and skin temperature when instructed and directed by the therapist. Cool skin is more indicative of vascular obstruction; warm to hot skin may indicate inflammation or infection. Abrupt onset of ischemic rest pain or sudden worsening of intermittent claudication may be due to thromboembolism and must be reported immediately.[14]

? PICTURE THE PATIENT

If people with intermittent claudication have normal-appearing skin at rest, exercising the extremity to the point of claudication usually produces marked pallor in the skin over the distal third of the extremity. This postexercise cutaneous ischemia occurs in both upper and lower extremities and is due to selective shunting of the available blood to the exercised muscle and away from the more distal parts of the extremity.

▶ PTA ACTION PLAN

Points to Ponder

- Fatigue beyond expectations during or after exercise is a red-flag symptom.
- Be on the alert for cardiac risk factors in older adults, especially females, and begin a conditioning program before an exercise program.
- Anyone being treated with both NSAIDs and angiotensin-converting enzyme inhibitors must be monitored closely during exercise for elevated BP.
- A person taking medications, such as beta blockers or calcium channel blockers, may not be able to achieve a target heart rate above 90 bpm. To determine a safe rate of exercise the heart rate should return to the resting level 2 minutes after stopping exercise.
- Make sure that a client with cardiac compromise has not smoked a cigarette or eaten a large meal just before exercise.
- A 3-lb or greater weight gain or gradual, continuous gain over several days, which results in swelling of the ankles, abdomen, and hands, combined with SOB, fatigue, and dizziness that persist despite rest, may be red-flag symptoms of CHF (Case Example 4.3).
- Watch for muscle pain, cramps, stiffness, spasms, and weakness that cannot be explained by arthritis, recent strenuous exercise, a fever, a recent fall, or other common causes in clients taking statins to lower cholesterol.

RECOGNIZING AND REPORTING PULMONARY RED FLAGS

For the client with neck, shoulder, or back pain at presentation, the possibility of a pulmonary cause requiring further evaluation by the PT should be considered. The most common pulmonary conditions to mimic those of the musculoskeletal system include pneumonia, pulmonary embolism (PE), pleurisy, pneumothorax, and pulmonary arterial hypertension.

The material in this chapter will assist the PTA in treating both the client with a known pulmonary problem while quickly recognizing the client with musculoskeletal signs and symptoms that may have an underlying systemic basis.

Signs and Symptoms of Pulmonary Disorders

Signs and symptoms of pulmonary disorders can be many and varied; the most common symptoms associated with pulmonary disorders are cough and dyspnea. Other manifestations include chest pain, abnormal sputum, hemoptysis, cyanosis, digital clubbing, altered breathing patterns, and chest pain.[15]

CASE EXAMPLE 4.3 **Congestive Heart Failure: Muscle Cramping and Headache**

A 74-year-old retired homemaker had a total hip replacement 2 days ago and remains an inpatient with complications related to congestive heart failure (CHF). She has a previous medical history of gallbladder removal 20 years ago, total hysterectomy 30 years ago, and surgically induced menopause with subsequent onset of hypertension. Her medications include intravenous furosemide (Lasix), digoxin, and potassium replacement.

During the initial physical therapy session the client complained of muscle cramping and headache but was able to complete the entire exercise protocol. Blood pressure (BP) was 100/76 mm Hg. Systolic measurement dropped to 90 mm Hg when the client moved from supine to standing. Pulse rate was 56 bpm with a pattern of irregular beats. Pulse rate did not change with postural change. Platelet count was 98,000 cells/mm³.

Result: With CHF the heart will try to compensate by increasing the heart rate. However, the digoxin is designed to increase cardiac output and lower heart rate. In normal circumstances, postural changes result in an increase in heart rate, but when digoxin is used, this increase cannot occur so the person becomes symptomatic. Most of the clients like this one are also taking beta blockers, which also prevent the heart rate from increasing when the BP drops.

In a clinical situation such as this one the response of vital signs to exercise must be monitored carefully and charted. Any unusual symptoms, such as muscle cramping and headaches, and any irregular pulse patterns must also be reported and documented.

Cough

As a physiologic response, cough occurs frequently in healthy people, but a persistent dry cough may be caused by a tumor, congestion, or hypersensitive airways (allergies). A productive cough with purulent sputum (yellow or green) may indicate infection, whereas a productive cough with nonpurulent sputum (clear or white) is nonspecific and indicates airway irritation. Rust-colored sputum may be a sign of pneumonia and should also be reported. Hemoptysis (coughing and spitting blood) can indicate a pathologic condition such as infection, inflammation, abscess, tumor, or infarction and must be brought to the PT's attention immediately.

Dyspnea

Dyspnea, or SOB, usually indicates hypoxemia but can be associated with emotional states, particularly fear and anxiety. Dyspnea when the person is lying down is called *orthopnea* and is caused by redistribution of body water. Fluid shift leads to increased fluid in the lung, which interferes with gas exchange and leads to orthopnea. In supine and prone positions the abdominal contents also exert pressure on the diaphragm, increasing the work of breathing and often limiting vital capacity.

If a client denies compromised breathing, the PTA should continue to look for functional changes as the client accommodates for difficulty breathing by reducing activity or exertion.

> ## ▶▶ PTA ACTION PLAN
>
> ### *Follow-Up Questions*
>
> - Do you ever have trouble catching your breath?
>   - *If yes*, how long have you had this problem? Is this a new problem?
>   - How often does it happen?
>   - If a chronic problem, ask: Does it seem to be getting better, worse, or staying the same?
> - Are your activities limited in any way because you don't have enough air or can't catch your breath?
> - How many blocks (feet) can you walk before you have to stop to catch your breath?
> - How many stairs can you climb before you have to stop to catch your breath?
> - Does your SOB occur at rest? At night? With activity?
> - Do you sit up to sleep at night? How many pillows do you sleep with at night?
> - Do you have any other symptoms of any kind when you are short of breath (e.g., dizziness, coughing, excessive sweating, chest pain or discomfort or musculoskeletal pain anywhere else in the body)?
> - Do you have a personal or family history of asthma? (obstruction of the lower airways)
> - Do you have a personal or family history of heart disease?
> - Have you been pushed or punched in the chest? Any trauma of any kind to the chest?
> - For females: Are you taking birth control pills? (Combine this information with status of tobacco use; remember that these are risk factors for pulmonary embolus.)

> ## ▶▶ PTA ACTION PLAN
>
> ### *What to Watch for*
>
> - If the client reports new onset of SOB and is tachypneic, diaphoretic, or cyanotic, immediate medical referral is advised. Any suspicion of anaphylaxis is also an emergency situation.

> - Measure the client's actual respiratory rate and pulse rate. Is the heart rate regular? Assess breath sounds.
> - Is the SOB constant or intermittent?
> - Check blood gas results and pulse oximetry levels if possible. Observe for cyanosis of the lips or nail beds. Assess mental status for confusion or increased confusion. These tests and measures will help identify possible hypoxia, requiring urgent care and/or oxygen supplementation.
> - Look for edema in the lower extremities (positional or dependent); this is a potential sign of pulmonary edema or CHF, particularly concerning in the presence of NSAID use. Ask about recent weight gain.

Cyanosis

See earlier discussion in this chapter.

Clubbing

See Chapter 3.

Altered Breathing Patterns[16]

Changes in the rate, depth, regularity, and effort of breathing occur in response to any condition affecting the pulmonary system. Breathing patterns can vary, depending on the neuromuscular or neurologic disease or trauma (Box 4.3). Breathing pattern abnormalities seen with head trauma, brain abscess, diaphragmatic paralysis of chest wall muscles and thorax (e.g., generalized myopathy or neuropathy), heat stroke, spinal meningitis, and encephalitis can include apneustic breathing, ataxic breathing, or Cheyne-Stokes respiration (CSR).

Apneustic breathing (gasping inspiration with short expiration) localizes damage to the midpons and is most commonly a result of a basilar artery infarct. *Ataxic*, or *Biot*, breathing (irregular pattern of deep and shallow breaths with abrupt pauses) is caused by disruption of the respiratory rhythm generator in the medulla.

CSR may be evident in the well older adults, as well as in compromised clients. The most common cause of CSR is severe CHF, but it can also occur with renal failure, meningitis, drug overdose, and increased intracranial pressure. CSR may be a normal breathing pattern in infants and older persons during sleep.

Exercise may induce pleural pain, coughing, hemoptysis, SOB, and/or other abnormal changes in breathing patterns. When asked if the client is ever short of breath, the individual may say "no" because he or she has reduced activity levels to avoid dyspnea (see the follow-up questions previously outlined in this section).

Pulmonary Pain Patterns[13]

The most common sites for referred pain from the pulmonary system are the chest, ribs, upper trapezius, shoulder, and thoracic spine. The first symptoms may not appear until the client's respiratory system is stressed by the addition of exercise during treatment with the PTA. On the other hand, the client may present with what appears to be primary musculoskeletal pain in any one of those areas.

BOX 4.3 Breathing Patterns and Associated Conditions

Hyperventilation
Anxiety
Acute head injury
Hypoxemia
Fever

Kussmaul Respirations
Strenuous exercise
Metabolic acidosis

Cheyne-Stokes
Congestive heart failure
Renal failure
Meningitis
Drug overdose
Increased intracranial pressure
Infants (normal)
Older people during sleep (normal)

Hypoventilation
Fibromyalgia syndrome
Chronic fatigue syndrome
Sleep disorder
Muscle fatigue

Muscle weakness
Malnutrition
Neuromuscular disease
Guillain-Barré
Myasthenia gravis
Poliomyelitis
Amyotrophic lateral sclerosis
Pickwickian or obesity hypoventilation syndrome
Severe kyphoscoliosis

Apneustic
Midpons lesion
Basilar artery infarct

Biot Respiration (Ataxia)
Exercise
Shock
Cerebral hypoxia
Heat stroke
Spinal meningitis
Head injury
Brain abscess
Encephalitis

From Ikeda B, Goodman CC, Fuller K: The respiratory system. In Goodman CC: *Pathology: implications for the physical therapist*, ed 3, St. Louis, 2009, Elsevier.

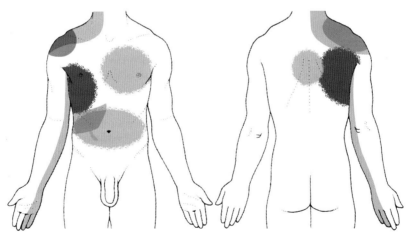

FIG. 4.1 A composite picture of the pain patterns associated with many different impairments of the pulmonary parenchyma including pleuritis, pneumothorax, pulmonary embolism, cor pulmonale, and pleurisy. No single individual will present with all of these patterns at the same time. A composite illustration gives an idea of the wide range of referred pain patterns possible with pulmonary diseases or conditions. Remember that viscerogenic pain patterns do not usually present as discrete circles or ovals of pain as depicted here. This figure is an approximation of what the therapist might expect to hear the client describe associated with a pulmonary problem.

Pulmonary pain patterns are usually localized in the substernal or chest region over involved lung fields that may include the anterior chest, side, or back. However, pulmonary pain can radiate to the neck, upper trapezius muscle, costal margins, thoracic back, scapulae, or shoulder. Shoulder pain may radiate along the medial aspect of the arm, mimicking other neuromuscular causes of neck or shoulder pain (Fig. 4.1).

❓ PICTURE THE PATIENT

Pulmonary pain usually increases with inspiratory movements, such as laughing, coughing, sneezing, or deep breathing, and the client notes the presence of associated symptoms, such as dyspnea (exertional or at rest), persistent cough, fever, and chills. Palpation and resisted movements will not reproduce the symptoms, which may get worse with recumbency, especially at night or while sleeping.

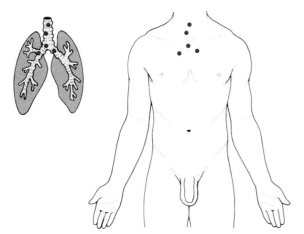

FIG. 4.2 Tracheobronchial pain is referred to sites in the neck or anterior chest at the same levels as the points of irritation in the air passages. The points of pain are on the same side as the areas of irritation.

Tracheobronchial Pain. Within the pulmonary system the trachea and large bronchi are innervated by the vagus trunks, whereas the finer bronchi and lung parenchyma appear to be free of pain innervation. Tracheobronchial pain is referred to sites in the neck or anterior chest at the same levels as the points of irritation in the air passages (Fig. 4.2). This irritation may be caused by inflammatory lesions, irritating foreign materials, or cancerous tumors.

Pleural Pain. The thoracic cavity is lined with pleura, or serous membrane. One surface of the pleura lines the inside of the rib cage (parietal) and the other surface covers the lungs (visceral). The parietal pleura is sensitive to painful stimulation, but the visceral pleura is insensitive to pain. Extensive disease may occur in the lung without occurrence of pain until the process extends to the parietal pleura. This explains why pathology of the lungs may be painless until obstruction or inflammation is enough to press on the parietal pleura.

Pleural irritation then results in sharp, localized pain that is aggravated by any respiratory movement. Clients usually note that the pain is alleviated by autosplinting (i.e., lying on the affected side), which diminishes the movement of that side of the chest (see further discussion of pleural pain in this chapter).[17]

Pleural pain is present in pulmonary diseases such as pleurisy, pneumonia, pulmonary infarct (when it extends to the pleural surface, thus causing pleurisy), tumor (when it invades the parietal pleura), and pneumothorax. Tumor, especially bronchogenic carcinoma, may be accompanied by severe, continuous pain when the tumor tissue, extending to the parietal pleura through the lung, constantly irritates the pain nerve endings in the pleura.

Diaphragmatic Pleural Pain. *Diaphragmatic pleurisy* resulting from pneumonia is common and refers sharp pain along the costal margins or upper trapezius, which is aggravated by any diaphragmatic motion, such as coughing, laughing, or deep breathing.

Stimulation of the peripheral portions of the diaphragmatic pleura results in sharp pain felt along the costal margins, which can be referred to the lumbar region by the lower thoracic

somatic nerves. Stimulation of the central portion of the diaphragmatic pleura results in sharp pain referred to the upper trapezius muscle and shoulder on the ipsilateral side of the stimulation (see Figs. 2.4 and 2.5 in Chapter 2).

There may be tenderness to palpation along the costal margins, and sharp pain occurs when the client is asked to take a deep breath. A change in position (sidebending or rotation of the trunk) does not reproduce the symptoms, which would be the case with a true intercostal lesion or tear.

Forceful, repeated coughing can result in an intercostal lesion in the presence of referred intercostal pain from diaphragmatic pleurisy, which can make differentiation between these two entities impossible without a medical referral and further diagnostic testing.

Pulmonary Embolism and Deep Venous Thrombosis

PE involves pulmonary vascular obstruction by a displaced thrombus (blood clot), an air bubble, a fat globule, a clump of bacteria, amniotic fluid, vegetations on heart valves that develop with endocarditis, or other particulate matter. Once dislodged, the obstruction travels to the blood vessels supplying the lungs, causing SOB, tachypnea (very rapid breathing), tachycardia, and chest pain.

The most common cause of PE is deep venous thrombosis (DVT) originating in the proximal deep venous system of the lower legs. The embolism causes an area of blockage, which then results in a localized area of ischemia known as a *pulmonary infarct*. The infarct may be caused by small emboli that extend to the lung surface (pleura) and result in acute pleuritic chest pain.

Risk Factors. Three major risk factors linked with DVT are blood stasis (e.g., immobilization because of bed rest, such as with burn clients, obstetric and gynecologic clients, and older or obese populations), endothelial injury (resulting from neoplasm, surgical procedures, trauma, or fractures of the legs or pelvis), and hypercoagulable states.

Other people at increased risk for DVT and PE include those with CHF; trauma or fracture of the arms, pelvis, or legs; recent surgery (especially hip, knee, and prostate surgery); age over 50 years; previous history of thromboembolism; cancer; infection; diabetes mellitus (DM); inactivity or obesity; pregnancy, clotting abnormalities; and oral contraceptive use.

▶▶ PTA ACTION PLAN

Prevention of Deep Venous Thrombosis and Pulmonary Embolism

Given the mortality of PE and the difficulties involved in its clinical diagnosis, prevention of DVT and PE is critical. A careful review of the Personal/Family History form (outpatient) or hospital medical chart (inpatient) may alert the PTA to the presence of factors that predispose a client to have a PE.

Although frequent changing of position, exercise, and early ambulation are necessary to prevent thrombosis and embolism, sudden and extreme movements should be avoided. Under no circumstances should the legs be massaged to relieve "muscle cramps," especially when the pain is located in the calf and the client has not been up and about.

Restrictive clothing and prolonged sitting or standing should be avoided. Elevating the legs should be accomplished with caution to avoid severe flexion of the hips, which will slow blood flow and increase the risk of new thrombi.

BOX 4.4 Signs and Symptoms of Pulmonary Embolisms and Deep Vein Thrombosis

Pulmonary Embolus
Dyspnea
Pleuritic (sharp, localized) chest pain
Diffuse chest discomfort
Persistent cough
Hemoptysis (bloody sputum)
Apprehension, anxiety, restlessness
Tachypnea (increased respiratory rate)
Tachycardia
Fever

Deep Venous Thrombosis
Unilateral tenderness or leg pain; dull ache or sensation of "tightness" in the area where the deep vein thrombosis is located
Unilateral swelling (difference in leg circumference)
Warmth
Subcutaneous venous distention (superficial thrombus)
Discoloration
Palpable cord (superficial thrombus)
Pain with placement around calf of blood pressure cuff inflated to 160–180 mm Hg

Unfortunately, at least half the cases of DVT are asymptomatic,[21] and up to one-third of all clients with apparent clinical appearance of DVT have no demonstrable DVT. A more sensitive and specific tool for predicting DVT is the Autar DVT Scale[23] (Table 4.2) or Wells Risk Assessment.

TABLE 4.2 Autar Deep Vein Thrombosis Scale

Category (Points)	Possible Score (Points)	Score
Age (years)	10–30	0
	31–40	1
	41–50	2
	51–60	3
	61+	4
Body mass index (wt kg)/(hgt m)	16–19	0
	20–25	1
	26–30	2
	31–40	3
	41+	4
Mobility	Ambulant	0
	Limited (walks with aids)	1
	Very limited (needs help)	2
	Chair bound	3
	Bed rest	4
Special DVT risk	Birth control pills (<35 years)	1
	Birth control pills (35 years/older)	2
	Pregnant/up to 6 weeks postpartum	3
Trauma risk factors (score only preoperatively; score only one item)	Head or chest	1
	Head and chest	2
	Spinal	2
	Pelvic	3
	Lower limb	4
Surgical risk factors (score only one item)	Minor surgery (<30 min)	1
	Major surgery	2
	Emergency major	3
	Pelvic, abdominal, or thoracic	3
	Orthopedic (below waist)	4
	Spinal	4
High-risk diseases	Ulcerative colitis	1
	Anemia (sickle cell, polycythemic, hemolytic)	2
	Chronic heart disease	3
	Myocardial infarction	4
	Malignancy	5
	Varicose veins	6
	Previous DVT or cardiovascular accident	7
Results based on total score	<6	No risk
	7–10	Low risk (<10%)
	11–14	Moderate risk (11%–40%)
	≥15	High risk (>40%)

DVT, Deep vein thrombosis.

Pulmonary Embolism. Signs and symptoms of PE are nonspecific and vary greatly, depending on the extent to which the lung is involved, the size of the clot, and the general condition of the client (Box 4.4).

Clinical presentation does not differ between younger and older persons. Dyspnea, pleuritic chest pain, and cough are the most common symptoms reported. Typical pleuritic chest pain is sudden in onset and aggravated by breathing.

The client may also report hemoptysis, apprehension, tachypnea, and fever (temperature as high as 39.5°C [103.5°F]). The presence of hemoptysis indicates that the infarction or areas of atelectasis have produced alveolar damage.

Deep Venous Thrombosis. Signs and symptoms of DVT include tenderness, leg pain, swelling (a difference in leg circumference of 1.4 cm in males and 1.2 cm in females is significant), and warmth. The PTA may also see subcutaneous venous distention, discoloration, and/or a palpable cord.[18]

Homan sign is an unreliable test to diagnose DVT. The PTA should be aware that using the Homan test to assess for DVT is no longer recommended or supported by evidence.[19-22] Homan sign is elicited by gentle squeezing of the affected calf or slow dorsiflexion of the foot on the affected side to elicit deep calf pain. In theory, the inflamed nerves in the veins within the muscle are compressed or stretched causing deep calf pain. Only about half of all clients with DVT experience pain and Homan sign.

▶▶ PTA ACTION PLAN

Important Update on Homan Sign

If the PTA observes the previously mentioned signs and symptoms and the Homan sign test has been used by the PT, the PTA should discuss the need for further medical testing options with the supervising therapist.

PTA ACTION PLAN

Points to Ponder

- Pulmonary pain can radiate to the neck, upper trapezius muscle, costal margins, thoracic back, scapulae, or shoulder.
- Shoulder pain caused by pulmonary involvement may radiate along the medial aspect of the arm, mimicking other neuromuscular causes of neck or shoulder pain.
- Pulmonary pain usually increases with inspiratory movements such as laughing, coughing, sneezing, or deep breathing.
- Shoulder pain that is relieved by lying on the involved side may be "autosplinting,"[17] a sign of a pulmonary cause of symptoms.
- Shoulder pain that is aggravated when lying supine (arm/elbow supported) may be an indication of a pulmonary cause of symptoms.

RECOGNIZING AND REPORTING GASTROINTESTINAL RED FLAGS

A great deal of new understanding of the GI system and its relationship to other systems has been discovered over the last decade. The GI tract has its own independent nervous system called the enteric nervous system, the only internal organ to have evolved its own nervous system.[24] For example, it is now known that the lining of the digestive tract from the esophagus through the large intestine is composed of millions of nerve cells that contain neuropeptides and their receptors. These substances, produced by nerve cells, are a key to the mind-body connection that contributes to the physical manifestation of emotions.[25,26]

In addition to the classic hormonal and neural negative feedback loops, there are direct actions of gut hormones on the dorsal vagal complex. The person experiencing a "gut reaction" or "gut feeling" may indeed be experiencing the direct effects of gut peptides on brain function.[27–29]

The association between the enteric system, the immune system, and the brain (now a part of the research referred to as psychoneuroimmunology) has been clearly established and forms an integral part of GI symptoms associated with immune disorders such as fibromyalgia, systemic lupus erythematosus, rheumatoid arthritis, chronic fatigue syndrome.[30]

Allowing undigested food or bacteria into the bloodstream sets in motion a chain of events as the immune system reacts. The body responds as if to an illness and expresses it in a number of ways such as a rash, diarrhea, GI upset, joint pain, migraines, and headache. The exact cause for these microscopic breaches remains unknown, but food allergies, too much aspirin or ibuprofen, certain antibiotics, excessive alcohol consumption, smoking, or parasitic infections may be implicated.

All of these associations and new findings support the need for the PTA to notify the PT of any GI symptoms present but previously unreported. This is especially important when considering the fact that GI tract problems can sometimes imitate musculoskeletal dysfunction.

PICTURE THE PATIENT

GI disorders can refer pain to the sternal region, shoulder and neck, scapular region, mid-back, lower back, hip, pelvis, and sacrum. This pain can mimic primary musculoskeletal or neuromuscular dysfunction, causing confusion.

The most common intraabdominal diseases that refer pain to the musculoskeletal system are those that involve ulceration or infection of the mucosal lining. Drug-induced GI symptoms can also occur with delayed reactions as much as 6 or 8 weeks after exposure to the medication. The most common occurrences are antibiotic colitis; nausea, vomiting, and anorexia from digitalis toxicity; and NSAID-induced ulcers.

Signs and Symptoms of Gastrointestinal Disorders

Any disruption of the digestive system can create symptoms such as nausea, vomiting, pain, diarrhea, and constipation. The bowel is susceptible to altered patterns of normal motility caused by food, alcohol, caffeine, drugs, physical and emotional stress, and lifestyle (e.g., lack of regular exercise, tobacco use). GI effects of chemotherapy include nausea and vomiting, anorexia, taste alteration, weight loss, oral mucositis, diarrhea, and constipation.

Symptoms, including pain, can be related to various GI organ disturbances and differ in character, depending on the affected organ. The most clinically meaningful GI symptoms reported in a physical therapy practice include the following:
- Abdominal pain
- Dysphagia
- Odynophagia
- GI bleeding (emesis, melena, red blood)
- Epigastric pain with radiation to the back
- Symptoms affected by food
- Early satiety with weight loss
- Constipation
- Diarrhea
- Fecal incontinence
- Arthralgia
- Referred shoulder pain
- Neuropathy

Abdominal Pain

Pain in the *epigastric region* occurs anywhere from the midsternum to the xiphoid process from the heart, esophagus, stomach, duodenum, gallbladder, liver, and other mediastinal organs. The client may report that the pain radiates around the ribs or straight through the chest to the thoracic spine at the T3–T6/7 anatomic levels.

There can be referred pain from the esophagus to the mid-back as well as from the mid-back to the esophagus. For example, esophageal dysfunction can present as anterior neck pain or mid-thoracic spine pain, and disk disease of the mid-thoracic spine can masquerade as esophageal pain.

Pain in the *periumbilical region* (T11 nerve distribution) occurs with impairment of the small intestine, pancreas, and appendix. Primary pain in the periumbilical region usually sends the client to a physician. However, pain around the umbilicus may be accompanied by low back pain. In the healthy adult who is not obese and does not have a protruding abdomen, the umbilicus is level with the disk located anatomically between the L3 and L4 vertebral bodies.

PICTURE THE PATIENT

The PTA may be treating someone with anterior abdominal and low back pain at the same level but with alternating presentation. In other words, first the client experiences periumbilical pain with or without associated GI signs and symptoms, then the painful episode resolves. Later, the client develops low back pain with or without symptoms but does not realize there is a link between these painful episodes. This is a red-flag scenario that an alert PTA may recognize.

Clients reporting pain in the *lower abdominal region* (even in the presence of low back pain) must always be encouraged to report this to their physician. The PTA records and reports these findings to the PT, who then either speaks to the client directly or instructs the PTA to recommend medical evaluation.

Any structure touching the respiratory diaphragm can refer pain to the shoulder, usually to the ipsilateral shoulder, depending on where the direct pressure occurs.

Referred pain to the musculoskeletal system can occur alone, without accompanying visceral pain, but usually visceral pain (or other symptoms) precedes the development of referred pain. The PTA will find that the client does not connect the two sets of symptoms or fails to report abdominal pain and GI symptoms to the PT when experiencing a painful shoulder or low back, thinking these are two separate problems.

Dysphagia

Dysphagia (difficulty swallowing) is the sensation of food catching or sticking in the esophagus. This sensation may occur (initially) just with coarse, dry foods and may eventually progress to include anything swallowed, even thin liquids and saliva.

Other possible GI causes of dysphagia include peptic esophagitis (inflammation of the esophagus) with stricture (narrowing), gastroesophageal reflux disease (GERD), and neoplasm (Case Example 4.4). Dysphagia may be a symptom of many other disorders unrelated to GI disease (e.g., stroke, Alzheimer disease, Parkinson disease). Certain types of drugs, including antidepressants, antihypertensives, and asthma drugs, can make swallowing difficult.

PTA ACTION PLAN

Prompt Attention Required

The presence of dysphagia requires prompt attention by the PT. Medical intervention may be necessary, but the PT will evaluate the situation and make the final determination.

Odynophagia

Odynophagia, or pain during swallowing, can be caused by esophagitis or esophageal spasm. Esophagitis may occur secondary to GERD, the herpes simplex virus, or fungus caused by the prolonged use of strong antibiotics. Pain after eating may occur with esophagitis or may be associated with coronary ischemia.

Gastrointestinal Bleeding

Occult (hidden) GI bleeding can appear as mid-thoracic back pain with radiation to the right upper quadrant. The PT should

CASE EXAMPLE 4.4 Esophageal Cancer

An obese 88-year-old female with a total knee replacement was referred for rehabilitation because of loss of motion, joint swelling, and persistent knee pain. She was accompanied to the clinic for each session by one of her three daughters. Over a period of 2 weeks, each daughter commented on how much weight the mother had lost.

When the physical therapist assistant (PTA) questioned the client if she had made any changes to her diet as a result of her decrease in activity, the patient complained of a loss of appetite and frequent difficulty in swallowing. The client had not said anything to her family about her swallowing difficulties because she "thought it was normal for someone her age."

The PTA discussed the weight loss and swallowing concerns with the supervising physical therapist (PT) immediately after the treatment session that day. Upon the client's return to the clinic for the next treatment, the PT encouraged the patient to contact her family doctor for evaluation of these red-flag symptoms and was subsequently diagnosed with esophageal cancer.

be alerted to any type of bleeding reported by the client. The PTA can ask about the presence of other signs such as blood in the vomit or stools. Coffee-ground emesis (vomit) may indicate a perforated peptic or duodenal ulcer.

Bloody diarrhea may accompany other signs of ulcerative colitis. Bright red blood usually represents pathology close to the rectum or anus and may be an indication of rectal fissures (e.g., history of anal intercourse) or hemorrhoids, but can also occur as a result of colorectal cancer.

Melena, or black, tarry stool, occurs as a result of large quantities of blood in the stool. When asked about changes in bowel function, clients may describe black, tarry stools that have an unusual, noxious odor. The odor is caused by the presence of blood, and the black color arises as the digestive acids in the bowel oxidize RBCs (e.g., bleeding esophageal varices, stomach, or duodenal ulceration). Melena is very sticky and does not clean well.

It may be necessary to ask about bowel smears on undergarments or difficulty getting wiped clean after a bowel movement. The following questions may guide the PTA in this area.

PTA ACTION PLAN

Follow-Up Questions

- I would like to ask a few questions that may not seem related to your shoulder (back, hip, pelvic) pain, but these are very important in finding out what is causing your symptoms.
  - Have you noticed any blood in your stools or change in the color or consistency of your bowel movements?
  - Do you have any trouble wiping yourself clean after a bowel movement?
  - Have you noticed any bowel smears on your underwear later after a bowel movement?

After going through these potentially embarrassing questions, it may be helpful to leave the client with this thought:
- If you do not know the answer right now or if you just have not noticed, please feel free to let me, the PT, or your physician know if you notice any changes.

The client should be asked about the presence of any blood in the stool to determine whether it is melenic (from the upper GI tract; ask about a history of NSAID use) or bright red (from the distal colon or rectum).

Bleeding from internal or external hemorrhoids (enlarged veins inside or outside the rectum), rectal fissures, or colorectal carcinoma can lead to bright red blood in the stools. Rectal bleeding from anal lesions or fissures can occur in the homosexual population who are sexually active. Females engaging in anal intercourse can also be affected. The PT may need to conduct a brief sexual history in some cases.

Reddish or mahogany-colored stools can occur from eating certain foods, such as beets, or significant amounts of red food coloring, but can also represent bleeding in the lower GI/ colon. Medications that contain bismuth (e.g., Kaopectate, Pepto-Bismol, Bismatrol, pink bismuth) can cause darkened or black stools, and the client's tongue may also appear black.

Epigastric Pain With Radiation

Epigastric pain perceived as intense or sharp pain behind the breastbone with radiation to the back may occur as a result of long-standing ulcers. For example, the client may be aware of an ulcer but does not relate the back pain to the ulcer. The alert PTA listening to the client's report of ongoing medical problems and developing symptoms can be valuable in recognizing red flags associated with the back pain.

 PICTURE THE PATIENT

Anyone with epigastric pain accompanied by a burning sensation that begins at the xiphoid process and radiates up toward the neck and throat may be experiencing heartburn. Other common symptoms may include a bitter or sour taste in the back of the throat, abdominal bloating, gas, and general abdominal discomfort.

Heartburn is often associated with GERD. It can be confused with angina or heart attack when accompanied by chest pain, cough, and SOB. A physician must evaluate and diagnose the cause of epigastric pain or heartburn.

Symptoms Affected by Food

Musculoskeletal pain that is increased or eliminated by eating or drinking should always be a red flag. For example, back, shoulder, or upper chest pain associated with gastric ulcers (located more proximally in the GI tract) may begin within 30 to 90 minutes after eating, whereas abdominal and/or low back pain associated with duodenal or pyloric ulcers (located distally beyond the stomach) may occur 2 to 4 hours after meals (i.e., between meals).

 PTA ACTION PLAN

Communication With the Physical Therapist

Anyone whose musculoskeletal pain is altered (increased or decreased) or eliminated by food should be reevaluated by the PT who may refer the individual for further medical evaluation. Anyone with musculoskeletal pain that is altered by food and has a previous history of cancer and nighttime pain must also be observed more closely by the PTA.

Early Satiety

Early satiety occurs when the client feels hungry, takes one or two bites of food, and feels full. The sensation of being full is out of proportion with the time of the previous meal and the initial degree of hunger experienced. This can be a symptom of obstruction, stomach cancer, gastroparesis (slowing down of stomach emptying), peptic ulcer disease, and other tumors.

Vertebral compression fractures can occur from a variety of disorders, including osteoporosis, and can result in severe spinal deformity. This deformity, along with severe back pain, can cause early satiety resulting in malnutrition.[31]

Constipation

Constipation is defined clinically as being a condition of prolonged retention of fecal content in the GI tract resulting from decreased motility of the colon or difficulty in expelling stool. Constipated clients with tender psoas trigger points (TrPs) may report anterior hip, groin, or thigh pain when the fecal bolus presses against the TrPs.[32]

People with low back pain may develop constipation as a result of muscle guarding and splinting that causes reduced bowel motility. Pressure on sacral nerves from stored fecal content may cause an aching discomfort in the sacrum, buttocks, or thighs.

Intractable constipation is called *obstipation* and can result in a fecal impaction that must be removed. Back pain may be the overriding symptom of obstipation, especially in older adults who do not have regular bowel movements or who cannot remember the last bowel movement was several weeks ago.

Changes in bowel habit may be a response to many other factors such as diet (decreased fluid and bulk intake), smoking, side effects of medication (especially constipation associated with opioids), acute or chronic diseases of the digestive system, extraabdominal diseases, personality, mood (depression), emotional stress, inactivity, prolonged bed rest, and lack of exercise.

Commonly implicated medications include narcotics, aluminum- or calcium-containing antacids (e.g., Alu-Tab, Basaljel, Tums, Rolaids), anticholinergics, tricyclic antidepressants, phenothiazines, calcium channel blockers, and iron salts.

 PTA ACTION PLAN

Reporting Constipation

Because many specific organic causes of constipation exist, it is a symptom that should be reported to the appropriate medical staff (e.g., PT, nursing). It is considered a red-flag symptom when clients with previously unreported or unexplained constipation have sudden and unaccountable changes in bowel habits or blood in the stools.

Diarrhea

Diarrhea, by definition, is an abnormal increase in stool frequency and liquidity. This may be accompanied by urgency, perianal discomfort, and fecal incontinence. The causes of diarrhea vary widely from one person to another, but food, alcohol, use of laxatives and other drugs, medication side effects, and travel may contribute to the development of diarrhea.

Acute diarrhea, especially when associated with fever, cramps, and blood or pus in the stool, can accompany invasive enteric infection. Chronic diarrhea associated with weight loss is more likely to indicate neoplastic or inflammatory bowel disease. Extraintestinal manifestations such as arthritis or skin or eye lesions are often present in inflammatory bowel disease. Any of these combinations of symptoms must be reported.

Drug-induced diarrhea is associated most commonly with antibiotics. Diarrhea may occur as a direct result of antibiotic use, and the GI symptom resolves when the drug is discontinued. Symptoms may also develop 6 to 8 weeks after first ingestion of an antibiotic. A more serious, less frequent antibiotic-induced colitis with severe diarrhea is caused by *Clostridium difficile.*

This anaerobic bacterium colonizes the colon of 5% of healthy adults and over 20% of hospitalized patients. Clients receiving enteral (tube) feedings are at higher risk for acquisition of *C. difficile* and associated severe diarrhea. *C. difficile* is the major cause of diarrhea in patients hospitalized for more than 3 days. It is spread in an oral-fecal manner and is readily transmitted from patient to patient by hospital personnel. Fastidious handwashing, use of gloves, and extremely careful cleaning of bathroom, bed linen, and associated items are helpful in decreasing transmission.[33]

For the client describing chronic diarrhea, the PT, when informed about the situation, may find it necessary to probe further about the use of laxatives as a possible contributor to this condition. The abuse of laxatives is common in the eating disorder populations (e.g., anorexia, bulimia).

PICTURE THE PATIENT

Laxative abuse contributes to the production of diarrhea and begins a vicious cycle because chronic laxative users experience excessive secretion of aldosterone and resultant edema when they attempt to stop using laxatives. This edema and increased weight force the person to continue to rely on laxatives.

Fecal Incontinence

Fecal incontinence may be described as an inability to control evacuation of stool and is associated with a sense of urgency, diarrhea, and abdominal cramping. Causes include partial obstruction of the rectum (cancer), colitis, and radiation therapy, especially in the case of females treated for cervical or uterine cancer. The radiation may cause trauma to the rectum that results in incontinence and diarrhea. Anal distortion resulting from traumatic childbirth, hemorrhoids, and hemorrhoidal surgery may also cause fecal incontinence.

Arthralgia

The relationship between "gut" inflammation and joint inflammation is well known but not fully understood. Many inflammatory GI conditions have an arthritic component affecting the joints. For example, inflammatory bowel disease (ulcerative colitis and Crohn's disease) is often accompanied by rheumatic manifestations; peripheral joint arthritis and spondylitis with sacroiliitis are the most common of these manifestations.[34–37]

The relationship between intestinal problems and joint involvement may also be explained by some type of "interface" between the bowel and the articular surface of joints.[38–41] It is hypothesized that an antigen crosses the gut mucosa and enters the joint, which sets up an immunologic response. Arthralgia with synovitis and immune-mediated joint disease may occur as a result of this immunologic response.[38]

PICTURE THE PATIENT

Joint arthralgia associated with GI infection is usually asymmetric, migratory, and oligoarticular (affecting only one or two joints). This type of joint involvement is termed reactive arthritis when triggered by microbial infection such as *C. difficile* from the GI (and sometimes genitourinary or respiratory) tract. Other accompanying symptoms may include fever, malaise, skin rash or other skin lesions, nail-bed changes (nails separate from the nail beds and become thin and discolored), iritis, or conjunctivitis.

The bowel and joint symptoms may or may not occur at the same time. Usually, this type of arthralgia is preceded 1 to 3 weeks by diarrhea, urethritis, regional enteritis (Crohn's disease), or other bacterial infection. The knees, ankles, shoulders, wrists, elbows, and small joints of the hands and feet (listed in order of decreasing frequency) are the peripheral joints affected most often.[42–44]

A large knee effusion is a common presentation, but some clients have joint pain with minimal or no signs of inflammation. Muscle atrophy occurs when a chronic condition is present; in which case, there will be a history of previous GI and joint involvement. Stiffness, pain, tenderness, and reduced range of motion may be present, but with proper medical intervention, there is no permanent deformity.

PTA ACTION PLAN
Follow-Up Questions

It is important for the PTA to have a discussion with the PT regarding possible signs or symptoms to be alert to when working with a patient who has joint pain of an unknown cause. A few possible follow-up questions the PTA can ask to gather more information for the PT include the following:
- Please describe the pattern of pain/symptoms from when you wake in the morning to when you go to sleep at night.
- How would you describe the joint stiffness or pain today? (e.g., sharp, dull, aching, stabbing, throbbing)

PTA ACTION PLAN
Points to Ponder

The PTA should also keep in mind that the PT might have to conduct an environmental or work history (occupation, military, exposure to chemicals) to identify a delayed reaction.

A dusky blue discoloration or erythema accompanied by exquisite tenderness is a sign of septic (infected) joint; ask about a recent history of infection of any kind anywhere in the body. All information gathered should be immediately reported to the supervising PT.

Shoulder Pain

Pain in the left shoulder (Kehr sign, or pain with pressure placed on the upper abdomen; Danforth sign, or shoulder pain with inspiration) can occur as a result of free air following laparoscopic surgery or blood in the abdominal cavity, usually from a ruptured spleen or retroperitoneal bleeding causing distention.

Retroperitoneum refers to a position external or posterior to the peritoneum, or the serous membrane lining the abdominopelvic walls. *Retroperitoneal organs* refer to viscera that lie against the posterior body wall and are covered by the peritoneum on the anterior surface only (e.g., the thoracic portion of the esophagus, pancreas, duodenal cap, ascending and descending colon, rectum).

A ruptured ectopic pregnancy with retroperitoneal bleeding into the abdominal cavity can also present as low abdominal and/or shoulder pain. Usually there is a history of sexual activity and missed menses in a female of reproductive age.

Perforated duodenal or gastric ulcers can leak gastric juices on the posterior wall of the stomach that irritate the diaphragm referring pain to the shoulder; although the stomach is on the left side of the body, the referral pattern is usually to the right shoulder.

The client may report some type of trauma or injury such as a sharp blow during an athletic event, a fall, or perhaps even a minor automobile accident causing pressure from the steering wheel. The client may not connect these seemingly unrelated events with the present shoulder pain.

? PICTURE THE PATIENT

Pancreatic cancer can refer pain to the shoulder and is often missed as the cause. Fluid in the pleural space as a result of pancreatitis can present as shoulder pain. When the head of the pancreas is involved, the client could have right shoulder pain, but more often it manifests as mid-back or mid-thoracic pain that is sometimes lateralized from the spine on either side. When the tail of the pancreas is diseased, pain can be referred to the left shoulder. Pain may also occur in the right shoulder when blood is present in the abdominal cavity as a result of liver trauma. Accumulation of blood in this area from a slow bleed of the spleen, liver, or stomach can produce bilateral shoulder pain.

Neuropathy

Numbness and weakness of the lower extremities have been reported as a result of vitamin B_{12} deficiency in the aging adult population or from thiamine deficiency after gastric bypass. Such events are infrequent but expected to increase as the number of gastric bypasses increases.[45] Symmetric paresthesias and ataxia associated with loss of vibration and position sense in the lower extremities may occur with vitamin B_{12} deficiency. Other symptoms associated with vitamin B_{12} deficiency can include irritability, memory loss, and dementia.

? PICTURE THE PATIENT

Besides neuropathy, presentation may include confusion, nystagmus, seizures, unsteady gait and ataxia, hearing loss, and lower limb hypotonia.[46] Symptoms may resolve with medical treatment.

▶ PTA ACTION PLAN
Points to Ponder

- GI disorders can refer pain to the sternum, neck, shoulder, scapula, low back, sacrum, groin, and hip.
- When the PT evaluates during early onset of referred pain, there is usually full and painless range of motion, but as time goes on, the PTA may notice muscle splinting and guarding as a result of pain. A component of motor nerve involvement will produce altered movements as well.
- The membrane that envelops organs (visceral peritoneum) is insensitive to pain so that, except in the presence of inflammation/ischemia, it is possible to have extensive disease without pain.
- Clients may not relate known GI disorders to current (or new) musculoskeletal symptoms.
- Sudden and unaccountable changes in bowel habits, blood in the stool, or vomiting red blood or coffee-ground vomitus are red-flag symptoms requiring medical follow-up.
- Antibiotics and NSAIDs are the drugs that most commonly induce GI symptoms.
- Epigastric pain radiating to the upper back, or upper back pain alone, can be the primary symptom of peptic ulcer, pancreatitis, or pancreatic carcinoma.
- Appendicitis and diseases of the intestines, such as Crohn's disease and ulcerative colitis, can cause abscess of the iliopsoas muscle, resulting in hip, thigh, or groin pain.
- Arthritis and migratory arthralgias occur in up to one-third of Crohn's disease cases.[37,47]

RECOGNIZING AND REPORTING HEPATIC RED FLAGS

As with many of the organ systems in the human body, the hepatic and biliary organs (liver, gallbladder, and common bile duct) can develop diseases that mimic primary musculoskeletal lesions. The liver has the vital task of maintaining the body's metabolic homeostasis with its 500 separate functions related to the digestive, endocrine, excretory, and hematologic systems.[48,49] The musculoskeletal symptoms associated with hepatic and biliary pathologic conditions are generally confined to the mid-back, scapular, and right shoulder regions. These musculoskeletal symptoms can occur alone (as the only presenting symptom) or in combination with other systemic signs and symptoms presented in this section.

Hepatic and Biliary Signs and Symptoms

The major causes of acute hepatocellular injury include hepatitis, drug-induced hepatitis, and ingestion of hepatotoxins. Only the red-flag signs and symptoms of liver or gallbladder diseases likely to be reported by patients or observed by the PTA are included in this section (Fig. 4.3).

❓ PICTURE THE PATIENT

Clinical Signs and Symptoms of Liver and Gallbladder Disease

Liver Disease
Gastrointestinal
- Sense of fullness of the abdomen
- Anorexia, nausea, and vomiting

Integumentary
- Skin color changes and nail-bed changes
- Pallor (often linked to cirrhosis or carcinoma)
- Jaundice
- Bruising
- Spider angioma
- Palmar erythema
- White nails of Terry; other nail-bed changes may be present

Hepatic
- Dark urine and light- or clay-colored stools
- Ascites (see Fig. 4.3)
- Edema and oliguria (reduced urine secretion in relation to fluid intake)
- Right upper quadrant abdominal pain

Musculoskeletal
- Musculoskeletal pain, especially right shoulder pain
- Myopathy (rhabdomyolysis in severe cases)

Neurologic
- Confusion
- Sleep disturbances
- Muscle tremors
- Hyperactive reflexes
- Asterixis (motor disturbance resembling body or extremity flapping)
- Bilateral carpal tunnel syndrome (CTS) (numbness, tingling, burning pain in thumb, index and middle fingers)
- Bilateral tarsal tunnel (tarsal tunnel characterized by pain around the ankle that extends to the palmar surfaces of the toes, made worse by walking)

Other
- Gynecomastia (enlargement of breast tissue in males)

Gallbladder Disease
Gastrointestinal
- Right upper abdominal pain
- Indigestion, nausea, feeling of fullness
- Excessive belching, flatulence (intestinal gas)
- Intolerance of fatty foods

Integumentary
- Jaundice (result of blockage of the common bile duct)
- Persistent pruritus (skin itching)

Musculoskeletal
- Sudden, excruciating pain in the midepigastrium with referral to the back and right shoulder (acute cholecystitis)
- Anterior rib pain (tip of rib 10, can also affect ribs 11 and 12)

Constitutional
- Low-grade fever, chills

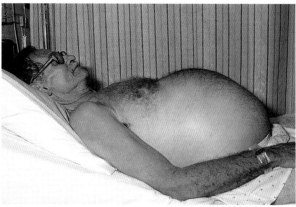

FIG. 4.3 Ascites is an abnormal accumulation of serous (edematous) fluid in the peritoneal cavity associated with liver impairment, especially the portal and hepatic venous hypertension that accompanies cirrhosis of the liver. This condition also may be associated with other disorders such as advanced congestive heart failure, constrictive pericarditis, cancer, chronic hepatitis, and hyperaldosteronism. Any condition affecting the peritoneum by producing increased permeability of the peritoneal capillaries and electrolyte disturbances can result in ascites. (From Swartz M: *Textbook of physical diagnosis: health and examination*, ed 6, Philadelphia, 2009, WB Saunders.)

Skin and Nail-Bed Changes

Skin and nail-bed changes associated with systemic diseases are discussed principally in Chapter 3 with brief reference here to those that are associated with impairment of the hepatic system. Primary clinical presentation of hepatic disease affecting the integumentary system includes jaundice, pallor, and orange or green skin in a White individual.

Change in skin tones may be visible in African American or Asian people, but these may only be observable to the affected individual or to those who know him or her well. In some situations, jaundice may be the first and only manifestation of disease. It is first noticeable in people of all skin colors in the sclera of the eye as a yellow hue when bilirubin reaches levels of 2 to 3 mg/dL. When the bilirubin level reaches 5 to 6 mg/dL, changes in skin color occur.

Other skin changes may include pruritus (itching), bruising, spider angiomas (see Fig. 3.6), and palmar erythema (see Fig. 3.4). *Spider angiomas* (arterial spider, spider telangiectasis, vascular spider), or branched dilations of the superficial capillaries resembling a spider in appearance (see Fig. 3.7), may be vascular manifestations of increased estrogen levels (hyperestrogenism). Spider angiomas and palmar erythema both occur in the presence of liver impairment as a result of increased estrogen levels normally detoxified by the liver.

Palmar erythema (warm redness of the skin over the palms, also called *liver palms*), caused by an extensive collection of arteriovenous anastomoses, is especially evident on the hypothenar and thenar eminences and pulps of the finger (see Fig. 3.4). The person may complain of throbbing, tingling palms. The soles of the feet may be similarly affected. Throbbing and tingling may be associated with these anastomoses.

Various forms of nail disease have been described in cases of liver impairment such as the white nails of Terry (see Fig. 3.3). Other nail-bed changes, such as white bands across the nail plate (leukonychia), clubbed nails (see Fig. 3.39), or koilonychia (see Fig. 3.35), can occur, but these are not specific to liver impairment and can develop in the presence of other diseases as well.

Musculoskeletal Pain

Musculoskeletal pain associated with the hepatic and biliary systems includes thoracic pain between the scapulae, right shoulder, right upper trapezius, right interscapular, or right subscapular areas (Fig. 4.4 and Table 4.3).

Referred shoulder pain may be the only presenting symptom of hepatic or biliary disease. Afferent pain signals from the superior ligaments of the liver and the superior portion of the liver capsule are transmitted by the phrenic nerves. Sympathetic fibers from the biliary system are connected through the celiac (abdominal) and splanchnic (visceral) plexuses to the hepatic fibers in the region of the dorsal spine (see Fig. 2.3).

Hepatic osteodystrophy, or abnormal development of bone, can occur in all forms of cholestasis (bile flow suppression) and hepatocellular disease, especially in the alcoholic person. Either osteomalacia or, more often, osteoporosis frequently accompanies bone pain from this condition. Vertebral wedging, vertebral crush fractures, and kyphosis can be severe.

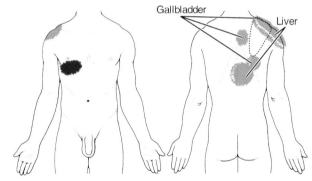

FIG. 4.4 The primary pain pattern from the liver, gallbladder, and common bile duct (*dark red*) presents typically in the midepigastrium or right upper quadrant of the abdomen. Innervation of the liver and biliary system is through the autonomic nervous system from T5 to T11. Liver impairment is primarily reflected through the ninth thoracic distribution. Referred pain (*light red*) from the liver occurs in the thoracic spine from approximately T7 to T10 and/or to the right of midline, possibly affecting the right shoulder (right phrenic nerve). Referred pain from the gallbladder can affect the right shoulder by the same mechanism. The gallbladder can also refer pain to the right interscapular (T4/5–T8) or right subscapular area.

TABLE 4.3 Referred Pain Patterns: Liver, Gallbladder, Common Bile Duct

Systemic Causes	Location (see Fig. 4.4)
Liver disease (abscess, cirrhosis, tumors, hepatitis)	Thoracic spine (T7–10; midline to the right) Right upper trapezius and shoulder
Gallbladder	Right upper trapezius and shoulder Right interscapular area (T4/5–8) Right subscapular area

Osteoporosis can be associated with primary biliary cirrhosis and primary sclerosing cholangitis. Painful osteoarthropathy may develop in the wrists and ankles as a nonspecific complication of chronic liver disease.

Rhabdomyolysis is a potentially fatal condition in which myoglobin and other muscle tissue contents are released into the bloodstream as a result of muscle tissue disintegration. This could occur with acute trauma (e.g., crush injuries, significant blunt trauma, high-voltage electrical burns, surgery,[50] severe burns, overexertion),[51,52] or in the case of liver impairment, from alcohol abuse or alcohol poisoning[53] or the use of cholesterol-lowering drugs called *statins* (e.g., simvastatin [Zocor], atorvastatin [Lipitor], rosuvastatin [Crestor], lovastatin [Mevacor], pravastatin [Pravachol]).[54,55]

? PICTURE THE PATIENT

Rhabdomyolysis is characterized by muscle aches, cramps, soreness, and weakness. It may be accompanied by other symptoms of respiratory muscle myopathy (impaired diaphragmatic function)[56] or liver or renal involvement. Laboratory testing will show a creatine kinase level more than 10 times the upper limit of normal.

Although the literature reports the incidence of this severe myopathy with statin use as about 0.1% to 2.0% in several studies,[57–59] therapists (and others) report seeing cases more often than the low percentage would suggest (up to 10% of all cases[60,61]). Any anatomic region can be affected, but the back and extremity musculoskeletal pain are the two areas of involvement reported most often.[62–65] Statin-associated myopathy has been reported as a result of physical activity.[66]

Statin-associated myopathy also appears to occur more often in people with complex medical problems and/or those taking illegal drugs (e.g., cocaine, heroin, LSD) or abusing prescription drugs (e.g., barbiturates and amphetamines).[67] Other risk factors that increase the chances of this condition include excessive alcohol use, being statin intolerant,[60] vitamin D deficient (in some but not all statins[68]), advancing age (over 80 years), recent history of surgery, and small physical stature.[54]

Neurologic Symptoms

Neurologic symptoms, such as confusion, sleep disturbances, muscle tremors, hyperreactive reflexes, and asterixis, may occur. When liver dysfunction results in increased serum ammonia and urea levels, peripheral nerve function can be impaired. Impaired neurotransmission leads to altered CNS metabolism and function. Symptoms of poor concentration and fatigue can result.

Asterixis is an outward sign of liver disease. Also called *flapping tremors* or *liver flap*, asterixis is described as the inability to maintain wrist extension with forward flexion of the upper extremities. It is tested by asking the client to actively hyperextend the wrist and hand with the rest of the arm supported on a firm surface or with the arms held out in front of the body (see Fig. 3.5).[69,70] The test is positive if quick, irregular extensions and flexions of the wrist and fingers occur. The PTA may observe asterixis when releasing the pressure in the arm cuff during BP readings.

Asterixis and numbness/tingling (the latter are misinterpreted as CTS) can occur as a result of this ammonia abnormality, causing an intrinsic nerve pathologic condition (Case Example 4.5). There are many potential causes of CTS, both musculoskeletal and systemic (Box 4.5). The PTA can watch carefully for any of the associated clinical presentations listed in Box 4.6.

 PTA ACTION PLAN

Tremors

There are many different types of tremors and causes for each one. The differential diagnosis usually requires medical evaluation.[72] The PT should be notified any time a patient or client demonstrates a previously undocumented movement disorder such as tremors. Nothing needs to be said to the patient/client about these tremors until the therapist is able to assess the individual and determine the next step in the evaluation process.

 PTA ACTION PLAN

Jaundice

Jaundice in the postoperative client is not uncommon, but it can be a potentially serious complication of liver damage that occurs following surgery and anesthesia. It is likely a condition that has already been observed by the supervising nursing and physical therapy staff but still something the PTA can discuss with the therapist in case there are any modifications required in the plan of care.

CASE EXAMPLE 4.5 Carpal Tunnel Syndrome From Liver Impairment

A 45-year-old truck driver was diagnosed by a hand surgeon as having bilateral carpal tunnel syndrome (CTS) and referred to physical therapy. A screening examination for a complete systems review was not performed by the physical therapist (PT) during the initial evaluation. During the fourth treatment session with the physical therapist assistant (PTA), the client commented that he was seeing an acupuncturist, who told him that liver disease was the cause of his bilateral CTS.

- "Describe your history of alcohol use." The client states his history does not include heavy use of alcohol.
- "Is there any drug use that could potentially harm your liver?" The client describes a long history of over-the-counter pain relievers and a short time of intravenous drug use in college.
- "Do you take cholesterol-lowering medication?" The client replies "yes."
- "Do you have any sleep disturbances?" The client replies "no."

The PTA reported the patient's comments to the supervising PT that afternoon after the client's session. The PT requested to see the patient for the next visit to complete further questioning to rule out liver or hepatic involvement. After further screening from the PT, it was decided that because his symptoms were bilateral and there is a known correlation between liver disease and CTS, the referring physician was notified of these findings.

The client was referred to his physician for evaluation, and a diagnosis of liver cancer was confirmed. Physical therapy for CTS was appropriately discontinued.

BOX 4.5 Causes of Carpal Tunnel Syndrome

Neuromusculoskeletal

Idiopathic
Cause unknown

Anatomic (Compression)
Small carpal canal, anomalous muscles/tendons
Basal joint (thumb) arthritis
Cervical disk lesions
Cervical spondylosis
Congenital anatomic differences or anatomic change in nerve or carpal tunnel (e.g., shape, size, volume of structures; presence of palmaris longus)
History of wrist surgery, especially previous carpal tunnel surgery
Injection: high pressure
Peripheral neuropathy
Poor posture (may also be associated with thoracic outlet syndrome [TOS])
Tendinitis
Trigger points
Tenosynovitis
TOS

Trauma/Exertional
Swelling, hemorrhage, scar, wrist fracture, carpal dislocation
Cumulative trauma disorders*
Repetitive strain injuries*
Vibrational exposure (jackhammer or other manual labor equipment)

Systemic
Chronic kidney disease (fluid imbalance)
Congestive heart failure (fluid imbalance)
Hemochromatosis
Leukemia (tissue infiltration)

Liver disease
Medications
- Nonsteroidal antiinflammatory drugs
- Oral contraceptives
- Statins
- Alendronate (Fosamax)
- Lithium
- Beta blocker
Obesity
Pregnancy (fluid retention)
Tumors (lipoma, hemangioma, ganglia, synovial sarcoma, fibroma, neuroma, neurofibroma)
Use of oral contraceptives
Vitamin deficiency

Endocrine
Acromegaly
Diabetes mellitus
Gout (deposits of tophi and calcium)
Hormonal imbalance (menopause; posthysterectomy)
Hyperparathyroidism
Hyperthyroidism (Graves disease)
Hypocalcemia
Hypothyroidism (myxedema)

Infectious Disease
Atypical mycobacterium
Histoplasmosis
Rubella
Sporotrichosis

BOX 4.5   Causes of Carpal Tunnel Syndrome—cont'd

Inflammatory
Amyloidosis
Arthritis (rheumatoid, gout, polymyalgia rheumatica)
Dermatomyositis
Gout/pseudogout
Scleroderma
Systemic lupus erythematosus

Neuropathic
Alcohol abuse
Chemotherapy (delayed, long-term effect)

Diabetes
Multiple myeloma (amyloidosis deposits)
Thyroid disease
Vitamin/nutritional deficiency (especially vitamin B_6; folic acid)
Vitamin toxicity

---

*The role of repetitive activities and occupational factors (e.g., hand use of any type and keyboard or computer work in particular) has been questioned as a direct cause of carpal tunnel syndrome (CTS) and remains under investigation; sufficient evidence to implicate hand use of any type linked with CTS remains unproven.[71]

Modified from Goodman CC and Snyder TK: *Differential diagnosis for physical therapists: screening for referral.* ed 3, Elsevier, Mosby, 2007, Saunders.

BOX 4.6   Evaluating Carpal Tunnel Syndrome Associated With Liver Impairment

For any client presenting with bilateral carpal tunnel syndrome:
- Ask about the presence of similar symptoms in the feet
- Ask about a personal history of liver or hepatic disease (e.g., cirrhosis, cancer, hepatitis)
- Look for a history of hepatotoxic drugs
- Look for a history of alcoholism
- Ask about current or previous use of statins (cholesterol-lowering drugs such as rosuvastatin [Crestor], atorvastatin [Lipitor], lovastatin [Mevacor], or simvastatin [Zocor])
- Look for other signs and symptoms associated with liver impairment
- Test for signs of liver disease
  - Skin color changes
  - Spider angiomas
  - Palmar erythema (liver palms)
  - Nail-bed changes (e.g., white nails of Terry, white bands, clubbing)
  - Asterixis (liver flap)

▶▶ PTA ACTION PLAN

Points to Ponder

- Primary signs and symptoms of liver diseases vary and can include GI symptoms, edema/ascites, dark urine, light- or clay-colored feces, and right upper abdominal pain.
- Skin changes associated with the hepatic system include pruritus, jaundice, pallor, orange or green skin, bruising, spider angiomas, and palmar erythema.
- Active, intense exercise should be avoided when the liver is compromised (jaundice or other active disease).
- Antiinflammatory and minor analgesic agents can cause drug-induced hepatitis. Nonviral hepatitis may occur postoperatively.
- When liver dysfunction results in increased serum ammonia and urea levels, peripheral nerve function is impaired. Flapping tremors (asterixis) and numbness/tingling (misinterpreted as CTS/tarsal tunnel syndrome) can occur.
- Musculoskeletal locations of pain associated with the hepatic and biliary systems include thoracic spine between scapulae, right shoulder, right upper trapezius, right interscapular, or right subscapular areas.

RECOGNIZING AND REPORTING ENDOCRINE-RELATED RED FLAGS

Whether a result of trauma or of insidious onset, a client's complaints of flank pain, low back pain, or pelvic pain may be of renal or urologic origin. Knowing the red-flag signs and symptoms of these systems will help the PTA quickly recognize what to document and report to the appropriate staff (nursing, PT) to ensure further evaluation and medical referral when it is appropriate.

Renal and urinary tract problems are primarily caused by inflammation, infection, and obstruction. Major risk factors for renal and urinary tract problems include the following:
- Age over 60 years
- Personal or family history of diabetes or hypertension
- Personal or family history of kidney disease, heart attack, or stroke
- Personal history of kidney stones, urinary tract infections (UTIs), lower urinary tract obstruction, or autoimmune disease
- African, Hispanic, Pacific Island, or Native American descent
- Exposure to chemicals (e.g., paint, glue, degreasing solvents, cleaning solvents), drugs, or environmental conditions

Urinary Tract Infections

All health care professionals including the PTA must be alert to the possibility of UTIs, especially in anyone with any of the risk factors listed. Upper UTIs include kidney or ureteral infections; lower UTIs include cystitis (bladder infection) or urethritis (urethral infection). Symptoms of UTI depend on the location of the infection in either the upper or lower urinary tract (although, rarely, infection could occur in both simultaneously) (Case Example 4.6).

Symptoms of upper urinary tract inflammations and infections are shown in Box 4.7. If the diaphragm is irritated, ipsilateral shoulder pain may occur. Signs and symptoms of renal impairment are also shown in Table 4.4; if present, they are significant symptoms of impending kidney failure.

A lower UTI occurs most commonly in females because of the short female urethra and the proximity of the urethra to the vagina and rectum. The rate of occurrence increases with age and

CASE EXAMPLE 4.6   Bladder Infection

A 55-year-old female came to the clinic with back pain associated with paraspinal muscle spasms. Pain was of unknown cause (insidious onset), and the client reported that she was "just getting out of bed" when the pain started. The pain was described as a dull aching that was aggravated by movement and relieved by rest (musculoskeletal pattern).

No numbness, tingling, or saddle anesthesia was reported, and the neurologic screening examination was negative. Sacroiliac testing was negative. Spinal movements were slow and guarded, with muscle spasms noted throughout movement and at rest. Because of her age and the insidious onset of symptoms, the physical therapist (PT) included a screening examination for medical disease.

This client was midmenopausal and was not taking any hormone replacement therapy. She had a bladder infection a month ago that was treated with antibiotics; tests for this were negative when she was evaluated and referred by her physician for back pain. Two weeks ago, she had an upper respiratory infection (a "cold") and had been "coughing a lot." There was no previous history of cancer.

The PT developed a plan of care that included local treatment to reduce paraspinal muscle spasms. The physical therapist assistant (PTA) documented and reported all appropriate observations noted during each treatment session. By the fifth treatment the PTA reported to the PT that the patient was not responding as expected. Because of her recent history of upper respiratory and bladder infections, the PT instructed the PTA to ask specific questions related to the presence of constitutional symptoms and changes in bladder function/urine color, force of stream, burning on urination, and so on. Occasional "sweats" (present sometimes during the day, sometimes at night) was the only red flag present. The combination of recent infection, failure to respond to treatment, and the presence of sweats suggested referral to the physician for early reevaluation.

The client did not return to the clinic for further treatment, and a follow-up telephone call indicated that she did indeed have a recurrent bladder infection that was treated successfully with a different antibiotic. Her back pain and muscle spasm were eliminated after only 24 hours of taking this new antibiotic.

BOX 4.7   Clinical Symptoms of Infectious/Inflammatory Urinary Tract Problems

Upper Urinary Tract (Kidney or Ureteral Infection)
Unilateral costovertebral tenderness
Flank pain
Ipsilateral shoulder pain
Fever and chills
Skin hypersensitivity (hyperesthesia of dermatomes)
Hematuria (blood [red blood cells] in urine)
Pyuria (pus or white blood cells in urine)
Bacteriuria (bacteria in urine)
Nocturia (unusual or increased nighttime need to urinate)

Lower Urinary Tract (Cystitis or Urethritis)
Urinary frequency
Urinary urgency
Low back pain
Pelvic/lower abdominal pain
Dysuria (discomfort, such as pain or burning during urination)
Hematuria
Pyuria
Bacteriuria
Dyspareunia (painful intercourse)

sexual activity since intercourse can spread bacteria from the genital area to the urethra. Chronic health problems, such as DM, gout, hypertension, obstructive urinary tract problems, and medical procedures requiring urinary catheterization, are also predisposing risk factors for the development of these infections.[73,74]

❓ PICTURE THE PATIENT

Older adults (both males and females) are at increased risk for UTI. They may present with nonspecific symptoms, such as loss of appetite, nausea, and vomiting; abdominal pain; or change in mental status (e.g., onset of confusion, increased confusion). Watch for predisposing conditions that can put the older client at risk for UTI. These may include DM or other chronic diseases (e.g., Alzheimer disease, Parkinson disease), immobility, reduced fluid intake, use of incontinence management products (e.g., pads, briefs, external catheters), indwelling catheterization, and previous history of UTI or kidney stones.

TABLE 4.4   Systemic Manifestations of Chronic Kidney Disease

System	Manifestation
General	Fatigue, malaise
Skin and nail beds	Pallor, ecchymosis, pruritus, dry skin and mucous membranes, thin/brittle nail beds, urine odor on skin, uremic frost (white urea crystals) on the face and upper trunk, poor wound healing
Skeletal	Osteomalacia, osteoporosis,* bone pain, myopathy, tendon rupture, fracture, joint pain, dependent edema
Neurologic	*CNS:* Recent memory loss, decreased alertness, difficulty concentrating, irritability, lethargy/sleep disturbance, coma, impaired judgment *PNS:* Muscle weakness, tremors, and cramping; neuropathies with restless leg syndrome, cramps, carpal tunnel syndrome, paresthesias, burning feet syndrome, pruritus (itching)
Eye, ear, nose, throat	Metallic taste in mouth, nosebleeds, uremic (urine-smelling) breath, pale conjunctiva, visual blurring
Cardiovascular	Hypertension, friction rub, congestive heart failure, pericarditis, cardiomyopathy, arrhythmia, Raynaud phenomenon
Pulmonary	Dyspnea, pulmonary edema, crackles (rales), pleural effusion
Gastrointestinal	Anorexia, nausea, vomiting, hiccups, gastrointestinal bleeding
Genitourinary	Decreased urine output and other changes in pattern of urination (e.g., nocturia)
Metabolic/endocrine	Dehydration, hyperkalemia, metabolic acidosis, hypocalcemia, hyperphosphatemia, fertility and sexual dysfunction (e.g., impotence, loss of libido, amenorrhea), hyperparathyroidism
Hematologic	Anemia, thrombocytopenia

*Bone demineralization leads to a condition called renal osteodystrophy.

CNS, Central nervous system; *PNS,* peripheral nervous system.

From Goodman CC, Snyder TE: *Differential diagnosis in physical therapy,* ed 3, Philadelphia, 2000, Saunders.

Urinary Incontinence

Urinary incontinence (UI) may be defined as a "complaint of involuntary urine loss."[75] There are currently eight categories of UI.[75] The two most common categories used to classify UI are as follows:

1. *Stress urinary incontinence* (SUI): complaint of involuntary loss of urine on effort or physical exertion or on sneezing or coughing. This occurs during activities that increase intraabdominal pressure.

2. *Urgency urinary incontinence* (UUI): complaint of involuntary loss of urine associated with urgency. Urgency is the report of a sudden compelling desire to urinate that is difficult to defer. UUI is often related to detrusor instability, a condition in which the bladder contracts at small volumes, often in response to triggers such as running water or arriving home. *Overactive bladder syndrome* (older terms include *hyperreflexive bladder* or *detrusor hyperreflexia*) is defined as "urinary urgency, usually accompanied by frequency and nocturia, with or without UUI, in the absence of UTI or other obvious pathology."[75]

Many people have more than one type of incontinence (most often SUI and UUI together), known as *mixed* UI.

Urinary incontinence is common, particularly in older adults. However, the actual prevalence greatly varies due to different definitions, study populations, and procedures. Prevalence is shown to increase with age and especially in women.[76] Yet the condition is poorly understood, underdiagnosed, and often inadequately treated. Many people are embarrassed to acknowledge that they are incontinent. Many incontinent adults do not seek any help for this problem, whereas others regard incontinence as part of the normal aging process.

Everyone should be asked if they have urinary incontinence, but especially perimenopausal or postmenopausal female, any female who has been pregnant, anyone (male or female) over the age of 60 years (earlier if prostate or bladder infection or cancer is evident), and any person with multiple risk factors should be screened for UI.

Risk Factors

A wide range of factors can contribute to the increased risk of developing UI (Box 4.8).[77] Some risk factors are more likely to lead to one type or another or several types of incontinence. The literature varies widely as to which risk factors are significant for different population groups.

Each type of UI has associated clinical manifestations. *UUI* is often caused by involuntary bladder (detrusor) spasms (also called detrusor overactivity [DO]) and is associated with both increased frequency and urgency. The pathophysiology of DO is not fully understood and may be related to irritated sensory signals from overactive pelvic floor muscles (PFMs), bacteria of UTI, fear of leaking, and other psychological factors.

Urge incontinence is characterized by leakage (sometimes large-volume accidents) after a sudden precipitant desire to urinate, such as trying to insert a key in the door, running hands under water (or hearing running water), thinking

---

BOX 4.8   Risk Factors for Urinary Incontinence

Obesity and Elevated Body Mass Index
- Age
- Pregnancy/multiple pregnancies; childbirth/delivery (vaginal or cesarean section); episiotomy; large gestational weight
- Cystocele or uterine prolapse
- Any pelvic surgery including hysterectomy for females, prostatectomy for males
- Diabetes mellitus
- Depression
- Constipation, fecal impaction
- Tobacco use
- Medications
  - Alpha-adrenergic blockers (antihistamines, decongestants)
  - Antihypertensives
  - Antiparkinsonian agents
  - Antipsychotics
  - Diuretics
  - Narcotic analgesics
  - Tranquilizers, sedatives
  - Tricyclic antidepressants
- History of recurrent urinary tract infections
- Bladder irritation (low fluid intake, caffeine, and possibly alcohol) [†]
- Loss of skills for toileting; decreased or impaired mobility
- Impaired cognitive function
- Race (White)
- Neurologic disorder (e.g., myelomeningocele, multiple sclerosis, brain injury, Parkinson disease)
- Cerebral palsy, spinal cord injury, stroke
- Psychogenic (e.g., childhood and/or adult sexual trauma for both males and females)
- Sexual experiences, emotional stress
- Frequent high-impact exercise*

*From Nygard I, et al: Exercise and incontinence, *Obstetr Gynecol* 75:848–851, 1990; Sherman RA, Davis GD, Wong MF: Behavioral treatment of exercise-induced urinary incontinence among female soldiers, *Military Med* 162:690–694, 1997.
[†] Bladder irritants are not likely to cause urinary incontinence without other contributing factors.
Source used for pharmacotherapy update: DiPiro JT, Talbert RL, Yee GC, et al., editors: *Pharmacotherapy: a pathophysiologic approach*, ed 8, New York, 2011, McGraw Hill.

---

about going to the bathroom, or passing by a bathroom. Some clinicians use the term *functional incontinence* to describe the consequence of chronic impairments of physical or cognitive function that make toileting in a timely fashion difficult (e.g., difficulty getting to the toilet on time, inability to manage pants zippers, forgetting how to get on and off the toilet).

SUI results from weakness or loss of tone in the PFM, internal urethral sphincter failure, hypermobility of the ureterovesical junction, or damage to the pudendal nerve (e.g., infection, tumor, childbirth) (Figs. 4.5 and 4.6). It is accompanied by leakage that is coincident with increases in intraabdominal pressure (e.g., coughing, sneezing, laughing, bending, high-impact physical activity, or exercise). A patient with mixed UI will exhibit signs of both UUI and SUI.

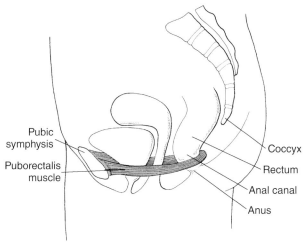

FIG. 4.5 Pelvic floor sling. The first layer of the pelvic floor is made up of the endopelvic fascia, one continuous body of connective tissue surrounding and supporting the pelvic organs (*not pictured*). The levator ani muscles (pelvic floor muscles) make up the second layer, forming a sling across the pelvic cavity from the pubis to the coccyx with openings to allow passage of the urethra, lower vagina, and anus. The puborectalis muscle (part of the levator ani muscle) works together with the pubococcygeus muscle (*not shown*, also part of the levator ani muscle) to support the pelvic viscera in both the male and female. (From Myers RS: *Saunders manual of physical therapy*, Philadelphia, 1995, Saunders.)

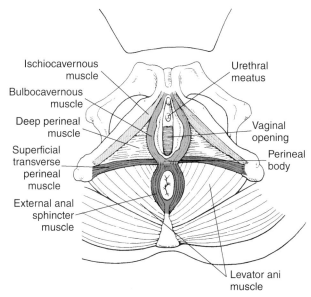

FIG. 4.6 Pelvic floor muscles. Third layer of the pelvic floor, sometimes referred to as the urogenital diaphragm or deep perineum. The deep transverse perineal muscle, external urethral sphincter, and enveloping fascia of the third layer are overlaid by the fourth (superficial) layer (perineum), including the bulbocavernous, ischiocavernous, superficial transverse perineal muscles, and the external anal sphincter and muscle. (From Myers RS: *Saunders manual of physical therapy*, Philadelphia, 1995, Saunders.)

Other clinical manifestations of UI depend on the type of incontinence and underlying pathology, but may include constant dribbling, frequency, urgency, nocturia, hesitancy, weak stream, or straining to void. Prolapsed bladder, uterus, and/or bowel may accompany or contribute to leakage, especially when caused by multiple pregnancies and deliveries.

> ▶▶ **PTA ACTION PLAN**
> ### Urinary Incontinence
>
> All PTAs can teach proper lifting techniques to minimize unnecessary increases in intraabdominal pressure, which could contribute to the occurrence of SUI and pelvic organ prolapse. Patients should be taught to contract the PFM before increased abdominal pressure (e.g., lifting, laughing, coughing, sneezing, vomiting). Anyone experiencing leaking during exercise should be reevaluated by the PT. A prescriptive PFM exercise program may be needed.

> ▶▶ **PTA ACTION PLAN**
> ### Follow-Up Questions
>
> Specific questions should be included in the intake history for all individuals to help bring this information to light, such as the following:
> - Do you leak urine when you lift, cough, sneeze, or stand up?
> - Do you get up at night to urinate (how often)?
> - Do you go to the bathroom more often than every 2 to 3 hours?
> - How much water do you drink in a waking day?
> - Are you constipated?

Kidney Stones

Kidney or ureteral stones are the second most likely urologic problem the PTA will encounter in the adult population. If a stone becomes wedged in the ureter, urine backs up, thus distending the ureter and potentially causing severe back pain. If a stone blocks the flow of urine, urine pressure may build up in the ureter and kidney, causing the kidney to swell (hydronephrosis). Unrecognized hydronephrosis can sometimes cause permanent kidney damage.[78]

The most characteristic symptom of renal or ureteral stones is sudden, sharp, severe pain. If the pain originates deep in the lumbar area and radiates around the side and down toward the testicle in the male and the bladder in the female, it is termed *renal colic. Ureteral colic* occurs if the stone becomes trapped in the ureter. Ureteral colic is characterized by radiation of painful symptoms toward the genitalia and thighs (Fig. 4.7).

Since the testicles and ovaries form in utero in the location of the kidneys and then migrate at full term following the pathways of the ureters, kidney stones moving down the pathway of the ureters cause pain in the flank. This pain radiates to the scrotum in males and the labia in females. For the same reason, ovarian or testicular cancer can refer pain to the back at the level of the kidneys.

Tumors of the Kidney or Bladder

Common symptoms of renal cancer are very similar to those of bladder cancer and require immediate referral for follow-up. These symptoms can include blood in the urine, pain in the side that does not go away, a lump or mass in the side or abdomen, weight loss, fever, and general fatigue or feeling of poor health.[79]

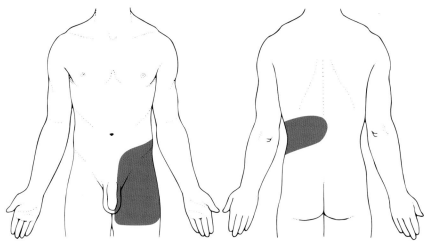

FIG. 4.7 Ureteral pain may begin posteriorly in the costovertebral angle. It may then radiate anteriorly to the ipsilateral lower abdomen, upper thigh, testes, or labium.

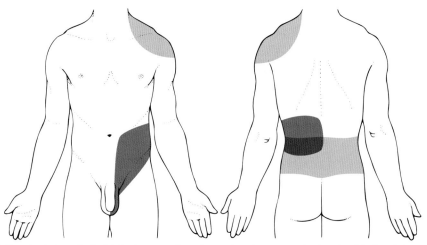

FIG. 4.8 Renal pain is typically felt in the posterior subcostal and costovertebral region (*dark red*). It can radiate across the low back (*light red*) and/or forward around the flank into the lower abdominal quadrant. Ipsilateral groin and testicular pain may also accompany renal pain. Pressure from the kidney on the diaphragm may cause ipsilateral shoulder pain.

⏩ PTA ACTION PLAN

Blood in the Urine

Renal tumors may present as a flank mass combined with unexplained weight loss, fever, pain, and hematuria. The presence of any amount of blood in the urine always requires notification of the PT with likely referral to a physician for further diagnostic evaluation. Blood in the urine is a primary symptom of urinary tract neoplasm.

Renal and Urologic Pain

Renal (kidney) pain (Fig. 4.8) is typically felt in the posterior subcostal and costovertebral regions, whereas ureteral pain is felt in the groin and genital area (see Fig. 4.7). With either renal pain or ureteral pain, radiation forward around the flank into the lower abdominal quadrant and abdominal muscle spasm with rebound tenderness can occur on the same side as the source of pain.[78]

Nerve fibers from the renal plexus are also in direct communication with the spermatic plexus; because of this close relationship, testicular pain may also accompany renal pain.[74,80] Neither renal nor urethral pain is altered by a change in body position. These are not typical musculoskeletal pain patterns and must be reported to the PT.

❓ PICTURE THE PATIENT

The typical renal pain sensation is aching and dull but can occasionally be a severe, boring type of pain. The constant dull and aching pain usually accompanies distention or stretching of the renal capsule, pelvis, or collecting system. This stretching can result from intrarenal fluid accumulation such as inflammatory edema, inflamed or bleeding cysts, and bleeding or neoplastic growths. Whenever the renal capsule is punctured, a dull pain can also be felt by the client. Ischemia of renal tissue caused by blockage of blood flow to the kidneys results in a constant dull or a constant sharp pain.

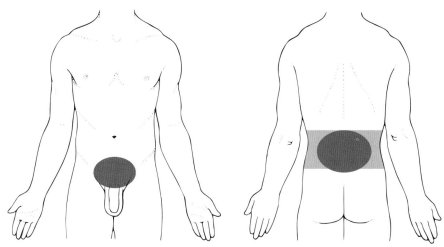

FIG. 4.9 *Left*, Bladder or urethral pain is usually felt suprapubically or ipsilaterally in the lower abdomen. This is the same pattern for gas pain from the lower gastrointestinal tract for some people. *Right*, Bladder or urethral pain may also be perceived in the low back area (*dark red*: primary pain center; *light red*: referred pain). Low back pain may occur as the first and only symptom associated with bladder/urethral pain, or it may occur along with suprapubic or abdominal pain or both.

BOX 4.9   Extraurologic Conditions Causing Urinary Tract Symptoms

Acute or chronic conditions affecting other viscera outside the urologic system can refer pain and symptoms to the upper or lower urinary tract. These can include the following:

- Perforated viscus (any large internal organ)
- Intestinal obstruction
- Cholecystitis (inflammation of the gallbladder)
- Pelvic inflammatory disease
- Tubo-ovarian abscess
- Ruptured ectopic pregnancy
- Twisted ovarian cyst
- Tumor (benign or malignant)

▶▶ PTA ACTION PLAN
Points to Ponder

- Change in color, consistency, smell, or reduced volume or flow of urine requires further assessment and change in urgency and frequency, and pain with urination requires further evaluation.
- Urinary incontinence is not a normal part of aging and should be evaluated by the PT carefully.
- Anyone with hypertension and/or diabetes (and/or other significant risk factors for renal disease) should be monitored carefully and consistently for any systemic signs and symptoms of renal impairment.
- People with diabetes are prone to complications associated with UTIs.

Ureteral obstruction (e.g., from a urinary calculus or "stone" consisting of mineral salts) results in distention of the ureter and causes spasm that produces intermittent or constant severe colicky pain until the stone is passed. Pain of this origin usually starts in the costovertebral angle and radiates to the ipsilateral lower abdomen, upper thigh, testis, or labium (see Fig. 4.7). Movement of a stone down a ureter can cause *renal colic*, an excruciating pain that radiates to the region just described and usually increases in intensity in waves of colic or spasm.[11,80]

Bladder or urethral pain is felt above the pubis (suprapubic) or low in the abdomen (Fig. 4.9). The sensation is usually characterized as one of urinary urgency, a sensation to void, and dysuria (painful urination). Irritation of the neck of the bladder or the urethra can result in a burning sensation localized to these areas, probably caused by the urethral thermal receptors.[11] See Box 4.9 for causes of pain outside the urogenital system that present like upper or lower urinary tract pain of either an acute or chronic nature.

Recognizing and Reporting Endocrine Red Flags

The musculoskeletal system is composed of a variety of connective tissue structures in which normal growth and development are influenced strongly and sometimes controlled by various hormones and metabolic processes. Alterations in these control systems can result in structural changes and altered function of various connective tissues, producing systemic and musculoskeletal signs and symptoms (Box 4.10).

Muscle Weakness, Myalgia, and Fatigue

Muscle weakness, myalgia, and fatigue may be early manifestations of thyroid or parathyroid disease, acromegaly, diabetes, Cushing syndrome, and osteomalacia.[11] Proximal muscle weakness associated with endocrine disease is usually painless and unrelated to either the severity or the duration of the underlying disease. The muscular system is sometimes but not always restored with effective treatment of the underlying condition.

Bilateral Carpal Tunnel Syndrome

Bilateral CTS, resulting from median nerve compression at the wrist, is a common finding in a variety of systemic and

BOX 4.10   Signs and Symptoms of Endocrine Dysfunction

Neuromusculoskeletal

Signs and symptoms associated with rheumatoid arthritis
Muscle weakness
Muscle atrophy
Myalgia
Fatigue
Carpal tunnel syndrome
Synovial fluid changes
Periarthritis
Adhesive capsulitis (diabetes)
Chondrocalcinosis
Spondyloarthropathy
Osteoarthritis
Hand stiffness
Arthralgia

Systemic

Excessive or delayed growth
Polydipsia
Polyuria
Mental changes (nervousness, confusion, depression)
Changes in hair (quality and distribution)
Changes in skin pigmentation
Changes in vital signs (elevated body temperature, pulse rate, increased blood pressure)
Heart palpitations
Increased perspiration
Kussmaul respirations (deep, rapid breathing)
Dehydration or excessive retention of body water

From Goodman CC, Fuller KS: Pathology: implications for the physical therapist, ed 3, Philadelphia, 2009, WB Saunders.

neuromusculoskeletal conditions[81–83] but especially with certain endocrine and metabolic disorders (see Box 4.5).[71] The fact that the majority of persons with CTS are females at or near menopause suggests that the soft tissues about the wrist could be affected in some way by hormones.[84–86] During pregnancy, hormonal fluctuations, fluid shifts, and musculoskeletal changes predispose females to CTS.[87]

Thickening of the transverse carpal ligament in certain systemic disorders (e.g., acromegaly, myxedema) may be sufficient to compress the median nerve. Any condition that increases the volume of the contents of the carpal tunnel (e.g., tumors,[88] calcium, and gouty tophi deposits[89,90]) can compress the median nerve.

⑦ PICTURE THE PATIENT

The signs and symptoms associated with CTS often include paresthesia, tingling, and numbness and/or pain (or burning pain) with cutaneous distribution of the median nerve to the thumb, index, middle, and radial half of the ring finger. Nocturnal paresthesia is a common complaint, and this discomfort causes sleep disruption. It can be partially relieved by shaking of the hand or changing wrist and hand position. Pain may radiate into the palm and up the forearm and arm.[91]

It should be noted that bilateral tarsal syndrome affecting the feet can also occur either alone or in conjunction with CTS of an endocrine (e.g., diabetes,[92] hypothyroidism) or other systemic origin (e.g., chemotherapy, ankylosing spondylitis,[93] rheumatoid arthritis), although from clinical experience the incidence of tarsal tunnel syndrome is not high. Bilateral median nerve neuritis can be characteristic of many systemic diseases, including rheumatoid arthritis, myxedema, localized amyloidosis, sarcoidosis, and infiltrative leukemia.[94,95]

A red flag is indicated whenever a client presents with bilateral symptoms. With bilateral CTS the PTA can ask a few follow-up questions to discern the need for consultation with the PT.

⏵⏵ PTA ACTION PLAN

Follow-Up Questions

By asking the following questions the PTA can gather some important information to take back to the PT. This information will help the PT to determine the appropriate plan for medical follow-up with the physician.

- Do you have any pain, numbness, or tingling in your feet? (peripheral neuropathy: diabetes, chronic alcohol use, liver impairment)
- Have you had any abdominal pain since the symptoms of CTS have come on? (liver impairment)
- Have you noticed any change in your energy level? Are you more fatigued than usual?
- Have you had any unusual weakness since you have had the CTS?
- Any recent, unintentional weight loss?
- Any nausea, vomiting, or other GI symptoms?
- Any recent swelling in the hands or feet?
- Any change in the color of your urine (cola colored)?
- Are you taking any medication to lower your cholesterol (e.g., Lipitor, Crestor, Zocor, Lescol, Mevacor)?

Periarthritis and Calcific Tendinitis

Periarthritis (inflammation of periarticular structures, including the tendons, ligaments, and joint capsule) and calcific tendinitis occur most often in the shoulders of people who have endocrine disease.[11,96,97] Physical therapy intervention may have a temporary palliative effect, but treatment of the underlying endocrine impairment is often needed to improve the clinical picture.

⏵⏵ PTA ACTION PLAN

Arthritis Does Not Improve With Treatment

The PTA should remain alert for clients who do not improve with treatment as expected and discuss this with the PT when a pattern of nonimprovement emerges.

Spondyloarthropathy and Osteoarthritis

Spondyloarthropathy (disease of joints of the spine) and osteoarthritis occur in individuals with various metabolic or endocrine diseases, including hemochromatosis (disorder of iron metabolism with excess deposition of iron in the tissues; also known as *bronze diabetes* and *iron storage disease*), ochronosis (metabolic disorder resulting in discoloration of body tissues caused by deposits of alkapton bodies), acromegaly, and DM.[98]

Neuromuscular Symptoms

Neuromuscular symptoms are among the most common manifestations of hypothyroidism (Box 4.11). Flexor tenosynovitis with stiffness often accompanies CTS in people with hypothyroidism. CTS can develop before other signs of hypothyroidism become evident. It is thought that this CTS arises from deposition of myxedematous tissue in the carpal tunnel area.[98] Acroparesthesias may occur as a result of median nerve compression at the wrist. The paresthesias are almost always located bilaterally in the hands. Most clients do not require surgical treatment because the symptoms respond to thyroid replacement.

Proximal muscle weakness sometimes accompanied by pain is common in clients who have hypothyroidism. As mentioned earlier, muscle weakness is not always related to either the severity or the duration of hypothyroidism and can be present several months before the diagnosis of hypothyroidism is made. Muscle bulk is usually normal; muscle hypertrophy is rare. Deep tendon reflexes (DTRs) are characterized by slowed muscle contraction and relaxation (prolonged reflex).

Characteristically, the muscular complaints of the client with hypothyroidism are aches and pains and cramps or stiffness. Involved muscles are particularly likely to develop persistent myofascial TrPs. Of particular interest to the therapist is the concept that clinically any compromise of the energy metabolism of muscle aggravates and perpetuates TrPs. Treatment of the underlying hypothyroidism is essential in eliminating the TrPs,[99] but research also supports the need for soft tissue treatment to achieve full recovery.[100]

▶▶ PTA ACTION PLAN

Hypothyroidism and Fibromyalgia

There appears to be an association between hypothyroidism and fibromyalgia syndrome (FMS).[101] Individuals with FMS and clients with undiagnosed myofascial symptoms may benefit from a medical referral for evaluation of thyroid function.[102–105]

Diabetes Mellitus

The classic clinical signs and symptoms of untreated or uncontrolled DM usually include one or more of the following:

- Polyuria: increased urination caused by osmotic diuresis
- Polydipsia: increased thirst in response to polyuria
- Polyphagia: increased appetite and ingestion of food (usually only in type 1)

BOX 4.11 Systemic Manifestations of Hypothyroidism

Central Nervous System Effects
Slowed speech and hoarseness
Anxiety, depression
Slow mental function (loss of interest in daily activities, poor short-term memory)
Hearing impairment
Fatigue and increased sleep
Headache
Cerebellar ataxia

Musculoskeletal Effects
Proximal muscle weakness
Myalgias
Trigger points
Stiffness, cramps
Carpal tunnel syndrome
Prolonged deep tendon reflexes (especially Achilles)
Subjective report of paresthesias without supportive objective findings
Muscular and joint edema
Back pain
Increased bone density
Decreased bone formation and resorption

Pulmonary Effects
Dyspnea
Respiratory muscle weakness
Pleural effusion

Cardiovascular Effects
Bradycardia
Congestive heart failure
Poor peripheral circulation (pallor, cold skin, intolerance to cold, hypertension)
Severe atherosclerosis; hyperlipidemias

Angina
Elevated blood pressure
Increased cholesterol, triglycerides, low-density lipoprotein
Cardiomyopathy

Hematologic Effects
Anemia
Easy bruising

Integumentary Effects
Myxedema (periorbital and peripheral)
Thickened, cool, and dry skin
Scaly skin (especially elbows and knees)
Carotenosis (yellowing of the skin)
Coarse, thinning hair
Intolerance to cold
Nonpitting edema of hands and feet
Poor wound healing
Thin, brittle nails

Gastrointestinal Effects
Anorexia
Constipation
Weight gain disproportionate to caloric intake
Decreased absorption of nutrients
Decreased protein metabolism (retarded skeletal and soft tissue growth)
Delayed glucose uptake
Decreased glucose absorption

Genitourinary Effects
Infertility
Menstrual irregularity
Heavy menstrual bleeding

From Goodman CC, Snyder T: *Differential diagnosis for physical therapists*, ed 5, St. Louis, 2013, Saunders.

- Weight loss in the presence of polyphagia; weight loss caused by improper fat metabolism and breakdown of fat stores (usually only in type 1)
- Fatigue and weakness
- Blurred vision
- Irritability
- Recurring skin, gum, bladder, or other infections
- Numbness/tingling in hands and feet
- Cuts/bruises that are difficult and slow to heal

▶ PTA ACTION PLAN

Reporting Clinical Signs and Symptoms

The presence of any of these (and especially a cluster of three or more) requires immediate reporting to the PT and documentation in the medical record.

Clients who have already been diagnosed with diabetes must be monitored carefully for change in their physical status and/or physical signs and symptoms that signal physical complications of this endocrine disorder. Infection and atherosclerosis are the two primary long-term complications of this disease and are the usual causes of severe illness and death in the person with diabetes.

Poorly controlled DM can lead to various tissue changes that result in impaired wound healing. Decreased circulation to the skin can further delay or diminish healing. Skin eruptions called *xanthomas* (see Fig. 3.19) may appear when high lipid levels (e.g., cholesterol and triglycerides) in the blood cause fat deposits in the skin over extensor surfaces such as the elbows, knees, back of the head and neck, and heels.[106]

Yellow patches on the eyelids are another sign of hyperlipidemia. These are red flags that medical treatment is required to normalize lipid levels. The importance of diet and exercise cannot be underestimated here. Consultation with the PT is necessary to review and potentially revise the plan of care.

Diabetic Neuropathy

Any new signs or symptoms of diabetic neuropathy or worsening of already present signs and symptoms require evaluation by the PT. Watch for any of the following associated with diabetic neuropathy.

Peripheral (Motor and Sensory)
- Sensory, vibratory impairment of the extremities
- Burning, stabbing, pain, or numbness of distal lower extremities
- Extreme sensitivity to touch
- Muscle weakness and atrophy (diabetic amyotrophy)
- Absence of distal DTRs (knee, ankle)
- Loss of balance
- CTS

Autonomic
- Gastroparesis (delayed emptying of the stomach)
- Constipation or diarrhea
- Erectile dysfunction (sex drive unaffected; sexual function decreased)
- UTIs; urinary incontinence
- Profuse sweating

- Lack of oil production, resulting in dry, cracked skin susceptible to bacteria and infection
- Pupillary adjustment restricted (difficulty seeing at night)
- Orthostatic hypotension

Exercise-Related Complications

Any exercise can improve the body's ability to use insulin. Exercise causes a decrease in the amount of insulin the pancreas releases because muscle contractions are increasing blood glucose uptake. For the person taking insulin, exercise adds to the effects of the insulin, dropping blood sugars to dangerously low levels. Exercise for the person with DM must be planned and instituted cautiously and monitored carefully because significant complications can result from exercise of higher intensity or longer duration.

Exercise-related complications can be prevented by careful monitoring of the client's blood glucose level before, during, and after strenuous exercise sessions. Safe levels are individually determined but usually fall between 100 and 250 mg/dL; between 250 and 300 mg/dL is considered the "caution zone."

▶ PTA ACTION PLAN

Guidelines for Exercise for Individuals With Diabetes Mellitus

As always, the PTA is required to communicate with the supervising PT and/or nurse responsible for the client prior to exercising an individual with known DM. The following recommendations are general guidelines and not necessarily "fasting levels" (unless the person has not eaten for the last 12 hours for some reason). Exceptions are common, depending on the type of exercise, training level of the participant, expected glycemic pattern, and whether the individual is using an insulin pump.

If the blood glucose level is between 250 and 300 mg/dL at the start of the exercise, the client may be experiencing a state of insulin deficiency. Exercise is likely to raise the blood sugars more; the exercise session should be postponed until the blood glucose level is under better control. Blood glucose levels of 300 mg/dL or higher indicate the blood sugar level is too high to exercise safely, putting the client at risk for ketoacidosis. Exercise should be postponed until the blood glucose level drops to a safe preexercise range (between 100 and 250 mg/dL, possibly up to 300 mg/dL as described).

If the blood glucose level is less than 100 mg/dL, a 10- to 15-g carbohydrate snack should be given and the glucose retested in 15 minutes to ensure an appropriate level. When in doubt, always check with the supervising nurse or therapist.

▶ PTA ACTION PLAN

Follow-Up With the Physical Therapist

The PTA needs to thoroughly communicate the reasons for postponing the exercise session for that treatment and document blood glucose levels as well as the patient's physical signs and/or symptoms in the medical record. The PTA should request instruction from the PT regarding the specific education appropriate for the client on the importance of monitoring blood glucose levels prior to completing the home exercise program.

Points to Ponder

It is very important to have the client avoid insulin injection to active extremities within 1 hour of exercise because insulin is absorbed much more quickly in an active extremity.

It is also important to know the type, dose, and time of the client's insulin injections so that exercise is not planned for the peak activity times of the insulin.

Clients with type 1 diabetes may need to reduce the insulin dose or increase food intake when initiating an exercise program. During prolonged activities a 10- to 15-g carbohydrate snack is recommended for each 30 minutes of activity. Activities should be promptly stopped with the development of any symptoms of hypoglycemia, and blood glucose should be tested. In addition, individuals with diabetes should not exercise alone. Partners, teammates, and coaches must be educated regarding the possibility of hypoglycemia and the way to manage it.

Insulin Pump During Exercise. People with type 1 diabetes (and some individuals with insulin-requiring type 2 diabetes) may be using an insulin pump. Continuous subcutaneous insulin infusion therapy, known as *insulin pump therapy*, can bring the hormonal and metabolic responses to exercise close to normal for the individual with diabetes.[107,108]

Although there are many benefits of pump use for active individuals with diabetes, there are a few drawbacks as well.[109-111] Exercise can speed the development of diabetic ketoacidosis when there is an interruption of insulin delivery, which can quickly become a life-threatening condition.

Other considerations include the effect of excessive perspiration or water on the infusion set (the needle into the skin at the infusion site gets displaced), ambient temperature (insulin degrades under extreme conditions of heat or cold), and the effect of movement or contact at the infusion site (this causes skin irritation).

Insulin pump users who have preexercise blood glucose levels less than 100 mg/dL may not need a carbohydrate snack because they can reduce or suspend base insulin levels during an activity. The insulin reductions and required level of carbohydrate intake needed depend on the intensity and duration of the activity.[109]

Insulin Pump

The PTA should become familiar with the features of each pump in use by clients. Knowledge of basic guiding principles for exercise with diabetes and general recommendations for insulin regimen changes is also helpful.

RECOGNIZING AND REPORTING METABOLIC DISTURBANCE RED FLAGS

The PTA is unlikely to observe someone with a primary musculoskeletal lesion that reflects an underlying metabolic disorder. However, many inpatients in hospitals and some outpatients may be affected by disturbances in acid-base metabolism and other specific metabolic disorders. Only those conditions that are likely to be encountered by the PTA are included in this section.

Dehydration

Causes of the loss of both water and solutes include hemorrhage, profuse perspiration (e.g., marathon runners), and loss of GI tract secretions (e.g., vomiting, diarrhea, draining fistulas, ileostomy). Postsurgical patients who have had joint replacements, hip fractures, multiple trauma, or neurosurgery often lose blood and become hypovolemic despite efforts to maintain their homeostasis through blood transfusion and fluid replacement.[112]

Points to Ponder

Individuals being treated for hypertension with diuretics to reduce volume excess may be at risk for too much dieresis resulting in dehydration. It is important to observe individuals who take diuretic therapy for clinical symptoms of fluid loss, dehydration, and potassium depletion.

It is also very important to check laboratory data for the potassium level in any client taking diuretics, particularly before exercise. Any value below the normal range (<3.5 mEq/L) is potentially dangerous and could result in a lethal cardiac arrhythmia even with moderate cardiovascular exercise.[113] Any concerns should be discussed with the PT before carrying out the planned intervention.

Severe losses of water or solutes (or both) can lead to dehydration and hypovolemic shock. It is important for the PTA to be aware of possible fluid losses or water shifts in any client who is already compromised by advanced age or by a situation, such as an ileostomy or tracheostomy, that results in a continuous loss of fluid. Because the response to fluid loss is highly individual, it is important to recognize the early clinical symptoms of fluid loss and to carefully monitor vital signs and clinical symptoms in clients who are at risk, especially the elderly, the very young, or the chronically ill.[114]

Athletes and normal adults may experience orthostatic hypotension when slightly dehydrated, especially when intense exercise increases the core body temperature. The normal vascular system can accommodate this effectively. Severe dehydration (usually in endurance athletes participating in extreme events,[115,116] but also in compromised older adults) may require immediate evaluation.

Early clinical signs and symptoms of dehydration or fluid loss include the following:
- Thirst
- Weight loss

As the condition worsens, other symptoms may include the following:
- Poor skin turgor
- Dryness of the mouth, throat, and face
- Absence of sweat
- Increased body temperature
- Low urine output
- Postural hypotension (increased heart rate by 10 bpm and decreased systolic or diastolic BP by 20 mm Hg when moving from a supine to a sitting position)
- Dizziness when standing

- Confusion
- Increased hematocrit

Clinical signs and symptoms of potassium depletion include the following:

- Muscle weakness
- Fatigue
- Cardiac arrhythmias
- Abdominal distention
- Nausea and vomiting

RECOGNIZING AND REPORTING RED FLAGS OF CANCER

Early Warning Signs

For many years the American Cancer Society has publicized seven warning signs of cancer, the appearance of which could indicate the presence of cancer and the need for a medical evaluation (Box 4.12). Awareness of these signals is useful, but it is generally agreed that these symptoms do not always reflect early curable cancer; nor does this list include all possible signs for the different types of cancer.

Other early warning signs can include rapid, unintentional weight loss in a short period of time (e.g., 10% of the person's body weight in 2 weeks), unusual changes in vital signs, frequent infections (e.g., respiratory or urinary), and night pain.[117] Bleeding is an important sign of cancer. Bleeding develops as a result of ulcerations in the central areas of the tumor or by pressure on or rupture of local blood vessels. As the tumor continues to grow, it may enlarge beyond its capacity to obtain necessary nutrients, resulting in revitalization of portions of the tumor.[118]

This process of invading and compressing local tissue, shutting off blood supply to normal cells, is called *necrosis*. Tissue

---

BOX 4.12   **Cancers Linked to Obesity, Diet, and Nutrition**
Mouth, pharynx, esophagus
Colon, rectum
Larynx
Breast
Lung
Ovary
Stomach
Endometrium
Pancreas
Cervix
Gallbladder
Prostate
Liver
Kidney
Uterus
Bladder

From American Institute for Cancer Research [AICR]: *Food, nutrition, and the prevention of cancer: a global perspective*, Washington, DC, 2007, AICR.

---

necrosis ultimately leads to secondary infection, severe hemorrhage, and the development of pain when regional sensory nerves become involved. Other symptoms can include pathologic fractures, anemia, and thrombus formation.

Lumps, Lesions, and Lymph Nodes

The PTA should take special note of "T," which is *thickening or lump in breast or elsewhere*. Clients often point out a subcutaneous lesion (often a benign lipoma) and ask what it is. The PTA cannot answer this question directly, but a baseline list of observations of the lump or lesion is important to gather for an accurate report back to the supervising therapist.

▶▶ PTA ACTION PLAN
Follow-Up Questions

When observing and assessing skin lesions, remember to always ask these three questions:
- How long have you had this area of skin discoloration/mole/spot (use whatever brief description seems most appropriate)?
- Has it changed in the past 6 weeks to 6 months?
- Has the PT examined this area (or have you discussed this with the PT)?

▶▶ PTA ACTION PLAN
Communication With the Physical Therapist

The PTA should document and report location, size, shape, consistency, mobility or fixation, and signs of tenderness of any new skin lesions or changes in previously documented lesions. For more details, see the discussion of "The Integumentary System: Skin and Nail Beds" in Chapter 3.

A clinically detectable tumor the size of a small pea already contains billions of cells. Most health care professionals trained in palpation will be able to feel a lesion below the skin when it is half that size.[119] All suspicious lumps, lesions, or palpable lymph nodes should be reported to the PT for further evaluation (Case Example 4.7).

Any lymph nodes that are hard, immovable, and nontender raise the suspicion of cancer, especially in the presence of a previous history of cancer. Keep in mind that lymph nodes can fluctuate over the course of 10 to 14 days. When making observations, look for a cluster of signs and symptoms, recent trauma (including recent biopsy), or a past history of chronic fatigue syndrome, mononucleosis, and allergies.[120] Record and report all findings.

Proximal Muscle Weakness

Proximal muscle weakness of unknown cause may be an early sign of cancer (Fig. 4.10). This syndrome of proximal muscle weakness is referred to as *carcinomatous neuromyopathy*. It is accompanied by changes in two or more DTRs (ankle jerk usually remains intact[121]). See further discussion in "Change in One or More Deep Tendon Reflexes" in this chapter.

Recognizing muscle weakness is not always easy. Sometimes, questions must be directed toward function to find out this information. If a client is asked whether he or she has any muscle weakness, difficulty getting up from sitting, trouble climbing stairs, or SOB, the answer may very well be negative on all accounts.

CASE EXAMPLE 4.7 Palpable and Observable Lymph Nodes

A 73-year-old female was referred to a physical therapy clinic by her oncologist with a diagnosis of cervical radiculopathy. She had a history of uterine cancer 20 years ago and a history of breast cancer 10 years ago.

Treatment included a hysterectomy, left radical mastectomy, radiation therapy, and chemotherapy. She has been cancer free for almost 10 years. Her family physician, oncologist, and neurologist all evaluated her before she was referred to the physical therapist (PT).

The examination and evaluation were performed by the PT. A plan of care was developed to include local treatment of the cervical radiculopathy symptoms. On the third treatment session the client reported to the physical therapist assistant (PTA) that no changes in her symptoms have occurred and that the "swelling" and pain are worse today. The PTA quickly made note of the size, shape, and tenderness of the area and immediately reported to the PT who then completed a follow-up assessment of the client's status.

The PT found obvious lymphadenopathy of the left cervical and axillary lymph nodes. When asked if the referring physician (or other physicians) saw the "swelling," she told the therapist that she had not disrobed during her medical evaluation and consultation.

The PT must ascertain whether or not the physician is already aware of the problem and has requested physical therapy as a palliative measure. Requesting the physician's dictation or notes from the examination is essential. Contact with the physician will be important soon after the records are obtained, either to confirm the request as palliative therapy or to report your findings and confirm the need for medical reevaluation. If it turns out that the physician is indeed unaware of these physical findings, it is best to send a problem list identified as "outside the scope of a physical therapist" when returning the client to the physician.

Critical Thinking Activity
- Could the PTA have done more prior to reporting to the PT?
- Was it necessary for the PTA to immediately report to the PT during this session? Why or why not?

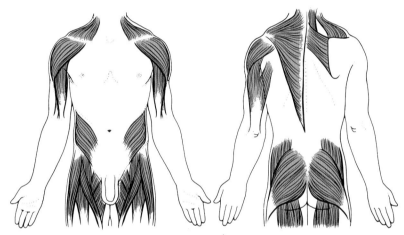

FIG. 4.10 Proximal muscle weakness can be observed clinically as a positive Trendelenburg test (usually present bilaterally) and abnormal manual muscle testing. It can also be observed functionally when the client has difficulty getting up from sitting or climbing stairs. As the weakness progresses, the client may have trouble getting into and out of a vehicle and/or the bathtub. Respiratory muscle weakness may be seen as shortness of breath or reported as altered activity to avoid dyspnea.

▶▶ PTA ACTION PLAN

Follow-Up Questions

The PTA should consider using these follow-up questions when it is necessary to further investigate the impairments leading to a person's loss of function:
- Do you have any trouble getting into and out of a chair?
- Are there any activities you would like to be able to do that you currently can't do?
- Are there any activities you used to be able to do that you can't do now?
- Are there activities you can do now that used to be much easier?
- Do you have any trouble going up and down stairs without stopping?
- Can you do all your grocery shopping without sitting down or stopping?
- Are you able to complete your household chores (e.g., make a meal, wash and dry clothes) without stopping?

Pain

Pain is rarely an early warning sign of cancer, even in the presence of unexplained bleeding. Night pain that is constant and intense (often rated 7 or higher on the Numeric Rating Scale) is a red flag. But not all people with musculoskeletal cancers experience night pain.[122]

Pain is usually the result of destruction of tissue or pressure on tissue caused by the presence of a tumor or lesion. The lesion or lesions must be of significant size or location to create pressure and/or occlusion of normal structures; pain will be dependent on the area of the body affected.

Acute and chronic cancer-related pain syndromes can occur in association with diagnostic and therapeutic interventions such as bone marrow biopsy, lumbar puncture, colonoscopy, percutaneous biopsy, and thoracentesis. Chemotherapy and radiation toxicities can result in painful peripheral neuropathies.

Likewise, many different chronic pain syndromes (e.g., tumor-related radiculopathy, phantom breast pain, postsurgical pelvic or abdominal pain, burning perineum syndrome, postradiation pain syndrome) can occur as a result of tumors or cancer therapy. The supervising PT can guide the PTA in recognizing pain patterns of concern that require reporting and further follow-up.

Change in One or More Deep Tendon Reflexes

When testing of DTRs is performed, the PTA will observe that some individuals have very brisk reflexes under normal circumstances; others are much more hyporeflexive.

Tumors (whether benign or malignant) can also press on the spinal nerve root, mimicking a disk problem. A lesion that is small enough can put just enough pressure to irritate the nerve root, resulting in a hyperreflexive DTR. A large tumor can obliterate the reflex arc, resulting in diminished or absent reflexes. Either way, changes in DTRs must be considered a red-flag sign (possibly of cancer[80]) that should be documented and further investigated by the PT.

Clinical Manifestations of Cancer Recurrence or Metastases

The PTA may be the first to see clinical manifestations of primary cancer but is more likely to see signs and symptoms of cancer recurrence or cancer metastasis. In general, the five most common sites of cancer metastasis are bone, lymph nodes, lung,

liver, and brain.[123,124] However, the PTA is most likely to observe signs and symptoms affecting one of the following systems:
- Integumentary
- Pulmonary
- Neurologic
- Musculoskeletal
- Hepatic

Each of these systems has a core group of most commonly observed signs and symptoms (Box 4.13).

Pulmonary

Pleural pain and dyspnea are two common symptoms of pulmonary compromise. When either or both of these pulmonary symptoms occur, look for increased symptoms with deep breathing and activity.

Ask about a productive cough with bloody or rust-colored sputum. Ask about new onset of wheezing at any time or difficulty breathing at night. Symptoms that are relieved by sitting up are indicative of pulmonary impairment and must be reported to the PT.

BOX 4.13 Signs and Symptoms of Metastases*

Integumentary
Any skin lesion or observable/palpable skin changes
Any observable or palpable change in nail beds (fingers or toes)
Unusual mole (use ABCDE method of assessment)
Cluster mole formation
Bleeding or discharge from mole, skin lesion, scar, or nipple
Tenderness and soreness around a mole; sore that does not heal

Musculoskeletal
May present as an asymptomatic soft tissue mass
Bone pain:
- Deep or localized
- Increased with activity
- Decreased tolerance to weightbearing; antalgic gait
- Does not respond to physical agents
Soft tissue swelling
Pathologic fractures
Hypercalcemia CNS
- Musculoskeletal
- Cardiovascular
- Gastrointestinal
Back or rib pain

Neurologic (Central Nervous System)
Drowsiness, lethargy
Headaches
Nausea, vomiting
Depression
Increased sleeping
Irritability, personality change
Confusion, increased confusion
Change in mental status, memory loss, difficulty concentrating

Vision changes (blurring, blind spots, double vision)
Numbness, tingling
Balance/coordination problems
Changes in deep tendon reflexes
Change in muscle tone for individual with previously diagnosed neurologic condition
Positive Babinski reflex
Clonus (ankle or wrist)
Changes in bowel and bladder function
Myotomal weakness pattern
Paraneoplastic syndrome

Pulmonary
Pleural pain
Dyspnea
New onset of wheezing
Productive cough with sputum tinged yellow, green, or rust color

Hepatic
Abdominal pain and tenderness
Jaundice
Ascites
Distended abdomen
Dilated upper abdominal veins
Peripheral edema
General malaise and fatigue
Bilateral carpal/tarsal tunnel syndrome
Asterixis (liver flap) (see Fig. 3.5)
Palmar erythema (liver palms) (see Fig. 3.4)
Spider angiomas (over the abdomen) (see Fig. 3.6)
Nail beds of Terry (see Fig. 3.3)
Right shoulder pain

* Seen most often in a physical therapy practice.
ABCDE, Asymmetry, border, color, diameter, evolving; *CNS,* central nervous system.

Neurologic

When tumors compress, impinge, or infiltrate any of the nerve plexuses, the primary sign is unrelenting pain (worse at night) followed by development of weakness. Watch for focal sensory disturbances or weakness in the distribution of the affected plexus or spinal cord segment involved. Brachial plexopathy most commonly occurs in carcinoma of the breast and lung; lumbosacral plexopathy is most common with colorectal and gynecologic tumors, sarcomas, and lymphomas.[125,126]

If a tumor is growing in the motor cortex, the client may develop isolated extremity weakness or hemiparesis. If the tumor is developing in the cerebellum, coordination may be affected with ataxia as an observable sign to be reported.

? PICTURE THE PATIENT

Two of the most common clinical manifestations of brain tumor are headache and personality change, but personality change is often attributed to depression, delaying the diagnosis of brain tumor. Tumors that affect the frontal lobes are most likely to produce personality changes (mentioned by the family to the PTA). Seizures occur in approximately one-third of persons with metastatic brain tumors. Any sign of seizure activity must be reported.

Whether from a primary cord tumor or a metastasis, compression of the cord with neck or back pain can be the first symptom of cancer.[127] Prostate, lung, and breast cancers are the most common tumors to metastasize to the spine, leading to epidural spinal cord compression, but lymphoma, multiple myeloma, and carcinomas of the colon or kidney and sarcomas can also result in spinal cord and nerve root compression.[128,129] The PTA may observe progressive pain that does not respond to therapy, possibly accompanied by stiffness, scoliosis, or other problems such as severe neurologic deficits.[130]

Peripheral neuropathy with loss of vibratory sense, proprioception, and DTRs is most often chemotherapy related (e.g., cisplatin, Taxol, vincristine). Numbness, tingling, and burning pain in the hands and feet and loss of balance and difficulties with mobility are common with this problem.[131] The PT should help the PTA understand the different types and etiology of peripheral neuropathy (e.g., chemotherapy-induced versus lymphedema-induced nerve compression) before planning treatment intervention.

Musculoskeletal

Bone pain, resulting from structural damage, rate of bone resorption, periosteal irritation, and nerve entrapment, is the most common complication of metastatic disease to the skeletal system. A history of sudden onset of severe pain usually indicates the complication of a pathologic fracture (a break in an already weakened bone). Pathologic fractures are the result of metastatic disease of primary cancers most often affecting the lung, prostate, and breast.

? PICTURE THE PATIENT

Bone pain is usually deep, intractable, and poorly localized, sometimes described as burning or aching and accompanied by episodes of stabbing discomfort (Case Example 4.8). The pain may be cyclic and progressive until it becomes constant. The pain is made worse by activity, especially weight-bearing activity. It is often worse at night, awakening the person; neither sleep nor lying down provides relief. Pain at night that is unrelieved by rest or change in position is a red flag that must be reported.

▶▶ PTA ACTION PLAN

Red Flags to Report

The PTA should watch for pain that does not respond to physical agents or other physical therapy intervention. Sometimes the client has some relief after the first few sessions of physical therapy, but pain returns and may even be worse than before. The PTA may think the chosen intervention has been unsuccessful and is at fault. Consider it a red flag whenever a client fails to improve or improves and then gets worse. Further evaluation by the PT is required under these circumstances.

CASE EXAMPLE 4.8 Uterine Cancer With Bone Metastasis

A 44-year-old slender, athletic female with isolated left knee pain of unknown cause was referred to physical therapy by her physician for a "strengthening program." She was actively involved in a variety of physical activities, including a co-ed baseball team, a hiking club, and church basketball intramurals, but she could not recall any specific injury, fall, or other impact to her leg. She had a pair of shoe orthotics prescribed by a podiatrist 5 years ago "to compensate for my excessive Q-angle."

Initial Evaluation Information

The physical therapy examination was unremarkable for any joint swelling, redness, or palpable warmth. There was point tenderness along the medial joint line and a palpable although asymptomatic plica. Joint integrity was intact, and all special tests were negative. The neurologic screening examination was also considered within normal limits, although muscle strength for the quadriceps and hamstrings was diminished by pain. Pain was present on weight-bearing activities but did not prevent the female from participating in all activities. There was no reported night pain, fever, or other associated signs and symptoms.

Without a definitive physical therapy diagnosis a treatment plan was outlined to include modalities for pain and a stretching and strengthening program.

Intervention

A week later, the client reports to the physical therapist assistant (PTA) that her pain level has escalated on the Numeric Rating Scale from 3 to 10 (on a scale from 1 to 10) with constant pain that has kept her awake at night for hours. When she returned to the physical therapy clinic, she was using crutches and was not bearing weight on the left leg. The PTA immediately requested that the physical therapist see the client for further examination because of the significant decline in status since her last session.

Results: Given the insidious onset of this joint pain and the rapidly progressive nature of the symptoms, this client was immediately sent back to her physician. A diagnosis of bone metastasis was made, with early-stage endometrial carcinoma appearing as an unusual, isolated skeletal lesion.

She was treated with aggressive multidisciplinary therapy, including limb salvage and physical therapy as part of her rehabilitation program. The early referral most likely contributed to her favorable prognosis and cancer-free status 2 years later.

Hepatic

Symptoms of hepatic manifestations of cancer observed by the PTA include bilateral CTS/tarsal tunnel syndrome, possibly accompanied by abdominal pain and tenderness with general malaise and fatigue. Right upper quadrant pain with possible referral to the right shoulder may also occur with or without CTS. A client presenting with shoulder or upper back pain may not think nausea and abdominal bloating are related in any way to the symptoms in the wrists and hands. It may be appropriate to ask about the presence of other GI signs and symptoms.

Recognizing When to Consult With the Physical Therapist

 PTA ACTION PLAN

Communication With the Physical Therapist

Guidelines for Immediate Attention

It is important for the PTA to understand that the PT is not responsible for diagnosing cancer. The primary goal in screening for cancer is to make sure the client's problem is within the scope of a PT's practice. In this regard, documentation of key findings and communication with the PT and physician are both very important.

- Presence of recently discovered lumps or nodules or changes in previously present lumps, nodules, or moles, especially in the presence of a previous history of cancer or when accompanied by carpal tunnel or other neurologic symptoms.
- Detection of a palpable, fixed, irregular mass in the breast, axilla, or elsewhere requires medical referral or a recommendation to the client to contact a physician for evaluation of the mass.
- Suspicious lymph node enlargement or lymph node changes; generalized lymphadenopathy.
- Presence of any of the early warning signs of cancer, including idiopathic muscle weakness accompanied by decreased DTRs.
- Any unexplained bleeding from any area (e.g., rectum, blood in urine or stool, unusual or unexpected vaginal bleeding, breast, penis, nose, ears, mouth, mole, skin, or scar).

Points to Ponder

- Whether you are working in an oncology setting or in a general practice with an occasional client, good resource information is available. Thorough, reliable, and up-to-date information about specific types of cancer, cancer treatments, and recent breakthroughs in cancer research is available from The Abramson Cancer Center of the University of Pennsylvania (Philadelphia) at http://oncolink.upenn.edu.
- Fifty percent of clients with persistent back pain from a malignancy have an identifiable preceding trauma or injury to account for the pain or symptoms. Always remember that clients may erroneously attribute symptoms to an event.
- The five most common sites of metastasis are the lymph nodes, liver, lung, bone, and brain.
- Lung, breast, prostate, thyroid, and the lymphatics are the primary sites responsible for most metastatic bone disease.
- Monitoring physiologic responses (vital signs) to exercise is important in the immunosuppressed population. Watch closely for early signs (dyspnea, pallor, sweating, and fatigue) of cardiopulmonary complications of cancer treatment.

REFERENCES

1. Bushnell BD: Perioperative medical comorbidities in the orthopaedic patient, *J Am Acad Orthop Surg* 16:216–227, 2008.
2. Hillman R: *Hematology in clinical practice*, ed 5, New York, 2011, McGraw-Hill.
3. Hoffman R: *Hematology: basic principles and practice*, ed 5, Philadelphia, 2008, Churchill-Livingstone.
4. Sostres C, Gargallo CJ, Lanas A: Nonsteroidal anti-inflammatory drugs and upper and lower gastrointestinal mucosal damage, *Arthritis Res Ther* 15(Suppl 3):s3, 2013.
5. Weber CG: *Clinical hematology-oncology 2013*, ed 12. In The clinical medicine series, 2013, Primary Care Software, Amazon Digital Series, Inc
6. Casciato DA: *Manual of clinical oncology*, ed 7, Philadelphia, 2012, Lippincott, Williams & Wilkins.
7. Goodman C, Helgeson K: *Exercise prescription for medical conditions: handbook for physical therapists*, Philadelphia, 2011, FA Davis.
8. van Mourik Y: Triage of frail elderly with reduced exercise tolerance in primary care (TREE). A clustered randomized diagnostic study, *BMC Public Health* 12:385, 2012. https://doi.org/10.1186/1471-2458-12-385
9. Connes P, Machado R, Hue O, Reid H: Exercise limitation, exercise testing and exercise recommendations in sickle cell anemia, *Clin Hemorheol Microcirc* 49(1–4):151–163, 2011.
10. Bonow RO: *Braunwald's heart disease: a textbook of medicine*, ed 9, Philadelphia, 2011, Saunders.
11. Goldman L, Schafer AI: *Goldman's Cecil medicine*, ed 24, Philadelphia, 2012, Saunders.
12. Fillit HM: *Brocklehurst's textbook of geriatric medicine*, ed 7, Philadelphia, 2010, Saunders.
13. Mason RJ: *Murray and Nadel's textbook of respiratory medicine*, ed 5, Philadelphia, 2010, Saunders.
14. Harward MP: *Medical secrets*, ed 5, St. Louis, 2012, Mosby.
15. Leslie KO, Wick MR: *Leslie & Wick: practical pulmonary pathology*, ed 2, Philadelphia, 2011, Saunders.
16. Frownfelter D, Dean E: *Cardiovascular and pulmonary physical therapy: evidence to practice*, ed 5, St. Louis, 2012, Mosby.
17. Scharf SM: History and physical examination. In Baum GL, Wolinsky E, editors: *Textbook of pulmonary diseases* ed 5, Boston, 1989, Little, Brown, pp 218.
18. Raskob GE, Silverstein F, Bratzler DW, et al: Surveillance for deep vein thrombosis and pulmonary embolism: recommendations from a national workshop, *Am J Prev Med* 38(4 Suppl):S502–509, 2010.
19. Le Gal G, Carrier M, Rodger M: Clinical decision rules in venous thromboembolism, *Best Pract Res Clin Hematol* 25:303–317, 2012.
20. Molloy W, English J, O'Dwyer R, et al: Clinical findings in the diagnosis of proximal deep venous thrombosis, *Ir Med J* 75:119–120, 1982.
21. Delis KT: Incidence, natural history, and risk factors of deep vein thrombosis in elective knee arthroscopy, *Thromb Haemost* 86(3):817–821, 2001.
22. Shah NB: 82-year-old man with bilateral leg swelling, *Mayo Clinic Proc* 85(9):859–862, 2010.
23. Yin HZ, Shan CM: The effect of nursing intervention based on Autar scale results to reduce deep venous thrombosis incidence in orthopaedic surgery patients, *Int J Nurs Sci* 2(2):178–183, 2015.
24. Spencer NJ, Hu H: Enteric nervous system: sensory transduction, neural circuits and gastrointestinal motility, *Nat Rev Gastroenterol Hepatol* 17(6):338–351, 2020.

25. Goldstein AM, Hofstra RMW, Burns AJ: Building a brain in the gut: development of the enteric nervous system, *Clin Genet* 83(4):307–316, 2013.

26. Pert C: Paradigms from neuroscience: when shift happens, *Mol Interv* 3(7):361–366, 2003.

27. Wood J: Enteric nervous system: brains-in-the-gut. In Said HM, editor: *Physiology of the gastrointestinal tract,* , 2018, Elsevier, pp 6e.

28. O'Hare A: Gut feelings: the potential of oral administration of therapeutic peptides to the brain, *Nanomedicine (Lond)* 7(7):946, 2012.

29. Burnet PW: Gut bacteria and brain function: the challenges of a growing field, *Proc Natl Acad Sci USA* 109(4):E175, 2012.

30. Moraes LJ, Miranda MB, Loures LF, et al: A systematic review of psychoneuroimmunology-based interventions, *Psychol Health Med* 23(6):635–652, 2018.

31. Ledlie J, Renfro M: Balloon kyphoplasty: one-year outcomes in vertebral body height restoration, chronic pain, and activity levels, *J Neurosurg (Spine I)* 98:36–42, 2003.

32. Travell JG, Simons DG: *Myofascial pain and dysfunction: the trigger point manual,* Baltimore, 1992, Williams & Wilkins. vol 2

33. Siegel JD, Rhinehart E, Jackson M, Chiarello L. Healthcare Infection Control Practices Advisory Committee: 2007 guideline for isolation precautions: preventing transmission of infectious agents in health care settings, *Am J Infect Control* 35(10):S65–S164, 2007.

34. Gracey E, Vereecke L, McGovern D, et al: Revisiting the gut-joint axis: links between gut inflammation and spondyloarthritis, *Nat Rev Rheumoatol* 16:415–433, 2020.

35. Gran JT, Husby G: Joint manifestations in gastrointestinal diseases, *Digest Dis* 10:295–312, 1992.

36. Huang V, Mishra R, Thanabalan R, Nguyen GC: Patient awareness of extraintestinal manifestations of inflammatory bowel disease, *J Crohns Colitis* 7(8):e318–e324, 2013.

37. Brakenhoff LK: The joint-gut axis in inflammatory bowel disease, *J Crohns Colitis* 4(3):257–268, 2010.

38. Baeten D: Influence of the gut and cytokine patterns in spondyloarthropathy, *Clin Exp Rheumatol* 20(6 Suppl 28):S38–S42, 2002.

39. Sieper J, Rudwaleit M, Braun J, van der Heijde D: Diagnosing reactive arthritis: role of clinical setting in the value of serologic and microbiologic assays, *Arthritis Rheum* 46:319, 2002.

40. Hvatum M, Kanerud L, Hällgren R, Brandtzaeg P: The gut-joint axis: cross reactive food antibodies in rheumatoid arthritis, *Gut* 55(9):1240–1247, 2006.

41. Rudwaleit M, Baeten D: Ankylosing spondylitis and bowel disease, *Best Pract Res Clin Rheumatol* 20(3):451–471, 2006.

42. van der Horst-Bruinsma IE, Nurmohamed MT: Management and evaluation of extra-articular manifestations in spondyloarthritis, *Ther Adv Musculoskelet Dis* 4(6):413–422, 2012.

43. van der Horst-Bruinsma IE: Comorbidities in patients with spondyloarthritis, *Rheum Dis Clin North Am* 38(3):523–538, 2012.

44. Yüksel I: Peripheral arthritis in the course of inflammatory bowel diseases, *Dig Dis Sci* 56(1):183–187, 2011.

45. Aluka KJ, Turner PL, Fullum TM: Guillain-Barré syndrome and postbariatric surgery polyneuropathies, *JSLS* 13(2):250–253, 2009.

46. Yasawy ZM, Hassan A: Post bariatric surgery acute axonal polyneuropathy: doing your best is not always enough, *Ann Indian Acad Neurol* 20(3):309–312, 2017.

47. D'Incà R, Podswiadek M, Ferronato A, et al: Articular manifestations in inflammatory bowel disease patients: a prospective study, *Dig Liver Dis* 41(8):565–569, 2009.

48. Peterson C: *The hepatic, pancreatic and biliary systems.* In *Goodman and Fuller's pathology: implications for the physical therapist,* ed 5, 2020, Elsevier.

49. Kumar V, Abbas AK, Aster JC: *Robbins basic patholgoy,* ed 9, 2013, Elsevier.

50. Baxter RE, Moore JH: Diagnosis and treatment of acute exertional rhabdomyolysis, *J Orthop Sports Phys Ther* 33(3):104–108, 2003.

51. Kumbhare D: Validity of serum creatine kinase as a measure of muscle injury produced by lumbar surgery, *J Spinal Disord Tech* 21(1):49–54, 2008.

52. Reese JM: Exertional rhabdomyolysis: attrition through exercise, a case series and review of the literature, *J Spec Oper Med* 12(3):52–56, 2012.

53. Su MS, Jiang Y, Yan XY, et al: Alcohol abuse-related severe acute pancreatitis with rhabdomyolysis complications, *Exp Ther Med* 5(1):189–192, 2013.

54. Lenfant C: ACC/AHA/NHLBI clinical advisory on the use and safety of statins, *Cardiol Rev* 20(4Suppl):9–11, 2003.

55. Alreja G, Inayatullah S, Goel S, Braden G: Rhabdomyolysis caused by an unusual interaction between azithromycin and simvastatin, *J Cardiovasc Dis Res* 3(4):319–322, 2012.

56. Chatham K: Suspected statin-induced respiratory muscle myopathy during long-term inspiratory muscle training in a patient with diaphragmatic paralysis, *Phys Ther* 89(3):1–10, 2009.

57. Newman CB, Palmer G, Silbershatz H, et al: Safety of atorvastatin derived from analysis of 44 completed trials in 9,416 patients, *Am J Cardiol* 92(6):670–676, 2003.

58. Newman CB: The safety and tolerability of atorvastatin 10 mg in the Collaborative Atorvastatin Diabetes Study (CARDS), *Diab Vasc Dis Res* 5(3):177–183, 2008.

59. Mareedu RK: Use of an electronic medical record to characterize cases of intermediate statin-induced muscle toxicity, *Prev Cardiol* 12(2):88–94, 2009.

60. Harris LJ: Clinical and laboratory phenotype of patients experiencing statin intolerance attributable to myalgia, *J Clin Lipidol* 5(4):299–307, 2011.

61. Janssen SP: Muscle problems due to statins: underestimated, *Ned Tijdschr Geneeskd* 154:A1684, 2010.

62. Tomlinson SS, Mangione KK: Potential adverse effects of statins on muscle, *Phys Ther* 85:459–465, 2005.

63. Buettner C: Prevalence of musculoskeletal pain and statin use, *J Gen Intl Medicine* 23:1182–1186, 2008.

64. Buettner C: Statin use and musculoskeletal pain among adults with and without arthritis, *Am J Med* 125(2):176–182, 2012.

65. Lasker SS: Myalgia while taking statins, *BMJ* 345:e5348, 2012.

66. Meador BM: Statin-associated myopathy and its exacerbation with exercise, *Muscle Nerve* 42(4):469–479, 2010.

67. Ballantyne CM, Corsini A, Davidson MH, et al: Risk for myopathy with statin therapy in high-risk patients, *Arch Intern Med* 163(5):553–564, 2003.

68. Gupta A, Thompson PD: The relationship of vitamin D deficiency to statin myopathy, *Atherosclerosis* 215(1):23–29, 2011.

69. Shawcross DL, Wendon JA: The neurological manifestations of acute liver failure, *Neurochem Int* 60(7):662–671, 2012.

70. Mendizabal M, Silva MO: Images in clinical medicine: asterixis, *N Engl J Med* 363(9):e14, 2010.

71. Lozano-Calderon S: The quality and strength of evidence for etiology: example of carpal tunnel syndrome, *J Hand Surg* 33A(4):525–538, 2008.

72. Alty JE, Kempster PA: A practical guide to the differential diagnosis of tremor, *Postgrad Med J* 87(1031):623–629, 2011.

73. Storme O, Saucedo JT, Garcia-Mora A, Dehesa-Davila M, Naber KG: Risk factors and predisposing conditions for urinary tract infection, *Ther Adv Urol* 11, 2019. 1756287218814382

74. Wein AJ: *Campbell-Walsh urology*, ed 10, Philadelphia, 2011, Saunders.

75. Haylen BT, de Ridder D, Freeman RM, et al: An International Urogynecological Association (IUGA)/International Continence Society (ICS) joint report on the terminology for female pelvic floor dysfunction, *Int Urogynecol J* 21:5–26, 2010.

76. Milsom I, Gyhagen M: The prevalence of urinary incontinence, *Climacteric* 22(3):217–222, 2019.

77. Stothers L, Friedman B: Risk factors for the development of stress urinary incontinence in women, *Curr Urol Rep* 12(5): 363–369, 2011.

78. Townsend CM: *Sabiston textbook of surgery*, ed 19, Philadelphia, 2012, Saunders.

79. Schmidt-Hansen M, Berendse S, Hamilton W: The association between symptoms and bladder or renal tract cancer in primary care: a systematic review, *Br J Gen Pract* 65(640):e769–e775, 2015.

80. Ferri FF: *Ferri's clinical advisor 2013*, St. Louis, 2013, Mosby.

81. Spahn G: Metaanalysis for the evaluation of risk factors for carpal tunnel syndrome (CTS) Part II. General factors, *Z Orthop Unfall* 150(5):516–524, 2012.

82. Spahn G: Metaanalysis for the evaluation of risk factors for carpal tunnel syndrome (CTS) Part I. General factors, *Z Orthop Unfall* 150(5):503–515, 2012.

83. Tseng CH: Medical and non-medical correlates of carpal tunnel syndrome in a Taiwan cohort of one million, *Eur J Neurol* 19(1): 91–97, 2012.

84. Phalen GS: The carpal tunnel syndrome: seventeen years' experience in diagnosis and treatment of six hundred and fifty-four hands, *J Bone Joint Surg* 48A(2):211–228, 1966.

85. Wluka AE, Cicuttini FM, Spector TD: Menopause, oestrogens, and arthritis, *Maturitas* 35(3):183–189, 2000.

86. Ferry S, Hannaford P, Warskyj M, et al: Carpal tunnel syndrome: a nested case-control study of risk factors in women, *Am J Epidemiol* 151(6):566–574, 2000.

87. Osterman M: Carpal tunnel syndrome in pregnancy, *Orthop Clin North Am* 43(4):515–520, 2012.

88. Chen CH: Unusual causes of carpal tunnel syndrome: space occupying lesions, *J Hand Surg Eur Vol* 37(1):14–19, 2012.

89. Sikkandar MF: Gouty wrist arthritis causing carpal tunnel syndrome: a case report, *Med J Malaysia* 67(3):333–334, 2012.

90. Hernández-Cortés P: Digital flexion contracture and severe carpal tunnel syndrome due to tophaceus infiltration of wrist flexor tendon: first manifestation of gout, *Orthopedics* 34(11):e797–e799, 2011.

91. Michlovitz S: Conservative interventions for carpal tunnel syndrome, *J Orthop Sports Phys Ther* 34(10):591–598, 2004.

92. Dellon AL: The four medial ankle tunnels: a critical review of perceptions of tarsal tunnel syndrome and neuropathy, *Neurosurg Clin N Am* 19(4):629–648, 2008.

93. Ozdemir O: Tarsal tunnel syndrome in a patient on long-term peritoneal dialysis: case report, *Turk Neurosurg* 17(4):283–285, 2007.

94. Sriwong PT, Sirasaporn P, Foochareon C, Srichompoo K: Median neuropathy at the wrist in patients with systemic sclerosis: two-year follow-up study, *Reumatologia* 56(5):294–300, 2018.

95. Katz JN: Clinical practice: carpal tunnel syndrome, *N Engl J Med* 346:1807, 2002.

96. Hsu JE: Current review of adhesive capsulitis, *J Shoulder Elbow Surg* 20(3):502–514, 2011.

97. Garcilazo C: Shoulder manifestations of diabetes mellitus, *Curr Diabetes Rev* 6(5):334–340, 2010.

98. Firestein GS: *Kelley's textbook of rheumatology*, ed 9, Philadelphia, 2012, Saunders.

99. Lowe JC, Honeyman-Lowe G: *The metabolic treatment of fibromyalgia*, Lafayette, 2000, McDowell Health Science Books.

100. Bazzichi L, Rossi A, Zirafa C, et al: Thryoid autoimmunity may represent a predisposition for the development of fibromyalgia? *Rheumatol Int* 32:335, 2012.

101. Lowe JC, Reichman AJ, Honeyman GS, et al: Thyroid status of fibromyalgia patients, *Clin Bull Myofascial Ther* 3(1):47–53, 1998.

102. Lowe JC, Reichman AJ, Yellin BA: A case-control study of metabolic therapy for fibromyalgia: long term follow-up comparison of treated and untreated patients, *Clin Bull Myofascial Ther* 3(1):65–79, 1998.

103. Bazzichi R, Rossi A, Zirafa C, et al: Thyroid autoimmunity may represent a predisposition for the development of fibromyalgia? *Rheumatol Int* 32(2):335–341, 2012.

104. Geenen R, Jacobs JW, Bijlsma JW: Evaluation and management of endocrine dysfunction in fibromyalgia, *Rheum Dis Clin North Am* 28(2):389–404, 2002.

105. Garrison RL, Breeding PC: A metabolic basis for fibromyalgia and its related disorders: the possible role of resistance to thyroid hormone, *Med Hypotheses* 61(2):182–189, 2003.

106. Habif TP: *Clinical dermatology*, ed 5, St. Louis, 2010, Mosby.

107. Yardley JE, Iscoe KE, Sigal RJ, et al: Insulin pump therapy is associated with less post-exercise hyperglycemia than multiple daily injections: an observational study of physically active type 1 diabetes patients, *Diabetes Technol Ther* 15(1):84–88, 2013.

108. Schmidt S: Effects of everyday life events on glucose, insulin, and glucagon dynamics in continuous subcutaneous insulin infusion-treated type 1 diabetes: collection of clinical data for glucose modeling, *Diabetes Technol Ther* 14(3):210–217, 2012.

109. Colberg SR, Walsh J: Pumping insulin during exercise: what healthcare providers and diabetic patients need to know, *Phys Sportsmed* 30(4):33–38, 2002.

110. Meneghini L: Practical aspects and considerations when switching between continuous subcutaneous insulin infusion and multiple daily injections, *Diabetes Technol Ther* 12(Suppl 1):S109–S114, 2010.

111. Alsaleh FM: Insulin pumps: from inception to the present and toward the future, *J Clin Pharm Ther* 35(2):127–138, 2010.

112. Swope R, Adams A: Prevention and treatment of orthostatic hypotension in the orthopedic patient population, *Orthopedics* 35(7):600–603, 2012.

113. Corbett J: *Laboratory tests and diagnostic procedures with nursing diagnoses*, ed 8, Upper Saddle River, 2012, Prentice Hall Health.

114. Roberts JR: *Clinical procedures in emergency medicine*, ed 5, Philadelphia, 2010, Saunders.

115. Scott JM, Esch BT, Lusina SJ, et al: Post-exercise hypotension and cardiovascular responses to moderate orthostatic stress in endurance-trained males, *Appl Physiol Nutr Metab* 33(2):246–253, 2008.

116. Asplund CA, O'Connor FG, Noakes TD: Exercise-associated collapse: an evidence-based review and primer for clinicians, *Br J Sports Med* 45(14):1157–1162, 2011.

117. Bope ET: *Bope & Kellerman: Conn's current therapy 2013*, Philadelphia, 2013, Saunders.

118. Walsh D: *Palliative medicine*, ed 1, Philadelphia, 2009, Saunders.

119. McGarvey CL: *Principles of oncology for the physical therapist,* Long Island, 2003, Stony Brook University.
120. Lester SC: *Manual of surgical pathology,* ed 3, Philadelphia, 2010, Saunders.
121. Abeloff MD: *Abeloff's clinical oncology,* ed 4, Philadelphia, 2008, Churchill Livingstone.
122. Slipman CW: Epidemiology of spine tumors presenting to musculoskeletal physiatrists, *Arch Phys Med Rehab* 84:492–495, 2003.
123. Riihimaki M, Thomsen H, Sundquist K, Sundquist J, Hemmink K: Clinical landscape of cancer metastases, *Cancer Med* 7(11):5534–5542, 2018.
124. National Cancer Institute: *Metastatic cancer: when cancer spreads.* https://www.cancer.gov/types/metastatic-cancer Accessed July 16, 2023.
125. Jaeckle KA: Neurological manifestations of neoplastic and radiation-induced plexopathies, *Semin Neurol* 24:385–393, 2004.
126. Jaeckle KA: Neurologic manifestations of neoplastic and radiation-induced plexopathies, *Semin Neurol* 30(3):254–262, 2010.
127. Jimi SI, Yasui Takaharu, Hotokezaka Masayuki, et al: Clinical features and prognostic factors of bone metastases from colorectal cancer, *Surg Today* 43(7):751–756, 2013.
128. Abrahm JL: Assessment and treatment of patients with malignant spinal cord compression, *J Support Oncol* 2:377–401, 2004.
129. Siemionow K: Identifying serious causes of back pain: cancer, infection, fracture, *Cleveland Clinic J Med* 75(8):557–566, 2008.
130. Uccello M: Osteoblastoma of cervical spine causing an unusual neck pain, *Eur Rev Med Pharmacol Sci* 16:17–20, 2012.
131. Hile ES: Persistent mobility disability after neurotoxic chemotherapy, *Phys Ther* 90(11):1649–1657, 2010.
132. Callahan L, Woods K: Cardiopulmonary responses to exercise in women with sickle cell anemia, *Am J Respir Crit Care Med* 165(9):1309–1316, 2002.

5

Recognizing and Reporting Red Flags in the Head, Neck, and Back

In the United States, back pain is one of the most common reasons individuals seek medical care.[1] It is estimated that almost half of all adults have reported an episode of acute low back pain (LBP) during their lifetime and 20% of those report frequent LBP.[2]

It has been suggested that mechanical LBP and leg pain with spinal causes compose approximately 97% of all cases.[3] Nonmechanical spinal disease can be attributed to neoplasm, infection, or inflammation in 1% of all cases with another 2% accounted for by visceral disorders (pelvic organs, gastrointestinal [GI] dysfunction, renal involvement, and abdominal aneurysms).[4]

Most cases of back pain in adults are related to age-related degenerative processes, physical loading, and musculoligamentous injuries. Many mechanical causes of back pain resolve within 1 to 4 weeks without serious problems. Fewer than 2% of individuals presenting with LBP present with significant neurologic involvement or other signs that require referral or imaging.[5] Up to 10% of LBP patients have no identifiable cause.[6]

Sacroiliac (SI) joint dysfunction can mimic LBP and diskogenic disease with pain referred below the knee to the foot. Studies show SI joint dysfunction is the primary source of LBP in 18% to 30% of people with LBP.[6-12] As always, when conducting a physical examination, the therapist must consider the possibility of a mechanical problem above or below the area of pain or symptom presentation.

A smaller number of people will develop chronic pain without organic pathology or they may have an underlying serious medical condition. The physical therapist (PT) and physical therapist assistant (PTA) must be aware that many different diseases can appear as neck pain, back pain, or both at the same time (Table 5.1). For example, rheumatoid arthritis affects the cervical spine early in the course of the disease but may go unrecognized at first.[13-16] Neck pain may be a feature of any disorder or disease that occurs above the shoulder blades; although rare, it can be a symptom of neoplasm or infection.[17]

In this chapter, general information is offered about back pain with a focus on clinical presentation, while keeping in mind risk factors and associated signs and symptoms typical of each visceral system capable of referring pain to the head, neck, and back. Neck and back pain may arise in the spine from infection, fracture, or inflammatory, metabolic, or neoplastic disorders.

In addition, LBP can be referred from abdominal or pelvic disease. Nonsteroidal antiinflammatory drug (NSAID) use is a typical cause of internal bleeding causing LBP. People most often taking NSAIDs have a history of inflammatory conditions such as osteoarthritis.

Although the incidence of back pain from NSAIDs is fairly low (i.e., the number of people on NSAIDs who develop GI problems and referred pain), the prevalence—the number seen in a physical therapy setting—is much higher.[18-20] In other words, PTs and PTAs are seeing a majority of people with arthritis or other inflammatory conditions who are taking one or more prescription and/or over-the-counter NSAIDs.[21]

Recognizing and reporting red-flag signs and symptoms is an important part of the PTA's role throughout the episode of care. The clues about the quality of pain, the age of the client, and the presence of systemic complaints or associated signs and symptoms indicate the need to consult with the PT.

GOODMAN MODEL FOR THE PHYSICAL THERAPIST ASSISTANT

Using the Goodman Screening Model modified for the PTA as presented in Chapter 1, we now apply each variable to clinical practice to aid the PTA in recognizing red and yellow flags associated with head, neck, and/or back pain/symptoms (see Box 1.2).

PAST MEDICAL HISTORY

A carefully taken, detailed medical history is essential for the recognition of systemic disease or medical conditions that may be causing integumentary, muscle, nerve, or joint symptoms. The history combined with the physical therapy examination provides essential clues for the therapist in determining the need for referral to a physician or other appropriate health care provider.

Likewise, the PTA must keep this information in mind so that new developing signs and/or symptoms, a significant change in clinical presentation, or failure to progress in treatment are recognized quickly and easily.

For example, a history of cancer is important, however long ago. If a client has had a low backache for years, progressive serious disease is unlikely. But 6 weeks to 6 months of increasing backache, often in an older client, may be a signal of lumbar metastases, especially in a person with a past history of cancer.

TABLE 5.1	**Viscerogenic Causes of Neck and Back Pain**		
	Cervical	**Thoracic/Scapular**	**Lumbar/Sacrum**
Cancer	Metastatic lesions (leukemia, Hodgkin disease) Cervical bone tumors Cervical cord tumors Lung cancer; Pancoast tumor Esophageal cancer Thyroid cancer	Mediastinal tumors Metastatic extension Pancreatic cancer Breast cancer Multiple myeloma	Primary bone tumors Neurogenic tumors (sacrum) Metastatic lesions Prostate cancer Testicular cancer Pancreatic cancer Colorectal cancer Multiple myeloma Lymphoma
Cardiovascular	Angina Myocardial infarction Aortic aneurysm Occipital migraine Cervical artery ischemia or dissection Arteritis	Angina Myocardial infarction Aortic aneurysm	Abdominal aortic aneurysm Endocarditis Myocarditis Peripheral vascular: • Postoperative bleeding from anterior spine surgery
Pulmonary	Lung cancer; Pancoast tumor Tracheobronchial irritation Chronic bronchitis Pneumothorax Pleuritis involving the diaphragm	Respiratory or lung infection Empyema Chronic bronchitis Pleurisy Pneumothorax Pneumonia	
Renal/urologic		Acute pyelonephritis Kidney disease	Kidney disorders: • Acute pyelonephritis • Perinephritic abscess • Nephrolithiasis • Ureteral colic (kidney stones) • Urinary tract infection • Dialysis (first-use syndrome) • Renal tumors
Gastrointestinal	Esophagitis Esophageal cancer	Esophagitis (severe) Esophageal spasm Peptic ulcer Acute cholecystitis Biliary colic Pancreatic disease	Small intestine: • Obstruction (neoplasm) • Irritable bowel syndrome • Crohn disease Colon: • Diverticular disease Pancreatic disease Appendicitis
Gynecologic			Gynecologic disorders: • Cancer • Retroversion of the uterus • Uterine fibroids • Ovarian cysts • Endometriosis • Pelvic inflammatory disease • Incest/sexual assault • Rectocele, cystocele • Uterine prolapse Normal pregnancy Multiparity
Infection	Vertebral osteomyelitis Meningitis Lyme disease Retropharyngeal abscess; epidural abscess (poststeroid injection)	Vertebral osteomyelitis Herpes zoster HIV Epidural abscess	Vertebral osteomyelitis Herpes zoster Spinal tuberculosis Candidiasis (yeast) Psoas abscess HIV

TABLE 5.1	Viscerogenic Causes of Neck and Back Pain—cont'd		
	Cervical	**Thoracic/Scapular**	**Lumbar/Sacrum**
Other	Osteoporosis	Osteoporosis	Osteoporosis
	Fibromyalgia	Fibromyalgia	Fibromyalgia
	Psychogenic (nonorganic causes)	Psychogenic (nonorganic)	Psychogenic (nonorganic)
	Fracture	Acromegaly	Fracture
	Rheumatoid:	Cushing syndrome	Cushing syndrome
	• Rheumatoid arthritis and atlantoaxial subluxation	Fracture	Type III hypersensitivity disorder (back/flank pain)
	• Psoriatic arthritis		Postregional anesthesia
	• Polymyalgia rheumatica		Ankylosing spondylitis
	• Ankylosing spondylitis		
	Viral myalgias		
	Cervical lymphadenitis		
	Thyroid disease		

HIV, Human immunodeficiency virus.

PTA ACTION PLAN

What to Watch for in the Patient/Client History

Watch for history of diabetes, immunosuppression, rheumatologic disorders, tuberculosis, and any recent infection (Case Example 5.1). A history of fever and chills with or without previous infection anywhere in the body may indicate a low-grade infection.[22,23]

Symptoms are likely to appear some time before striking physical signs of disease are evident and before laboratory tests are useful in detecting disordered physiology. Thus an accurate and sufficiently detailed history provides historical clues that can be significant in determining when the PTA should contact the PT with concerns and observations.

The PTA should be aware of any history of motor vehicle accident, blunt impact, repetitive injury, sudden stress caused by lifting or pulling, or trauma of any kind. Even minor falls or lifting when osteoporosis is present can result in severe fracture in older adults. Anyone who cannot bear weight through the legs and hips should be reevaluated by the PT immediately.[24]

PTA ACTION PLAN

Points to Ponder

Surgery of any kind can result in infection and abscess leading to hip, pelvic, abdominal, and/or LBP.[25] A recent history of spinal procedures (e.g., fusion, diskectomy, kyphoplasty, vertebroplasty) can be followed by back pain, motor impairment, and/or neurologic deficits when complicated by hematoma, infection, bone cement leakage, or subsidence (graft or instrumentation sinking into the bone).[26] Infection following spinal epidural injection is an infrequent but potentially serious complication.[27,28]

PTA ACTION PLAN

Follow-Up Questions for New Onset of Pain or Other Symptoms

A few key questions to ask might include:
• What do you think caused this pain/symptom?
• When did the pain (numbness, weakness, stiffness) start?
• Have you ever had this type of problem before?

• Have you ever had back surgery, seen a chiropractor (or other health care professional), or had injection therapy for this problem?
The PTA can document the new symptoms or change in clinical presentation and provide the PT with any supplementary details gained from asking a few additional questions.

RISK FACTOR ASSESSMENT

Understanding who is at risk and what the risk factors are for various illnesses, diseases, and conditions will help the PTA recognize early on the need for further evaluation by the PT and possibly make suggestions regarding education and prevention as part of the plan of care. Educating clients about their risk factors is a key element in risk factor reduction.

Risk factors vary, depending on family history, previous personal history, and disease, illness, or condition present. For example, risk factors for heart disease will be different from risk factors for osteoporosis or vestibular/balance problems. When it comes to the musculoskeletal system, risk factors such as heavy nicotine use, injection drug use, alcohol abuse, diabetes, history of cancer, or corticosteroid use may be important.

PTA ACTION PLAN

Risk Factors to Discuss With the PT

Always discuss with the PT the patient's medications and potential for adverse side effects causing muscular, joint, neck, or back pain. Long-term use of corticosteroids can lead to vertebral compression fractures (Case Example 5.2). Fluoroquinolones (antibiotics) can cause tendinopathy.[29–31] Headache is a common side effect of many medications.

Age is a risk factor for many systemic, medical, and viscerogenic problems. The risk of certain diseases associated with back pain increases with advancing age (e.g., osteoporosis, aneurysm, myocardial infarction [MI], cancer). The red-flag ages for serious spinal pathology are patients under the age of 20 or over the age of 50. The highest likelihood of vertebral fracture occurs in females aged 75 years or older.[32]

CASE EXAMPLE 5.1 **Bilateral Facial Weakness**

A 79-year-old female was in a rehabilitation facility following a stroke with resultant left hemiplegia. She told the physical therapist assistant (PTA) that she was starting to have some new symptoms in her face. She could not smile on her "good" side and was having trouble closing her eyes, which was not a problem after her stroke.

Clinical Presentation: There were no apparent changes in hearing, sensation, or motor control of the right arm. The PTA notified the therapist of the patient's new complaints and discussed the need for a new neurologic screening examination. The therapist conducted the neurologic examination and found the following results.

Cranial Nerve VII: The client was unable to raise and lower either eyebrow or close the eyes tightly; there was bilateral facial drooping; as reported, the client was unable to smile with the right side of her face.

There was no change in sensory or motor findings from the initial evaluation post–cerebral vascular accident. However, the therapist found that deep tendon

reflexes were absent in both arms and both legs. There were no other significant neurologic changes from the initial evaluation.

The therapist reviewed the Special Questions to Ask: Neck or Back (Pain Assessment and General Systemic) to look for any other screening questions and asked about a recent history of infection. The client reported a mild upper respiratory infection 2 weeks ago. There were no other obvious red-flag findings.

Result: The therapist reported the new episode of signs and symptoms to the physician. Red flags observed included bilateral symptoms, absent muscle stretch reflexes, and recent history of infection. A medical evaluation was carried out, and a diagnosis of Guillain-Barré syndrome was made. The client continued to get worse with involvement of the respiratory muscles, foot drop, and numbness in the hands and feet.

A new episode of care was initiated to include physical therapy to strengthen facial musculature and prevent atrophy on the right side and to prevent pneumonia from respiratory muscle involvement.

CASE EXAMPLE 5.2 **Corticosteroid Use**

A 73-year-old male was referred to a physical therapist (PT) by his family practitioner for evaluation of middle-to-low back pain that started when he stepped down from a curb. He was not experiencing radiating pain or sciatica and appeared to be in good general health. His medical history included bronchial asthma treated with oral corticosteroids and an abdominal hernia repaired surgically 10 years ago. There were no diagnostic imaging tests ordered.

Clinical Presentation: Vital signs were measured and appeared within normal limits for the client's age. There were no constitutional symptoms, no fever present, and no other associated signs or symptoms reported.

There was a marked decrease in thoracic and lumbar range of motion from T10 to L1 and tenderness throughout this same area. No other objective findings were noted despite a careful screening examination.

The client was treated by the PT/physical therapist assistant (PTA) team conservatively over a 2-week period, but there were no changes in his painful symptoms and no improvement in spinal movement. A second therapist in the same clinic was consulted for a reevaluation without significant differences in findings. Several suggestions were made for alternative treatment techniques.

During a session with the PTA 1 week later, it was determined that there has been no change in client symptoms, so the PTA appropriately notified the PT of the client's need to be reevaluated.

What is the Next Step?
Using Table 5.1, the PT and PTA can scan down the Thoracic/Scapular and Lumbar columns for any screening clues. Prostate and testicular cancers are listed along

with metastatic lesions. Given the client's age, questions should be asked about a past history of cancer and any associated urinary signs and symptoms.

The PT and PTA discuss that cardiovascular causes of back pain are also possible because of the client's age. The PT reviewed the past medical history and risk factors and asked about signs and symptoms associated with angina, myocardial infarction, and aneurysm.

The therapist can continue to review Table 5.1 for potential pulmonary and gastrointestinal causes of this client's back pain and further instructed the PTA to ask the client questions regarding possible risk factors and past history. The PTA recorded all positive findings and reported back to the PT, who then decided to conduct a final Review of Systems.

Result: In this case the client's age, lack of improvement with a variety of treatment techniques, lack of diagnostic imaging studies to rule out fracture or infection, and history of long-term corticosteroid use necessitated a return to the referring physician for further medical evaluation.

Long-term corticosteroid therapy and radiation therapy for cancer are risk factors for ischemic or avascular necrosis. Hip or back pain in the presence of these factors should be examined carefully.

Radiographic testing demonstrated ischemic vertebral collapse as a result of chronic corticosteroid administration. Diffuse osteopenia and a compression fracture of the 10th thoracic vertebral body were also mentioned in the medical report.

This case is a great example that demonstrates the PT/PTA team approach and that allows the PTA to directly learn from the PT in the clinic.

As with all decision-making variables, a single risk factor may or may not be significant and must be viewed in context of the whole patient/client presentation. Some other possible health risk factors the PTA should keep in mind include age; body mass index; occupation; lifestyle (sedentary); exposure to radiation, toxins, or chemicals; and overseas travel.

Routine screening for osteoporosis, hypertension, incontinence, cancer, vestibular or balance problems, and other potential problems can be a part of the PT's practice. Therapists can instruct the PTA in providing patients with information on disease prevention, wellness, and promotion of healthy lifestyles.

The PT and PTA may work together in offering wellness education as part of primary prevention.

CLINICAL PRESENTATION

During the treatment process the PTA will begin to get a more complete idea of the client's overall clinical presentation. Assessment of pain and symptoms is often a large part of the picture. Characteristics of pain, such as onset, description, duration, pattern, aggravating and relieving factors, and associated signs and symptoms are presented in Chapter 2. Reviewing the comparison in Table 2.1 will assist the PTA in recognizing red-flag systemic versus musculoskeletal presentation of signs and symptoms.

Effect of Position

When seen early in the course of symptoms, neck or back pain of a systemic, medical, or viscerogenic origin is usually accompanied by full and painless range of motion (ROM) without limitations. When the pain has been present long enough to cause muscle guarding and splinting, subsequent biomechanical changes may occur.

Typically, systemic back pain or back pain associated with other medical conditions is not relieved by rest or recumbency (lying down). In fact, the bone pain of metastasis or myeloma tends to be more continuous, progressive, and prominent when the client is recumbent.

💡 PICTURE THE PATIENT

In particular, visceral diseases, such as pancreatic neoplasm, pancreatitis, and posterior penetrating ulcers, often have a systemic backache that causes the client to curl up, sleep in a chair, or pace the floor at night.

Beware of the client with acute backache who is unable to lie still. Almost all clients with regional or nonspecific backache seek the most comfortable position (usually recumbency) and stay in that position. In contrast, individuals with systemic backache tend to keep moving trying to find a comfortable position.

▶▶ PTA ACTION PLAN

Reporting Back Pain

Back pain that is unrelieved by rest or change in position or pain that does not fit the expected mechanical or neuromusculoskeletal pattern red flags should be documented and reported to the PT. When the symptoms cannot be reproduced, aggravated, or altered in any way during the treatment session, the therapist should be notified.

Night Pain

Pain at night can signal a serious problem such as tumor, infection, or inflammation. Long-standing night pain unaltered by positional change suggests a space-occupying lesion such as a tumor.

Systemic back pain may get worse at night, especially when caused by vertebral osteomyelitis, septic diskitis, Cushing disease, osteomalacia, primary and metastatic cancer, Paget disease, ankylosing spondylitis, or tuberculosis of the spine (see further discussion of "Night Pain" in Chapter 2).

Associated Signs and Symptoms

Some situations may be appropriate for the PTA to ask the client about the presence of additional signs and symptoms. Signs and symptoms associated with systemic disease or other medical conditions are often present but go unidentified, either because the client does not volunteer the information or the therapist does not ask. In other situations, new signs and symptoms have developed since the patient was first evaluated by the PT.

▶▶ PTA ACTION PLAN

Follow-Up Question

To assess for associated signs and symptoms the PTA can ask the following:
- Are there any other symptoms anywhere else in your body that you haven't told me or your therapist? They do not have to be related to your back pain or symptoms.

The client with back pain and bloody diarrhea or the person with mid-thoracic or scapular pain in the presence of nausea and vomiting may not think the two symptoms are related. If the chief complaint of back, neck, shoulder, or other musculoskeletal pain is the only focus and no one asks about the presence of symptoms anywhere else, an important diagnostic clue may be overlooked.

Other possible associated symptoms may include fatigue, dyspnea, sweating after only minor exertion, and GI symptoms (also see Box 4.1 for a more complete list of possible associated signs and symptoms).

REVIEW OF SYSTEMS

Chapter 4 showed how the Review of Systems provides the PT with one final step in the screening process that may bring to light important clues. Sometimes it is also helpful for the PTA to step back and look at the big picture. Clusters of associated signs and symptoms usually accompany the pathologic state of each organ system (see Box 4.1).

Sometimes the progression of disease is gradual or follows the initial physical therapy evaluation. It may be appropriate to ask some general questions about fevers, excessive weight gain or loss, and appetite loss. Medications should be considered and reviewed for possible adverse side effects. The PTA may be the first one to see a suspicious pattern and bring this to the PT's attention.

▶▶ PTA ACTION PLAN

Watching for Yellow and Red Flags

Throughout the interview the PTA must remain alert to any yellow (caution) or red (warning) flags that may signal the need for further assessment by the PT. The PTA may want to ask the therapist if any yellow or red flags are currently present and what to watch for in terms of continued progression or new onset of symptoms that should be reported.

Yellow-Flag Findings

Yellow flags are indicators that findings may be present requiring special attention but not necessarily immediate action.[33] One of the primary yellow-flag findings that is important in individuals with LBP, in terms of prognosis, is the presence of psychosocial risk factors (e.g., work, attitudes and beliefs, behaviors, affective presentation).[34–38] The presence of these yellow flags suggests a poor response to traditional intervention and the need to address the underlying psychosocial aspects of health and healing.[39,40]

Work

In particular, the belief that pain is harmful (resulting in fear-avoidance behavior) and the belief that all pain must be gone before going back to work and/or normal, daily activities contribute to yellow (psychosocial) warning flags. Poor work history, unsupportive work environment, and belief that work is harmful all fall under the category of yellow work flags.[33]

Beliefs

People with chronic LBP who demonstrate yellow-flag beliefs also have an increased risk for poor prognosis. This category includes catastrophizing, thinking the worst, a belief that pain is uncontrollable, poor compliance with exercise, low educational background, and the expectation of a quick fix for pain.

Behaviors

Beliefs extend into behaviors such as passive attitude toward rehabilitation, use of extended rest, reduced activity, increased intake of alcohol and other drugs to "manage" the pain, and avoidance or withdrawal from daily and/or social activities.

Affective Presentation

Depressed mood, irritability, and heightened awareness of bodily sensations along with anxiety represent affective psychosocial yellow flags (also prognostic of poor outcome for chronic LBP). Other affective yellow flags include feeling useless and not needed, disinterest in outside activities, and lack of family or personal support systems.

PTA ACTION PLAN
Responding to Yellow Flags

The PTA may want to ask the PT for specific ways to work with individuals who may demonstrate psychosocial risk factors or other behaviors to suggest fear avoidance. The PTA's observations may provide enough information for the PT to consider referral to a mental health professional for that individual.

The PTA's role in this area is critical since waiting until someone develops chronic pain (approximately 3 months) may be too late; the window of opportunity to prevent chronicity will have passed, by definition. Therefore, in anyone with persistent pain, formal exploration of yellow flags should occur no later than 2 months after onset of pain, and possibly by the end of the first month. A practical clinical approach would be to look for yellow-flag issues at the 1-month follow-up appointment.[41]

The PTA's knowledge of these time lines may help guide when to probe further with the patient/client and when to discuss these issues with the therapist. Some simple but effective questions may include the following:
- What do you understand is the cause of your back pain?
- What are you doing to cope with your symptoms?
- Do you expect to get back to work after treatment?
- (Alternate): Do you expect to fully return to work?

If possible, the PTA should discuss his/her plan for engaging the patient/client in this particular conversation with the primary PT. It is important for the PTA to keep the PT up to date and aware of the intent to follow through on observed yellow-flag issues.

Red-Flag Signs and Symptoms

Each condition (e.g., infection, malignancy, fracture) will likely have its own predictive risk factors. For example, three red flags associated with fracture are prolonged use of corticosteroids, age older than 70 years, and significant trauma.[42]

Individuals with serious spinal pathology almost always have at least one red flag that can be missed when everyone believes the client's symptoms are the result of mechanical-induced back pain.

Five red flags have been identified for vertebral fractures in clients presenting with acute LBP: age over 70 years, female sex, major trauma, pain and tenderness, and a distracting painful injury.[43] Older females, especially older adults who have used corticosteroids, are predisposed to osteoporosis and increased risk of fracture from even minor trauma.[44]

PICTURE THE PATIENT

Red flags for possible malignancy causing LBP include advancing age, significant recent weight loss, previous malignancy, and constant pain that is not relieved by positional change or rest and that is present at night, disturbing the person's sleep. Poor response to the PTA's plan of care is an additional red flag when dealing with musculoskeletal spine pain.[45]

PTA ACTION PLAN
Recognizing Most Common Red Flags Associated With Back Pain

The PTA can watch for the most common red flags associated with back pain of a systemic origin or other medical condition (Box 5.1) and report these to the therapist. Red flags requiring reevaluation include back pain or symptoms that are not improving as expected, steady pain irrespective of activity, symptoms that are increasing, or the development of new or progressive neurologic deficits such as weakness, sensory loss, reflex changes, bowel or bladder dysfunction, or myelopathy.[43]

Cancer as a cause of LBP is unlikely when the affected individual is younger than 50 years old, has no prior history of cancer, has no unexplained or unintended weight loss, and responds to conservative care.[4] The therapist should be aware that some recommended red flags have high false-positive rates when used in isolation.[42]

The PTA can always ask the therapist if it is possible or probable that there may be a serious systemic disease or medical condition causing the individual's pain. Other areas to discuss might include whether there is neurologic compromise that might require surgical intervention or social or psychological distress that may amplify or prolong pain?

Pediatric Red Flags

Evidence suggests that backache is a frequent finding in children and adolescents and is seldom associated with serious pathology.[47–49] However, back pain in children and adolescents is still considered a red flag, especially in young children[50] and/or if the pain has been present for more than 6 weeks because of the concern for infection or neoplasm.[51] A recent history of viral illnesses may be linked to myalgias and diskitis.[50,52]

Early detection of spine fractures in children is difficult because there may be a lack of reported symptoms and the vertebrae are still cartilaginous, so x-ray findings may not be diagnostic. A history of a fall or some other trauma to the spine is a red flag. Most common causes of back pain in children are listed in Box 5.2.

Recognizing Red Flags in Children

Children are less likely to report associated signs and symptoms and must be interviewed carefully. Ask about any other joint involvement, any swelling, changes in ROM, and the presence of any constitutional and GI symptoms.

BOX 5.1 Most Common Red Flags Associated With Back Pain of Systemic Origin

- Age less than 20 years or over 50 years (malignancy)*
- Age over 70 years (fracture)*
- Previous history of cancer*
- Constitutional symptoms (e.g., fever, chills, unexplained weight loss)*
- Failure to improve with conservative care (usually over 4–6 weeks)*
- Recent urinary tract infection, blood in urine (or stools), difficulty with urination
- History of injection drug use
- Immunocompromised condition (e.g., prolonged use of corticosteroids, transplant recipient, autoimmune diseases)
- Pain not relieved by rest or recumbency
- Severe, constant nighttime pain
- Progressive, neurologic deficit; saddle anesthesia; urinary or fecal incontinence
- Back pain accompanied by abdominal, pelvic, or hip pain
- History of falls or trauma (assess for fracture, osteoporosis, domestic violence, alcohol use)
- Significant morning stiffness with limitation in all spinal movements (ankylosing spondylitis or other inflammatory disorder)
- Skin rash (inflammatory disorder [e.g., Crohn's disease, ankylosing spondylitis])

* Recommendations made on the use of red flags for serious pathology have come under scrutiny in recent years. The first five red flags listed here have proven reliability and validity. The presence of any of these signals the need for additional medical evaluation (e.g., radiographs and simple blood tests) to detect cancer.[46]

Points to Ponder

Children presenting with back pain are very different from adults with the same problem; children are less likely than adults to report symptoms when there is no organic cause for the complaint.[53] Eighty-five percent of children with back pain lasting more than 2 months have a diagnosable lesion.[54] Children with persistent reports of LBP must be evaluated and reevaluated by the physician until a diagnosis is reached; x-rays and laboratory values are needed.

Location of Pain and Symptoms

There are many ways to view head, neck, and back pain. Pain can be divided into anatomic location of symptoms (i.e., where the pain is located): cervical, thoracic, scapular, lumbar, and SI joint/sacral (see Table 5.1). For example, intrathoracic disease refers more often to the neck, mid-thoracic spine, shoulder, and upper trapezius areas. Visceral disease of the abdomen and/or pelvis is more likely to refer pain to the low back region.

Headache

The PTA may hear the client report pain and/or see symptoms affecting the face, scalp, or skull. Headaches are a frequent complaint from adults and children. It may not be the primary reason for receiving physical therapy, but it is often mentioned when asked if there are any other symptoms of any kind elsewhere in the body.

The brain itself does not feel pain because it has no pain receptors. Most often the headache is caused by an extracranial disorder and is considered "benign." Headache pain is related to pressure on other structures such as blood vessels, cranial nerves, sinuses, and the membrane surrounding the brain. Serious causes have been reported in 1% to 5% of the total cases, most often attributed to tumors, brain abscess, and infections of the central nervous system (CNS).[55–57]

BOX 5.2 Causes of Back Pain in Children

Inflammatory Conditions
Diskitis (most common before age 6)
Vertebral osteomyelitis
Spinal abscess
Nonspinal infections (e.g., pancreatitis, pyelonephritis)
Rheumatoid arthritis (cervical spine involved most often)
Reiter syndrome
Psoriatic arthritis
Ankylosing spondylitis (presents during adolescence)
Inflammatory bowel disease

Developmental Conditions
Spondylolysis
Spondylolisthesis
Scheuermann syndrome
Scoliosis (especially left thoracic)

Trauma
Muscle strain

Vertebral stress or compression fracture
Overuse syndrome
Physical abuse

Neoplastic Disease
Leukemia
Hodgkin disease
Non-Hodgkin lymphoma
Ewing sarcoma (primary)
Osteogenic sarcoma (osteosarcoma) (primary)
Rhabdomyosarcoma (rare; skeletal metastasis)

Other
Mechanical (hip and pelvic anomalies, upper cervical spine instability)
Herniated disk
Psychosomatic (conversion reaction)
Benign tumors (osteoid osteoma)
After lumbar puncture
Juvenile osteoporosis

(From Kliegman RM editor: *Nelson's essentials of pediatrics*, ed 5, Philadelphia, 2006, WB Saunders.)

BOX 5.3   Clinical Signs and Symptoms of Major Headache Types

Migraine

Can be headache free

Migraines with headache are often described as throbbing or pulsating

Often one sided (unilateral); often around or behind one eye

Associated with nausea, vomiting

Light and/or sound sensitivity (photophobia and phonophobia)

Common triggers:

- Alcohol
- Food
- Hormonal changes
- Hunger
- Lack of sleep
- Perfume
- Stress
- Medications
- Environmental factors (e.g., pollutants, air pressure changes, temperature)

May be preceded by prodromal symptoms:

- Visual changes (aura): described as spots, balloons, lights, colors
- Motor weakness
- Dizziness
- Paresthesias (numbness/tingling)
- Confusion

Facial pallor; cold hands and feet

History of headaches in childhood; family history of migraines

Tension

Described as dull pressure

Sensation of band or vise around the head; sometimes described as a painful, "tight" scalp

Headache pain is bilateral or global (entire head)

Muscular tenderness or soreness in soft tissues of the upper cervical spine

Not usually accompanied by associated signs and symptoms

May get worse with loud sounds or bright lights

Current diagnosis or history of anxiety, depression, or panic disorder

Cervicogenic

Pain starts in the occipital region and spreads anteriorly toward the frontal area

Usually bilateral

Pain intensity fluctuating from mild to severe

Often made worse by neck movements or sustained postures

Decreased neck range or motion

Forward head posture

Trigger points or tender points in muscles

Cervical muscle weakness or dysfunction

Can resemble migraines with throbbing pain, nausea, phonophobia, photophobia

History of trauma (e.g., whiplash), disk disease, or arthritis may be helpful

---

Together, the PT and PTA often provide treatment for cervicogenic headaches (CGHs). This type of headache is defined as referred pain in any part of the head (e.g., musculoskeletal tissues innervated by these nerve roots) caused by spondylitic, fibrotic, or vascular compression or compromise of cervical nerves (C1–4).[58] CGHs are frequently associated with postural strain or chronic tension,[59] acute whiplash injury, intervertebral disk disease, or progressive facet joint arthritis (e.g., cervical spondylosis, cervical arthrosis) (Box 5.3).

💡 PICTURE THE PATIENT

Clients with posttraumatic brain injury, postwhiplash injury, or postconcussion injury often report headache pain. A constellation of other symptoms are often present such as dizziness, memory problems, difficulty concentrating, irritability, fatigue, sensitivity to noise, depression, anxiety, and problems with making judgments. Symptoms may resolve in the first 4 to 6 weeks following the injury but can persist for months to years, causing permanent disability.[60,61]

Headache can be a symptom of neurologic impairment, hormonal imbalance, neoplasm, side effect of medication,[62] or other serious condition (Box 5.4). Headache may be the only symptom of hypertension, cerebral venous thrombosis, or impending stroke.[63,64] Sudden, severe headache is a classic symptom of temporal vasculitis (arteritis), a condition that can lead to blindness if not recognized and treated promptly. Headache is a common and persistent symptom following traumatic (open or closed) head injury.[65]

▶▶ PTA ACTION PLAN

Assessing Headaches

Remember to assess and monitor vital signs (pain intensity, heart rate, blood pressure) in anyone complaining of a headache and report the symptoms and the findings to the therapist. Keep in mind that stress and inadequate coping are risk factors for persistent headache. Posttraumatic stress disorder and intimate partner violence occur among a large number of females with chronic or persistent headache patterns.[66]

Headache can be part of anxiety, depression, panic disorder, and substance abuse.[67,68] Headaches have been linked with excessive caffeine consumption or withdrawal in children, adolescents, and adults.[69] Having an opportunity to discuss the whole client (emotional, physical, psychological, spiritual) with the therapist, including possible risk factors for current and developing symptoms, can help direct and guide necessary changes in the PTA's plan of care.

Cancer. The greatest concern is always whether a brain tumor is causing the headaches. Only a minority of individuals who have headaches have brain tumors. Risk factors include occupational exposure to gases and chemicals and history of cranial radiation therapy for fungal infection of the scalp or for other types of cancer. A previous history of cancer, even long past history, is a red flag for insidious onset of head and occipital neck pain.

💡 PICTURE THE PATIENT

Although primary head and neck cancers can cause headaches, more likely problems are neck pain, facial pain, and/or numbness in the face, ear, mouth, and lips. Other signs and symptoms can include sore throat, dysphagia, a

BOX 5.4 Systemic Origins of Headache

Cancer
Primary neoplasm
Chemotherapy; brain radiation

Cardiovascular
Migraine
Ischemia (atherosclerosis; vertebrobasilar insufficiency; internal carotid artery dysfunction)
Cerebral vascular thrombosis
Arteriovenous malformation
Subarachnoid hemorrhage
Giant cell arteritis; vascular arteritis; temporal vasculitis
Hypertension
Febrile illnesses
Hypoxia
Systemic lupus erythematosus

Pulmonary
Obstructive sleep apnea
Hyperventilation (e.g., associated with anxiety or panic attacks)

Renal/Urologic
Kidney failure; renal insufficiency
Dialysis (first-use syndrome)

Gynecologic
Pregnancy
Dysmenorrhea

Neurologic
Postseizure
Disorder of cranium, cranial structures (e.g., nose, eyes, ears, teeth, neck)
Cranial neuralgia (e.g., trigeminal, Bell palsy, occipital, Herpes zoster, optic neuritis)
Brain abscess
Hydrocephalus

Other
History of physical or sexual abuse
Side effect of medications
Allergens/toxins (environmental or food)
Overuse of medications (analgesic rebound effect)
Psychogenic/psychiatric disorder
Substance abuse/withdrawal (drugs and/or alcohol)
Caffeine use/withdrawal
Candidiasis (yeast)
Trauma (e.g., cervicogenic headache, fracture, eating disorders with forced vomiting)
Infection (e.g., meningitis, sinusitis, syphilis, tuberculosis, sarcoidosis, herpes)
Postdural puncture
Scuba diving
Hantavirus
Paget disease (when skull is affected)
Hypoglycemia
Fibromyalgia
Temporomandibular joint dysfunction

chronic ulcer that does not heal, a lump in the neck, and persistent or unexplained bleeding. Color changes in the mouth known as leukoplakia (white patches) or erythroplakia (red patches) may develop in the oral cavity as a premalignant sign.[70,71]

Cancer recurrence is not uncommon within the first 3 years after treatment for cancers of the head and neck; often these cancers are not diagnosed until an advanced stage because of neglect on the part of the affected individual. Cervical spine metastasis is most common with distant metastases to the lungs, although any part of the body can be affected.[72]

Tension-type or migraine headaches can occur with tumors. Rapidly growing tumors are more likely to be associated with headache and will eventually present with other signs and symptoms such as visual disturbances, seizures, or personality changes.[73,74] Headaches associated with brain tumors occur in up to half of all cases and are usually bioccipital or bifrontal, intermittent, and of increasing duration. Presence of tumor headache varies, depending on size, location, and type of tumor.[75]

? PICTURE THE PATIENT

The headache is worse on awakening, because of differences in CNS drainage in the supine and prone positions, and usually disappears soon after the person arises. It may be intensified or precipitated by any activity that increases intracranial pressure, such as straining during a bowel movement, stooping, lifting heavy objects, or coughing.

Often, the pain can be relieved by taking aspirin, acetaminophen, or other moderate painkillers. Vomiting with or without nausea (unrelated to food) can occur in people with brain tumors and often accompanies headaches when there is an increase in intracranial pressure. If the tumor invades the meninges, the headaches will be more severe.

Migraines. Migraine headaches are often accompanied by nausea, vomiting, and visual disturbances, but the pain pattern is also often classic in description. Age is a yellow (caution) flag because migraines generally begin in childhood to early adulthood. Migraines can first occur in an individual beyond the age of 50 (especially in perimenopausal or menopausal females); advancing age makes other types of headaches more likely. A family history is usually present, suggesting a genetic predisposition in migraine sufferers. In addition to the typical clinical presentation, there are usually normal examination results.

? PICTURE THE PATIENT

Migraines can present with paralysis or weakness of one side of the body, mimicking a stroke. When present, associated signs and symptoms offer the best yellow- or red-flag warnings. For example, throbbing headache with unexplained diaphoresis and elevated blood pressure may signal a significant cardiovascular event. Daytime sleepiness, morning headache, and reports of snoring may point to obstructive sleep apnea. Headache-associated visual disturbances or facial numbness raises the suspicion of a neurologic origin of symptoms. Box 5.5 lists other red flags.

BOX 5.5   Red-Flag Signs and Symptoms Associated With Headache

The physical therapy assistant should watch for any of the following red flags and report them to the therapist.

- Headache that awakens the individual or is present upon awakening (e.g., hypertension, tumor)
- Headache accompanied by documented elevated blood pressure changes
- Insidious or new onset of headache (less than 6 months)
- New onset of headache with associated neurologic signs and symptoms (e.g., confusion, dizziness, gait or motor disturbances, fatigue, irritability or mood changes)
- New onset of headache accompanied by constitutional symptoms (e.g., fever, chills, sweats) or stiff neck (infection, arteritis)
- Episodes of "blacking out" during headache (seizures, hemorrhage, tumor)
- Sudden severe headache accompanied by flu-like symptoms, aching muscles, jaw pain when eating, and visual disturbances (temporal arteritis)
- No previous personal or family history of migraine headaches

Cervical Spine

Neck pain is very common and has many mechanical and systemic causes. Neck and shoulder pain and neck and upper back pain often occur together, making it more difficult to sort out cause and effect. Traumatic and degenerative conditions of the cervical spine, such as whiplash syndrome and arthritis, are the major primary musculoskeletal causes of neck pain.[76,77] There may be a history of motor vehicle accident or trauma of any kind, including domestic violence.

Cervical or neck pain with or without radiating arm pain or symptoms may be caused by a local biomechanical dysfunction (e.g., shoulder impingement, disk degeneration, facet dysfunction) or a medical problem (e.g., infection, tumor, fracture). Referred pain presenting in these areas from a systemic source may occur from infectious disease, such as vertebral osteomyelitis, or from cancer, cardiac, pulmonary, or abdominal disorders (see Table 5.1).

Rheumatoid arthritis is often characterized by polyarthritic involvement of the peripheral joints, but the cervical spine is often affected early on (first 2 years) in the course of the disease. Deep aching pain in the occipital, retroorbital, or temporal areas may be present with pain referred to the face, ear, or subocciput from irritation of the C2 nerve root. Some clients may have atlantoaxial (AA) subluxation and report a sensation of the head falling forward during neck flexion or a clunking sensation during neck extension as the AA joint is reduced spontaneously. Symptoms of cervical radiculopathy are common with AA joint involvement.[13,77]

Radicular symptoms accompanied by weakness, coordination impairment, gait disturbance, bowel or bladder retention or incontinence, and sexual dysfunction can occur whenever cervical myelopathy occurs, whether from a mechanical or medical cause. Cervical spondylotic myelopathy has been verified as a potential cause of LBP as well.[78,79]

? PICTURE THE PATIENT

Indicators of cervical myelopathy include the following:
- Neck pain and/or shoulder pain, stiffness
- Wide-based clumsy, uncoordinated gait

- Loss of hand dexterity
- Paresthesias in one or both arms or hands
- Visible change in handwriting
- Difficulty manipulating buttons or handling coins
- Hyperreflexia
- Lhermitte sign (electric shock sensation down spine/arms with neck flexion/extension)
- Urinary retention followed by overflow incontinence (severe myelopathy)
- LBP[78]

▶▶ PTA ACTION PLAN

Recognizing and Reporting Important Clinical Findings in the Cervical Spine

Any report of difficulty or pain with swallowing should be reported to the therapist. Observe for any deviation of the trachea to either side. Torticollis of the sternocleidomastoid muscle may be a sign of underlying thyroid involvement. Anterior neck pain that is worse with swallowing and turning the head from side to side may be present with thyroiditis. Ask about associated signs and symptoms of endocrine disease (e.g., temperature intolerance; hair, nail, and skin changes; joint or muscle pain) and a previous history of thyroid problems.

Thoracic Spine

Possible musculoskeletal sources of thoracic pain include muscle strain, vertebral or rib fracture, zygapophyseal joint arthropathy,[80] active trigger points, spinal stenosis, costotransverse and costovertebral joint dysfunction, ankylosing spondylitis, intervertebral disk herniation, intercostal neuralgia, diffuse idiopathic skeletal hyperostosis, and T4 syndrome.[81] Shoulder impingement and mechanical problems in the cervical spine can also refer pain to the thoracic spine.[82]

Systemic origins of musculoskeletal pain in the thoracic spine (Table 5.2) are usually accompanied by constitutional symptoms and other associated symptoms. Often, these additional symptoms develop after the initial onset of back pain, and the client may not relate them to the back pain and therefore may fail to mention them.

The close proximity of the thoracic spine to the chest and respiratory organs requires asking about pleuropulmonary symptoms in anyone with back pain of unknown cause or past medical history of cancer or pulmonary problems. Thoracic pain can also be referred from the kidney, biliary duct, esophagus, stomach, gallbladder, pancreas, and heart.[83]

Thoracic aortic aneurysm, angina, and acute MI are the most likely cardiac causes of thoracic back pain. Usually, there is a cardiac history and associated signs and symptoms such as weak or thready pulse, extremely high or extremely low blood pressure, or unexplained perspiration and pallor.[84]

Tumors occur most often in the thoracic spine because of its length, the proximity to the mediastinum, and direct metastatic extension from lymph nodes with lymphoma, breast, or lung cancer. The client may report symptoms typical of cancer. Tumor involvement in the thoracic spine may produce ischemic damage to the spinal cord or early cord compression since the ratio of canal diameter to cord size is small, resulting in rapid deterioration of neurologic status.

TABLE 5.2   Systemic Origins of Pain in the Thoracic Spine

Systemic Origin	Location	Neuromusculoskeletal
Cardiac		• Trauma (including motor vehicle accident, domestic violence, assault)
Myocardial infarct	Mid-thoracic spine	• Muscle strain; overuse from repetitive motions
Aortic aneurysm	Thoracic spine; thoracolumbar spine	• Degenerative disk disease; disk calcification or other disk lesions
Angina	Mid-thoracic spine; radiating down from shoulder (usually left side)	• Spinal stenosis • Rib syndromes or zygapophyseal joint disorders (e.g., costovertebral [rib] dysfunction, slipping rib syndrome, 12th rib syndrome, osteoarthritis, costovertebral or costotransverse joint hypomobility) • Thoracic outlet syndrome • Trigger points: Trapezius (middle), multifidi, rotators, rectus abdominis, latissimus dorsi, rhomboids, infraspinatus, serratus posterior • Vertebral or rib fracture or dislocation • Bone or soft tissue ossification (e.g., spinal ligaments, bone spurs) • Psychogenic (e.g., anxiety, depression, somatoform disorders) • Scoliosis; spinal deformity; Scheuermann disease • Scapular dyskinesia
Pulmonary		
Basilar pneumonia	Right upper back	
Empyema	Scapula	
Pleurisy	Scapula	
Pneumothorax	Ipsilateral scapula	
Renal		
Acute pyelonephritis	Costovertebral angle (posterior)	
Gastrointestinal		
Esophagitis	Mid-back between scapulae	
Peptic ulcer: Stomach/duodenal	6th through 10th thoracic vertebrae	
Gallbladder disease	Mid-back between scapulae; right upper scapula or subscapular area	
Biliary colic	Right upper back; mid-back between scapulae or subscapular areas	
Pancreatic carcinoma	Mid-thoracic or lumbar spine	
Inflammatory/Infectious		
Rheumatoid arthritis Ankylosing spondylitis Osteomyelitis Pott disease (tuberculosis of the spine) Spinal abscess or infection	Variable locations	
Cancer		
Primary: Osteoid osteoma, spinal canal, spinal nerve roots *Metastases:* Breast cancer, lung cancer, thyroid cancer, Hodgkin disease, esophageal cancer, skin cancer	Variable locations	
Other		
Acromegaly	Mid-thoracic or lumbar spine	
Breast cancer	Mid-thoracic spine or upper back	
Osteoporosis	Variable locations	
Paget disease of bone	Variable locations	
Pregnancy	Variable locations	
Blood disorders (sickle cell disease)	Variable locations	

Peptic ulcer can refer pain to the mid-thoracic spine between T6 and T10. A history of NSAID use, report of blood in the stools, and change in pain or bowel function as a result of eating food should be reported to the therapist.[85]

Scapula

Most causes of scapular pain occur along the vertebral border and result from various primary musculoskeletal lesions. However, cardiac, pulmonary, renal, and GI disorders can cause scapular pain. Table 5.2 indicates possible causes and locations of referred pain patterns to the scapular/mid-thoracic area.

Lumbar Spine

LBP is very prevalent in the adult population, affecting up to 80% of all adults sometime in their lives. In most cases, acute symptoms resolve within a few weeks to a few months. Individuals reporting persistent pain and activity limitation must be reevaluated by the PT.

As Table 5.1 shows, there is a wide range of potential systemic and medical causes of LBP. Older adults with more comorbidities are at increased risk for LBP. Bone and joint diseases (inflammatory and noninflammatory), lung and heart diseases, and enteric diseases top the list of conditions contributing to LBP in older adults.[9,86]

▶▶ PTA ACTION PLAN

Points to Ponder

Pain referred to the lumbar spine and low back region from the pelvic and abdominal viscera may come directly from the organ structures, but some experts suspect the referred pain pattern is really produced by irritation of the posterior abdominal wall by pus, blood, or leaking enzymes. If that is the case, the pain is not referred but rather arises directly from the anterior aspect of the back.[33]

Sacrum/Sacroiliac

The most common etiology of serious pathology in this anatomic region comes from the spondyloarthropathies (diseases of the joints of the spine) such as ankylosing spondylitis, Reiter syndrome, psoriatic arthritis, and arthritis associated with chronic inflammatory bowel (enteropathic) disease.[87]

💡 PICTURE THE PATIENT

In addition to back pain, these rheumatic diseases usually include a constellation of associated signs and symptoms, such as fever, skin lesions, anorexia, and weight loss that alert the PTA to the need for consultation with the therapist.

Spondyloarthropathy is characterized by morning pain accompanied by prolonged stiffness that improves with activity. There is limitation of motion in all directions and tenderness over the spine and SI joints. The most significant finding in ankylosing spondylitis is that the client has night (back) pain and morning stiffness as the two major complaints, but asymmetric SI involvement with radiation into the buttock and thigh can occur.[77]

▶▶ PTA ACTION PLAN

Follow-Up Questions

Anyone under the age of 45 with low back, hip, buttock, and/or sacral pain lasting more than 3 months should be asked these four questions:
* Do you have morning back *stiffness* that lasts more than 30 minutes?
* Does the back pain wake you up during the second half of the night?
* Does the pain alternate from one buttock to the other (shift from side to side)?
* Does rest relieve the pain?

There is a 70% sensitivity and 81% specificity for inflammatory back pain if two of the four questions are positive. Sensitivity reflects an accurate test showing that the person does have inflammation (true positive). Sensitivity drops to 33% if three of the four questions are answered positively, but the specificity increases to nearly 100% (test accurately shows the condition is not present; true negative).[88]

Sources of Pain and Symptoms

Besides anatomic location of pain just discussed, this symptom can be associated with the source of symptoms (what is causing the problem?). It could be any of the following:
* Viscerogenic
* Neurogenic
* Vasculogenic
* Spondylogenic
* Psychogenic

Specific symptoms and characteristics of pain (frequency, intensity, duration, description) help the PTA recognize potential sources of back pain (Table 5.3). The PTA should be alert for the report of any associated signs and symptoms that might indicate the presence of any one (or more) of these sources.

Viscerogenic

Visceral pain is not usually confused with pain originating in the head, neck, and back because a sufficient number of specific symptoms and signs are often present to localize the problem correctly. The unusual presentation of systemic disease will make it more difficult to recognize.

LBP is more likely to result from disease in the abdomen and pelvis than from intrathoracic disease, which usually refers pain to the neck, upper back, and shoulder. Disorders of the GI, pulmonary, urologic, and gynecologic systems can cause stimulation of sensory nerves supplied by the same segments of the spinal cord, resulting in referred back pain.[90] Back pain can be associated with distention or perforation of organs, gynecologic conditions, or gastroenterologic disease. Pain can occur from compression, ischemia, inflammation, or infection affecting any of the organs (Fig. 5.1).

Referred pain can also originate in organs that share pain innervation with areas of the lumbosacral spine. Colicky pain is associated with spasm in a hollow viscus. Severe, tearing pain with sweating and dizziness may originate from an expanding abdominal aortic aneurysm (AAA). Burning pain may originate from a duodenal ulcer.

TABLE 5.3   Neck and Back Pain: Symptoms and Possible Causes

Symptom	Possible Cause
Night pain unrelieved by rest or change in position; made worse by recumbency; back pain, scoliosis, sensory, and motor deficits in adolescents[89]	Tumor
Fever, chills, sweats	Infection
Unremitting, throbbing pain	Aortic aneurysm
Abdominal pain radiating to mid-back; symptoms associated with food; symptoms worse after taking NSAIDs	Pancreatitis, gastrointestinal disease, peptic ulcer
Morning stiffness that improves as day goes on	Inflammatory arthritis
Leg pain increased by walking and relieved by standing	Vascular claudication
Leg pain increased by walking, unaffected by standing but sometimes relieved by sitting or prolonged rest	Neurogenic claudication
"Stocking glove" numbness	Referred pain, nonorganic pain
Global pain	Nonorganic pain
Long-standing back pain aggravated by activity	Deconditioning
Pain increased by sitting	Diskogenic disease
Sharp, narrow band of pain radiating below the knee	Herniated disk
Chronic spinal pain	Stress/psychosocial factors (unsatisfying job, fear-avoidance behavior, work or family issues, attitudes and beliefs)
Back pain dating to specific injury or trauma	Strain or sprain, fracture; failed back surgery
Back pain in athletic teenager[24]	Abnormal development, trauma; epiphysitis; juvenile diskogenic disease; hyperlordosis; spondylosis, spondylolysis, or spondylolisthesis
Exquisite tenderness over spinous process	Tumor, fracture, infection
Back pain preceded or accompanied by skin rash	Inflammatory bowel disease

NSAIDs, Nonsteroidal antiinflammatory drugs.
(Modified from Nelson BW: A rational approach to the treatment of low back pain, *J Musculoskelet Med* 10(5):75, 1993.)

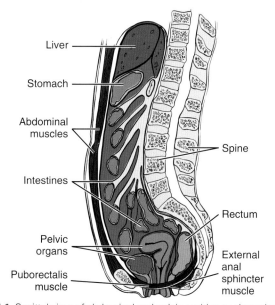

FIG. 5.1 Sagittal view of abdominal and pelvic cavities to show the proximity of viscera to the spine. The abdominal muscles and muscles of the pelvic floor provide anterior and inferior support, respectively. Any dysfunction of the musculature can alter the relationship of the viscera; likewise, anything that impacts the viscera can affect the dynamic tension and ultimately the function of the muscles. Pathology of the organs can refer pain through shared pathways or by direct distention as a result of compression from inflammation and tumor.

Labels in figure: Liver, Stomach, Abdominal muscles, Intestines, Pelvic organs, Puborectalis muscle, Spine, Rectum, External anal sphincter muscle

Muscle spasm and tenderness along the vertebrae may be elicited in the presence of visceral impairment. For example, spasm on the right side at the 9th and 10th costal cartilages can be a symptom of gallbladder problems. The spleen can cause tenderness and spasm at the level of T9 through T11 on the left side. The kidneys are more likely to cause tenderness, spasm, and possible cutaneous pain or sensitivity at the level of the 11th and 12th ribs.

▶▶ PTA ACTION PLAN

Staying Alert to Clusters of Signs and Symptoms

Vital signs, including body temperature, must be taken and recorded for any client older than 50 with back pain, especially with insidious onset or unknown cause. Careful questioning can elicit important information that the client withheld, thinking it was irrelevant to the problem, such as LBP alternating with abdominal pain at the same level or back pain alternating with bouts of bloody diarrhea. The PTA should remain alert for any clusters of signs and symptoms that may suggest involvement of a particular system. The information in Box 4.1 can be very helpful in recognizing the possibility of a visceral source of symptoms that should be reported to the therapist.

Neurogenic

Neurogenic pain is not easily differentiated. Radicular pain results from irritation of axons of a spinal nerve or neurons in the dorsal root ganglion, whereas referred pain results from activation of nociceptive free nerve endings (nociceptors) in somatic or visceral tissue.[91]

Neurologic signs are produced by conduction block in motor or sensory nerves, but conduction block does not cause pain. Thus, even in a client with back pain and neurologic signs, whatever causes the neurologic signs is not causing the back pain by the same mechanism. Therefore finding the cause of the neurologic signs does not always identify the cause of the back pain.[41]

Conditions such as radiculitis may cause both pain and neurologic signs, but in that case the pain occurs in the lower limb (not in the back) or in the upper extremity (not in the neck). If root inflammation also happens to involve the nerve root sleeve, neck or back pain might also arise. In such a case the individual will have three problems each with a different mechanism: neurologic signs resulting from conduction block, radicular pain resulting from nerve root inflammation, and neck or back pain resulting from inflammation of the dura.[41]

The presence of mechanical pain does not always rule out serious spinal pathology. For example, neurogenic pain can be caused by a metastatic lesion applying pressure or traction on any of the neural components. Positive neural dynamic tests do not reveal the underlying cause of the problem (e.g., tumor versus scar tissue restriction). The therapist must rely on history, clinical presentation, and the presence of any neurologic or other associated signs and symptoms to make a determination about the need for medical referral. Any information the PTA can provide along these lines may bring the problem to light sooner.

Sciatica alone or sciatica accompanying back pain is an important but unreliable symptom. Although 90% of cases of sciatica are caused by a herniated disk,[92] the other 10% must be kept in mind. For example, diabetic neuropathy can cause nerve root irritation. Prostatic metastases to the lumbar and pelvic regions or other neoplasms of the spine can create a clinical picture that is indistinguishable from sciatica of musculoskeletal origin. This similarity may lead to long and serious delays in diagnosis. The PTA's reported observations may help facilitate an earlier diagnosis.

Spinal stenosis caused by a narrowing of the vertebral (spinal) canal, lateral recess, or intervertebral foramina may produce neurogenic claudication (Fig. 5.2). The canal tends to be narrow at the lumbosacral junction, and the nerve roots in the cauda equina are tightly packed. Pressure on the cauda equina from tumor, disk protrusion, spinal fracture or dislocation, infection, or inflammation can result in cauda equina syndrome, which is a neurologic medical emergency.[93,94]

PICTURE THE PATIENT

Clinical signs and symptoms of cauda equina syndrome include the following:
- LBP
- Unilateral or bilateral sciatica
- Saddle anesthesia; perineal hypoesthesia
- Change in bowel and/or bladder function (e.g., difficulty initiating flow of urine, urine retention, urinary or fecal incontinence, constipation, decreased rectal tone and sensation)

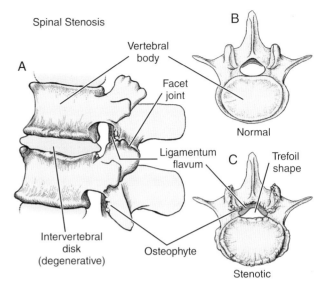

FIG. 5.2 Spinal stenosis. (A) Aging causes a loss of disk height and compression of the vertebral body. The bone attempts to cushion itself by forming a lip or extra rim around the periphery of the end-plates. This lipping can extend far enough to obstruct the opening to the vertebral canal. At the same time, the ligamentum flavum begins to hypertrophy or thicken and osteophytes (bone spurs) develop. Degenerative disease can cause the apophyseal (facet) joints to flatten out or become misshapen. Any or all of these variables can contribute to spinal stenosis. (B) Normal, healthy vertebral body with a widely open vertebral canal. (C) Stenotic spine from a variety of contributing factors. Many clients have all of these changes, but some do not. The presence of pathologic changes is not always accompanied by clinical symptoms.

- Sexual dysfunction:
  - Males: erectile dysfunction (inability to attain or sustain an erection)
  - Females: dyspareunia (inability to have an orgasm)
- Lower extremity motor weakness and sensory deficits; gait disturbance
- Diminished or absent lower extremity deep tendon reflexes (patellar, Achilles)

PICTURE THE PATIENT

Recognizing the difference between vascular and neurogenic pain patterns can be very challenging (Table 5.4). This is especially true in the treatment of unusual cases of sciatica or back pain with leg pain. The client with a neurogenic source of back pain may develop a characteristic pattern of symptoms, with back pain; discomfort in the buttock, thigh, or leg; and numbness and paresthesia in the leg developing after the person walks a few hundred yards (neurogenic claudication).[84] The person may be forced to stop walking and obtain relief after long periods of rest. The pattern of symptoms is similar to that of intermittent claudication associated with vascular insufficiency, the major differences being immediate response to rest and position of the spine (see Figs. 5.2 and 5.3). Position of the spine (e.g., flexion, extension, side bending, or rotation) does not affect symptoms of a cardiac origin.[23]

Vasculogenic

Pain of a vascular origin may be mistaken for pain from a wide variety of musculoskeletal, neurologic, and arthritic disorders. Conversely, in a client with known vascular disease, a primary musculoskeletal disorder may go undiagnosed (e.g., diskogenic disease, spinal cord tumor, peripheral neuritis, arthritis of the

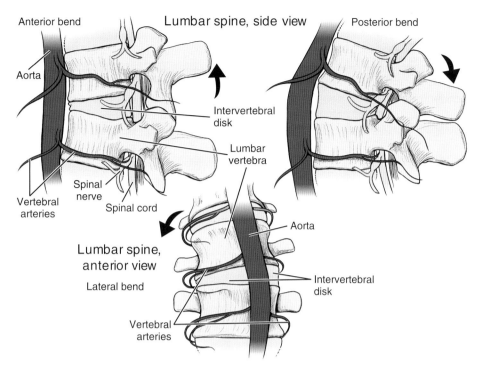

FIG. 5.3 Vascular supply is not compromised by position of the spine, so there is usually no change in back pain that is vascular induced with change of position. Forward bend, extension, and side bending do not aggravate or relieve symptoms. Rather, increased activity requiring increased blood supply to the musculature is more likely to reproduce symptoms; likewise, rest may relieve the symptoms. Watch for a lag time of 3–5 min after the start of activity or exercise before symptoms appear or increase as a sign of a possible vascular component.

TABLE 5.4 Back Pain: Vascular or Neurogenic?

Vascular	Neurogenic
Throbbing	Burning
Diminished, absent pulses	No change in pulses
Trophic changes (skin color, texture, temperature)	No trophic changes; look for subtle strength deficits (e.g., partial foot drop, hip flexor or quadriceps weakness; calf muscle atrophy)
Pain present in all spinal positions	Pain increases with spinal extension, decreases with spinal flexion
Symptoms with standing: No	Symptoms with standing: Yes
Pain increases with activity; promptly relieved by rest or cessation of activity	Pain may respond to prolonged rest

BOX 5.6 Clues to Recognizing and Reporting Vasculogenic Pain

Pain of a vascular origin may be:
- Described as "throbbing"
- Accompanied by leg pain that is relieved by standing still or rest
- Accompanied by leg pain that is described as "aching, cramping, or tired"
- Present in all spinal positions and increased by exertion
- Accompanied by a pulsing sensation in abdomen or palpable abdominal pulse
- Caused by a back injury (lifting) in someone with known heart disease or past history of aneurysm
- Accompanied by pelvic, leg, or buttock pain
- Presented as arm pain when working with the arms overhead
- Accompanied by temperature changes in the extremities
- An early or late complication of lumbar surgery (ask about a history of previous spine surgery)

💡 PICTURE THE PATIENT

Vascular back pain may be described as "throbbing" and almost always is increased with any activity that requires greater cardiac output and is diminished or even relieved when the workload or activity is stopped. A "throbbing" headache may be a vascular headache from a variety of causes.

hip) because all symptoms are attributed to cardiovascular insufficiency.

Vasculogenic pain can originate from both the heart (viscera) and the blood vessels (soma), primarily peripheral vascular disease (PVD). Back pain has been linked to atherosclerotic changes in the posterior wall of the abdominal aorta in older adults.[95] The PTA can rely on special clues to help recognize and report vasculogenic-induced pain (Box 5.6).

Atherosclerosis and the resulting peripheral arterial disease are the underlying causes of most vascular back pain. Often, the client history will reveal significant cardiovascular risk factors such as smoking, hypertension, diabetes, advancing age, or elevated serum cholesterol. Older age is an important red flag when assessing for pain of a vasculogenic origin. Most often, clients with back pain and any of the vascular clues listed are middle aged and older. A personal or family history of heart disease is a second red flag. Continuous mid-thoracic pain can be a symptom of MI, especially in a postmenopausal female with a positive family history of heart disease.[22]

Spondylogenic

Bone tenderness and pain on weightbearing usually characterize spondylogenic back pain (or the symptoms produced by bone lesions). Associated signs and symptoms may include weight loss, fever, deformity, and night pain. Numerous conditions are capable of producing bone pain, but the most common pathologic disorders are fracture from any cause, osteomalacia, osteoporosis, Paget disease, infection, inflammation, and metastatic bone disease (Case Example 5.3).[96–101]

? PICTURE THE PATIENT

The acute pain of a *compression fracture* superimposed on chronic discomfort, often in the absence of a history of trauma, may be the only presenting symptom. The client may recall a "snap" associated with mild pain, or there may have been no pain at all after the "snap." More intense pain may not develop for hours or until the next day. Other symptoms include paraspinal muscle spasms, loss of height, and kyphoscoliosis.

Back pain over the thoracic or lumbar spine that is intensified by prolonged sitting, standing, and the Valsalva maneuver may resolve after 3 or 4 months as the fractures of the vertebral bodies heal. Clients who undergo kyphoplasty or vertebroplasty may experience immediate pain relief.[102]

Psychogenic

Psychogenic pain is observed in the client who has anxiety that amplifies or increases the person's perception of pain. Depression has been implicated in many painful conditions as the primary underlying problem. The prevalence of depression in physical therapy patients being treated for LBP has been reported as high as 26%.[103] There is a concern that depression may go unrecognized or be inappropriately managed. Asking about depression can be done quickly and easily with the following two questions:

- During the past month, have you been bothered often by feeling down, depressed, or hopeless?
- During the past month, have you been bothered often by little interest or pleasure in doing things?

This two-question tool has proved to have a 96% sensitivity (test accurately shows the person does have depression) and 57% specificity (test accurately shows the condition is not present).[104,105] A positive response to either or both of these questions should be reported to the PT for further evaluation.

? PICTURE THE PATIENT

Anxiety, depression, and panic disorder can lead to muscle tension, more anxiety, and then to muscle spasm. Signs and symptoms of these conditions are listed in Table 2.6. The client who is unable to concentrate on anything except the symptoms and who reports that the symptoms interfere with every activity may need a psychological/psychiatric referral.

The client may use words to describe painful symptoms characterized as "emotional." Recognizing these descriptors will help the PTA recognize the possibility of an underlying psychological or emotional etiology. An "exploding" or "vicious" headache, "agonizing" neck pain, or "punishing" backache are all potential descriptors of psychogenic origin that should be discussed with the therapist.

CASE EXAMPLE 5.3   Osteoporosis

A 59-year-old male has been evaluated by the physical therapist (PT) for mid-thoracic back pain that seemed to come on gradually over the last few weeks and was starting to make his job as a janitor more difficult. He reported no other symptoms (i.e., no neck, chest, or arm pain).

Past medical history was without incident. The client had never missed a day of work because of illness, never been hospitalized, and had no previous history of surgery. He has a 40-pack/year history of smoking and "throws back a few beers" every night (a six-pack daily for the last 15 years).

Initial Evaluation Information
Clinical Presentation: Postural examination revealed a significant thoracic kyphosis with limited passive and active extension to neutral. Range of motion in the lumbar spine was within normal limits and was normal in the hip and knee. Neurologic screening examination was normal. Local tenderness was palpable in the mid-thoracic paraspinal and rhomboid muscles with evidence of erythema and swelling.

The physical therapy plan of care indicated by the PT directs the physical therapist assistant (PTA) to initiate use of electric and thermal modalities for treatment of muscular pain, tension, and swelling. The PT educated the client on the need for him to return to his primary physician for an x-ray of the thoracic spine as

soon as possible. An x-ray would be a good idea in this case before beginning a program of back extension exercises or applying any manual therapy.

Current Clinical Presentation on Second Treatment Session: The client reports that he has not had time to make an appointment for the x-ray. The client could take a deep breath without increasing his pain but not without setting off a long series of coughing. There was an increase in local tenderness palpable in the mid-thoracic paraspinal and rhomboid muscles with an increase in evidence of erythema and swelling.

Group Discussion
What are the red flags?

Should the PTA continue with the plan today before checking with and reporting the findings to the PT?

Red flags include age and a significant history of tobacco and alcohol abuse. All three are risk factors for reduced bone mass and fracture. Osteopenia and osteoporosis are often overlooked in males and occur more often than previously believed.[96–100] Thirty percent of osteoporotic fractures occur in males.[101]

Prior to treating this patient, the PTA should report to the PT that the client has not had an x-ray yet and that there is a change in physical observations of skin and pain today.

Recognizing and Reporting Red Flags of Cancer

Cancer is a possible cause of referred pain. Tumors of the spine reportedly account for anywhere between 0.1% and 12% of patients with back pain seen in a general medical practice.[106] Autopsy reports show up to 70% of adults who die of cancer have spinal metastases; up to 14% exhibit clinically symptomatic disease before death.[107]

Most reports place malignancy as a source of LBP in less than 1% of primary care patients.[108] Brain tumors (e.g., meningioma) in the motor cortex can present as LBP; abnormal symptom behavior and atypical responses to treatment may be observed and represent red flags for consultation with the therapist.[109] Head and neck pain from cancer is discussed earlier in this chapter (see the "Headache" section).

Multiple myeloma is the most common primary malignancy involving the spine, often resulting in diffuse osteoporosis and pain with movement that is not relieved while the person is recumbent. Back pain with radicular symptoms can develop with spinal cord compression. There can be a long period of development (5–20 years) with a chronic presentation of LBP.[110]

Past Medical History

Prompt identification of malignancy is important, starting with knowledge of previous cancers. Past history of cancer anywhere in the body is a red-flag warning that careful assessment is required. Always ask clients who deny a previous personal history of cancer about any previous chemotherapy or radiation therapy.

Early recognition and intervention do not always improve prognosis for survival from metastatic cancer, but they do reduce the risk of cord compression and paraplegia. It is important to remember that the history can be misleading. For example, almost 50% of clients with back pain from a malignancy have an identifiable (or attributable) antecedent injury or trauma.[111]

It is unclear if this is a coincidence or merely reflective of weakness in the musculoskeletal system leading to loss of balance and strength and ultimately an injury. If the trauma results in significant injury (e.g., fracture), the underlying cancer is usually identified right away. However, if soft tissue injury does not necessitate an x-ray or other imaging study, the underlying oncologic cause may go undetected. Once again the PTA may be the first to recognize the cluster of clinical signs and symptoms and/or red-flag findings to suggest a more serious underlying pathology.

Red Flags and Risk Factors

A combination of age (50 years or older), previous history of cancer, unexplained weight loss, and failure to improve after 1 month of conservative care has a reported sensitivity of 100%.[108] Of these four red flags a previous history of cancer is the most informative.[112]

Until now, the text has emphasized advancing age as a key red flag, but back pain at a young age (younger than 20 years old) may be considered a red flag as well. As a general rule, persistent backache resulting from extraspinal causes is rare in children. Mechanical back pain in children is possibly linked with heavy backpacks,[113,114] sports, and sedentary lifestyle. However,

primary bone cancer occurs most often in adolescents and young adults, hence the addition of this red flag: age younger than 20 years. Bones of the appendicular skeleton (limbs) are affected more than the spine in this age group, but secondary metastases to the vertebrae can occur.

> ### ❓ PICTURE THE PATIENT
>
> Clinical signs and symptoms of oncologic spine pain include the following:
> - Severe weakness without pain
> - Weakness with full range
> - Sciatica caused by metastases to bones of pelvis, lumbar spine, or femur
> - Pain (nonmechanical) does not vary with activity or position (intense, constant); night pain
> - Skin temperature differences from side to side
> - Progressive neurologic deficits[115]
>   - Sensory changes in myotome/dermatome pattern
>   - Decreased motor function
>   - Radiculopathy (rapid onset)
>   - Myelopathy or cauda equina syndrome
> - Positive percussive tap test to one or more spinous process
> - Occipital headache, neck pain, palpable external mass in neck or upper torso
> - Cervical pain or symptoms accompanied by urinary incontinence
> - Look for signs and symptoms associated with other visceral systems (e.g., GI, genitourinary [GU], pulmonary, gynecologic)

Clinical Presentation

For most oncologic causes of back pain, the thoracic and lumbosacral areas are affected. Pain and dysfunction in the lumbosacral area may be caused by direct spread of cancer from the abdomen or pelvic areas. When the lumbar spine is affected by metastases, it is usually from breast, lung, prostate, or kidney neoplasm. GI cancer, myelomas, and lymphomas can also spread to the spine via the paravertebral venous plexus. This thin-walled and valveless venous system probably accounts for the higher incidence of metastases in the thoracic spine from breast carcinoma and in the lumbar region from prostatic carcinoma.

Back pain associated with cancer is usually constant, intense, and worse at night or with weight-bearing activities; however, vague, diffuse back pain can be an early sign of non-Hodgkin lymphoma and multiple myeloma. Pain with metastasis to the spine may become quite severe before any radiologic manifestations appear.[107]

Back pain associated with malignant retroperitoneal lymphadenopathy from lymphomas or testicular cancers is characterized as persistent, poorly localized LBP present at night but relieved by forward flexion.[116,117] Pain may be so excruciating while lying down that the person can sleep only while sitting in a chair hunched forward over a table.

Neoplasm (whether primary or secondary) may interfere with the sympathetic nerves; if so, the foot on the affected side is warmer than the foot on the unaffected side. Paresis in the absence of nerve root pain suggests a tumor. Severe weakness without pain can be a red-flag sign of spinal metastases.

A short period of increasing central backache in an older person is always a red-flag symptom, especially if there is a previous history of cancer. The pain spreads down both lower limbs in a distribution that does not correspond with any one nerve root level. Bilateral sciatica then develops, and the back pain becomes worse.

X-rays do not show bone destruction from metastatic lesions until the lytic process has destroyed 30% to 50% of the bone. It cannot be assumed that metastatic lesions do not exist in the client with a past medical history of cancer now presenting with back pain and "normal" x-rays.[46,118,119]

Associated Signs and Symptoms

Clinical signs and symptoms accompanying back pain from an oncologic cause may be system related (e.g., GI, GU, gynecologic, spondylogenic), depending on where the primary neoplasm is located and the location of any metastases.

The PTA can always ask about the presence of constitutional symptoms and symptoms anywhere else in the body and then take vital signs as part of the assessment and data collection processes. Unexplained weight loss is a common feature in anyone with tumors of the spine. Review the red flags in Box 5.1 and conduct a Review of Systems to identify any clusters of signs and symptoms.

Recognizing and Reporting Cardiac Red Flags

Vascular pain patterns originate from two main sources: cardiac (heart viscera) and peripheral vascular (blood vessels). The most common referred cardiac pain patterns seen in a physical therapy practice are angina, MI, and aneurysm.

Pain of a cardiac nature referred to the soma is based on multisegmental innervation. For example, the heart is innervated by the C3 through T4 spinal nerves. Pain of a cardiac source can affect any part of the soma (body) also innervated by these levels. This explains why someone having a heart attack can experience jaw, neck, shoulder, arm, upper back, or chest pain. See Chapter 2 for an in-depth discussion of the origins of viscerogenic pain patterns affecting the musculoskeletal system.

On the other hand, pain and symptoms from a peripheral vascular problem are determined by the location of the underlying pathology (e.g., aortic aneurysm, arterial or venous obstruction). Peripheral vascular patterns are reviewed later in this chapter.

Angina

Angina may cause chest pain radiating to the anterior neck and jaw, sometimes appearing only as neck and/or jaw pain and misdiagnosed as temporomandibular joint dysfunction. Postmenopausal females are the most likely candidates for this type of presentation. If the jaw pain is steady, lasts a long time, or is worst when first waking up in the morning, the individual may be grinding teeth while sleeping. However, jaw pain that comes and goes with physical activity or stress may be a symptom of angina.[84]

Angina and/or MI can appear as isolated mid-thoracic back pain in males or females. There is usually a lag time of 3 to 5 minutes between increase in activity and onset of musculoskeletal symptoms caused by angina. This lag time is an important red flag to ask about or assess.

Myocardial Ischemia

Heart disease and MI, in particular, can be completely asymptomatic. In fact, sudden death occurs without any warning in many MIs. Back pain from the heart (cardiac pain pattern) can be referred to the anterior neck and/or mid-thoracic spine in both males and females.[120]

When pain does present, it may look like one of the patterns shown in Fig. 5.4. Some associated signs and symptoms usually appear, such as unexplained perspiration (diaphoresis), nausea, vomiting, pallor, dizziness, or extreme anxiety. Age and past medical history are important red flags for MI as a possible cause of musculoskeletal symptoms. Vital sign assessment is a key clinical assessment.

Abdominal Aortic Aneurysm

On occasion, an AAA can cause severe back pain (Fig. 5.5). An aneurysm is an abnormal dilation in a weak or diseased arterial wall causing a saclike protrusion. Prompt medical attention is imperative because rupture can result in death. Aneurysms can occur anywhere in any blood vessel, but the two most common places are the aorta and cerebral vascular system. AAAs occur most often in males in the sixth or seventh decade of life.[121]

Risk Factors. The major risk factors for AAA include older age, male sex,[122] smoking, and family history.[123–126] Although the underlying cause is most often atherosclerosis, aging athletes involved in weightlifting are at increased risk for tears in the arterial wall, resulting in an aneurysm. There is often a history of intermittent claudication and decreased or absent peripheral pulses. Other risk factors include congenital malformation and vasculitis. Often the presence of these risk factors remains unknown until an aneurysm becomes symptomatic.[127]

Clinical Presentation. Pain presents as deep and boring in the midlumbar region. The pattern is usually described as sharp, intense, severe, or knife-like in the abdomen, chest, or anywhere in the back (including the sacrum). The location of the symptoms is determined by the location of the aneurysm (see Fig. 5.5).

Most aortic aneurysms affect the abdominal rather than thoracic aorta and occur just below the renal arteries.[128] The client will be hypertensive if the renal artery is occluded as well. Peripheral pulses may be diminished or absent. Other historical clues of coronary disease or intermittent claudication of the lower extremities may be present.

▶▶ PTA ACTION PLAN

Working With Patients Who Have or Are at Risk for Aortic Aneurysm

Monitoring vital signs is important, especially among exercising senior adults. Teaching proper breathing and abdominal support without using a Valsalva maneuver is important in any exercise program, but especially for those clients at increased risk for aortic aneurysm.

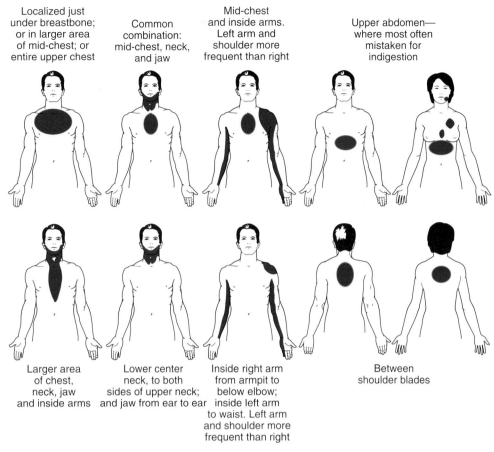

Localized just under breastbone; or in larger area of mid-chest; or entire upper chest

Common combination: mid-chest, neck, and jaw

Mid-chest and inside arms. Left arm and shoulder more frequent than right

Upper abdomen— where most often mistaken for indigestion

Larger area of chest, neck, jaw and inside arms

Lower center neck, to both sides of upper neck; and jaw from ear to ear

Inside right arm from armpit to below elbow; inside left arm to waist. Left arm and shoulder more frequent than right

Between shoulder blades

Most common warning signs of heart attack

- Uncomfortable pressure, fullness, squeezing or pain in the center of the chest (prolonged)
- Pain that spreads to the throat, neck, back, jaw, shoulders, or arms
- Chest discomfort with lightheadedness, dizziness, sweating, pallor, nausea, or shortness of breath
- Prolonged symptoms unrelieved by antacids, nitroglycerin, or rest

Atypical, less common warning signs (especially women)

- Unusual chest pain (quality, location, e.g., burning, heaviness; left chest), stomach or abdominal pain
- Continuous mid-thoracic or interscapular pain
- Continuous neck or shoulder pain (not shown in Fig. 5.4)
- Pain relieved by antacids; pain unrelieved by rest or nitroglycerin
- Nausea and vomiting; flu-like manifestation without chest pain/discomfort
- Unexplained intense anxiety, weakness, or fatigue
- Breathlessness, dizziness

FIG. 5.4 Early warning signs of a heart attack. Multiple segmental nerve innervations account for varied pain patterns possible. A female can experience any of the various patterns described but is just as likely to develop atypical symptoms of pain as depicted here. (From Goodman CC, Snyder TK: Differential diagnosis for physical therapists. *Screening for Referral.* ed 4, Mosby Saunders, 2007, Elsevier.)

❓ PICTURE THE PATIENT

Clinical signs and symptoms of impending rupture or actual rupture of the aortic aneurysm include the following:

- Rapid onset of severe neck or back pain (buttock, hip, and/or flank pain possible)
- Pain may radiate to chest, between the scapulae, or to posterior thighs
- Pain is not relieved by change in position
- Pain is described as "tearing" or "ripping"
- Other signs: cold, pulseless lower extremities, blood pressure differences between arms (>10 mm Hg diastolic)

The US Preventive Services Task Force (USPSTF) updated its guidelines for medical screening for AAA in 2019. The new guidelines recommend ultrasound screening for males ages 65 to 75 years who have ever smoked as a one-time screening evaluation.[129] The PTA/PT team should discuss and advise males in this age group who have ever smoked to discuss their risk for AAA with their primary care physician. The cost-effectiveness of routine screening in females for AAA is still under investigation by the USPSTF.

The PTA working in an orthopedic or acute care setting must be aware that aortic damage (not an aneurysm but a *pseudoaneurysm*) can occur with any anterior spine surgery (e.g., spinal fusion, spinal fusion with cages). Blood vessels are moved out of the way and can be injured during surgery. If the client (usually a postoperative inpatient) has internal bleeding from this complication, the following may occur:

- Distended abdomen
- Changes in blood pressure
- Changes in stool
- Possible back and/or shoulder pain

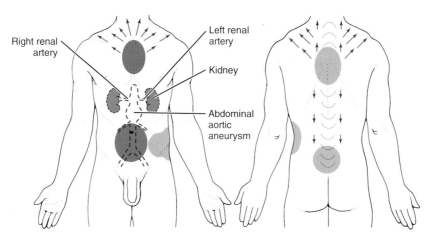

FIG. 5.5 Most aortic aneurysms (>95%) are located just below the renal arteries and extend to the umbilicus, causing low back pain. Chest pain (*dark red*) associated with thoracic aneurysms may radiate (*arrows*) to the neck, interscapular area, shoulders, lower back, or abdomen. Early warning signs of an impending rupture may include an abdominal heartbeat when lying down (*not shown*) or a dull ache in the midabdominal left flank or lower back (*light red*).

▶▶ PTA ACTION PLAN
Communication With the Physical Therapist

In such cases the client's recent history of anterior spinal surgery accompanied by any of these symptoms is enough justification for the PTA to notify the PT, nurse, or medical staff of concerns. Monitoring postoperative vital signs in these clients is essential.

Recognizing and Reporting Peripheral Vascular Red Flags

Most PTAs are very familiar with the signs and symptoms of PVD affecting the extremities, including both arterial and venous disease. PVD can also cause back pain. The location of the pain or symptoms is determined by the location of the pathology (Fig. 5.6).

❓ PICTURE THE PATIENT

With obstruction of the aortic bifurcation the client may report back pain alone, back pain with any of the following features, or any of these signs and symptoms alone (Table 5.5):
• Bilateral buttock and/or leg pain or discomfort
• Weakness and fatigue of the lower extremities
• Atrophy of the leg muscles
• Absent lower extremity pulses
• Color and/or temperature changes in the feet and lower legs

Symptoms are often (but not always) bilateral because the obstruction occurs before the aorta divides (i.e., before it becomes the common iliac artery and supplies each leg separately). Frequently, someone with symptomatic atherosclerotic disease in one blood vessel has similar pathology in other blood vessels as well. Over time, there may be a progression of symptoms as the disease worsens and blood vessels become more and more clogged with plaque and debris.

With obstruction of the iliac artery the client is more likely to present with pain in the low back, buttock, and/or leg of the affected side and/or numbness in the same area(s). Obstruction of the femoral artery can result in thigh and/or calf pain, again with distal pulses diminished or absent.[130]

Ipsilateral calf/ankle pain or discomfort (intermittent claudication) occurs with obstruction of the popliteal artery and is a common first symptom of PVD.

▶▶ PTA ACTION PLAN
Recognizing PVD Associated With Back Pain

When working with adults over the age of 50 who present with back pain of unknown cause and mild-to-moderate elevation of blood pressure, the PTA should consult with the therapist about the possibility of PVD.

Back Pain: Vascular or Neurogenic?

The medical differential diagnosis is difficult to make between back pain of a vascular versus neurogenic origin. Sometimes clients are referred to physical therapy to help make the differentiation (Case Example 5.4).

Frequently, vascular and neurogenic claudication occurs in the same age group (over 60, and often even more after age 70), and they coexist in the same person with an overlap of symptoms of each. The PTA should look for several major differences, but especially response to rest (i.e., activity pain), position of the spine, and the presence of any trophic (skin) changes (see Table 5.4 and Table 7.1).

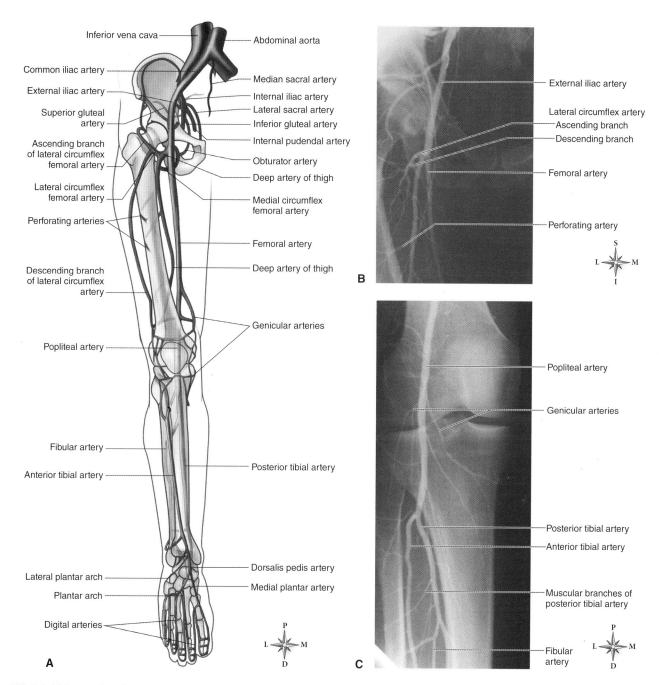

FIG. 5.6 Major arteries of the lower extremity. (A) Diagram of major arteries of lower extremity. (A) Diagram of major arteries of lower extremity. Anterior view of the right hip and leg. (B) Femoral arteriogram. Contrast material passing through the external iliac artery in the abdomen has entered the femoral artery and its branches in the thigh. (C) Popliteal arteriogram. (Patton KT, Thibodeau GA, Hutton A: Chapter 29: Blood vessels. *Anatomy and Physiology, International Edition*, 2019, Elsevier.)

🔎 PICTURE THE PATIENT

Vascular-induced back and/or leg pain or discomfort is alleviated by rest and usually within 1 to 3 minutes. Conversely, activity (usually walking) brings on the symptoms within 1 to 3, sometimes 3 to 5, minutes. The position of comfort for someone with back pain associated with spinal stenosis is usually lumbar flexion. The client may lean forward and rest the hands on the thighs or lean the upper body against a table or cupboard. Neurogenic-induced symptoms often occur immediately with use of the affected body part and/or when adopting certain positions. The client may report the pain is relieved by prolonged rest or not at all.

⏩ PTA ACTION PLAN

Recognizing Vascular and Neurogenic Back Pain

What is the effect of changing the position of the spine on pain of a vascular nature? Are the vascular structures compromised in any way by forward bending, side bending, or backward bending (see Fig. 5.3)? Are we asking the diseased heart or compromised blood vessels to supply more blood to this area? If the PTA understands these concepts, recognizing red flags requiring consultation with the therapist will be much easier.

TABLE 5.5   Back and Leg Pain From Arterial Occlusive Disease*

Site of Occlusion	Signs and Symptoms

Aortic bifurcation	• Sensory and motor deficits
	  • Muscle weakness and atrophy
	  • Numbness (loss of sensation)
	  • Paresthesias (burning, pricking)
	  • Paralysis
	• Intermittent claudication (pain or discomfort relieved by rest): bilateral buttock and/or leg, low back, gluteal, thigh, calf
	• Cold, pale legs with decreased or absent peripheral pulses

Iliac artery	• Intermittent claudication (pain or discomfort in the buttock, hip, thigh of the affected leg; can be unilateral or bilateral; relieved by rest) • Diminished or absent femoral or distal pulses • Impotence in males
Femoral and popliteal artery	• Intermittent claudication (pain or discomfort; calf and foot; may radiate) • Leg pallor and coolness • Dependent rubor • Blanching of feet on elevation • No palpable pulses in ankles and feet • Gangrene
Tibial and common peroneal artery	• Intermittent claudication (calf pain or discomfort; feet occasionally) • Pain at rest (severe disease); possibly relieved by dangling leg • Same skin and temperature changes in lower leg and foot as described above • Pedal pulses absent; popliteal pulses may be present

*The location of discomfort, pain, or other symptoms is determined by the location of the pathology (arterial obstruction).

From Goodman CC, Fuller KS: *Pathology: implications for the physical therapist*, ed 4, Philadelphia, 2014, WB Saunders.

For example, it is not likely that movements of the spine will reproduce back pain of a vascular origin. What about back pain of a neurogenic cause? Forward bending opens the vertebral canal (vertebral foramen), giving the spinal cord (through L1) additional space. This is important in preventing painful symptoms when spinal stenosis is present as a cause of neurogenic claudication.

Recognizing and Reporting Pulmonary Red Flags

Many potential pulmonary causes of back pain exist. The lungs occupy a large area of the upper trunk with an equally large anterior and posterior thoracic area where pain can be referred. The most common conditions known to refer pulmonary pain to the somatic areas are pleuritis, pneumothorax, pulmonary embolus, cor pulmonale, and pleurisy.

Past Medical History

A recent history of one of these disorders in a client with neck, shoulder, chest, or back pain raises a red flag of suspicion. In keeping with the model for recognizing red flags the PTA should be alert to (1) past medical history, (2) risk factors, (3) clinical presentation, and (4) associated signs and symptoms (Box 5.7).

Clinical Presentation

Pulmonary pain patterns vary in their presentation based in part by the lobe(s) or segment(s) involved and by the underlying pathology. Several different pain patterns are possible (see Fig. 4.1).

Autosplinting is considered a valuable red flag of possible pulmonary involvement.[131] Autosplinting occurs when the client prefers to lie on the involved side. Because pain of a pulmonary source is referred from the ipsilateral side, putting pressure on the involved lung field reduces respiratory movements and therefore reduces pain. It is uncommon for a person with a true musculoskeletal problem to find relief from symptoms by lying on the involved side.

⏩ PTA ACTION PLAN

Reporting Back Pain Associated With Respiratory Movements

The PTA can watch for anyone with back pain who has a suspicious history or respiratory symptoms at the same time they are experiencing back pain. If respiratory movements (e.g., deep breathing, laughing, or coughing) reproduce or increase painful symptoms, document and report this information.

Keep in mind that although reproducing pain or increased pain on respiratory movements is considered a hallmark sign of pulmonary involvement, symptoms of pleural, intercostal, muscular, costal, and dural origin all increase with coughing or deep inspiration.

Forceful coughing from an underlying pulmonary problem can cause an intercostal tear, which can be palpated. Even if some symptoms can be reproduced with palpation, the problem may still be pulmonary induced, especially if the cause is repeated, forceful coughing from a pulmonary etiology.

❓ PICTURE THE PATIENT

Pancoast tumors of the lung may invade the roots of the brachial plexus causing entrapment as they enlarge, appearing as pain in the C8–T1 region, possibly mimicking thoracic outlet syndrome. Other signs may include wasting of the muscles of the hand and/or Horner syndrome with unilateral constricted pupil, ptosis, and loss of facial sweating.[121]

Associated Signs and Symptoms

Assessing for associated signs and symptoms will usually bring to light important red flags to help the PTA recognize

CASE EXAMPLE 5.4   Spinal Stenosis

A 68-year-old female with a long history of degenerative arthritis of the spine was referred to physical therapy for conservative treatment toward a goal of improving function despite her painful symptoms. She was a nonsmoker with no other significant previous medical history.

Her symptoms were diffuse bilateral lumbosacral back pain into the buttocks and thighs, which increased with walking or any activity and did not subside substantially with rest (except for prolonged rest and immobility).

Initial Evaluation Information
Clinical Presentation: On examination, this client moved slowly and with effort, complaining of the painful symptoms described. There was no tenderness of the sacroiliac joint or sciatic notch but a subjective report of tenderness over L4–L5 and L5–S1. The tap test was negative; the client reported mild diffuse tenderness. There was no palpable step-off or dip of the spinous processes for spondylolisthesis and no paraspinal spasm, but a marked right lumbar scoliosis was noted. The client reported knowledge of scoliosis since she was a child.

A neurologic screening examination revealed normal straight leg raise and normal sensation and reflexes in both lower extremities. Motor examination was unremarkable for an inactive 68-year-old female. Dorsalis pedis and posterior tibialis pulses were palpable but weak bilaterally.

Current Clinical Presentation on Fourth Treatment Session: The client reports to the physical therapist assistant (PTA) compliance with her home program, but her symptoms are persisting and are actually worse today. The

PTA assessed the client's vital signs and asked for more specific information regarding the increase in pain to determine a possible connection to her movement patterns. The PTA notices that a complete review of systems has not been conducted to date and makes note of this to discuss with the physical therapist (PT).

What is the Appropriate Action of the PTA Today?
Document all observations. Notify the PT of progressive worsening of client's symptoms. Discuss the need to reevaluate the client's movement dysfunction and report on the selected interventions provided to date.

In this case the client's age, negative neurologic screening examination, and diminished lower extremity pulses suggested to the PT that a second look for vascular cause of symptoms was needed.

A peripheral vascular screening examination was completed. The bike test was also administered, but the results were unclear with increased pain reported in both extension and flexion.

Result: The patient returned to her physician with a report of these findings. Further testing showed that in addition to degenerative arthritis of the lumbosacral spine, there was secondary stenosis and marked aortic calcification, indicating a vascular component to her symptoms.

Surgery was scheduled: an L4–L5 laminectomy with fusion, iliac crest bone graft, and decompression foraminotomies. Postoperatively, the client subjectively reported 80% improvement in her symptoms with an improvement in function, although she was still unable to return to work.

BOX 5.7   Screening for Pulmonary-Induced Neck or Back Pain

History
Previous history of cancer (any kind, but especially lung, breast, bone cancer, myeloma, lymphoma)
Previous history of recurrent upper respiratory infection (URI) or pneumonia
Recent scuba diving, accident, trauma, or overexertion (pneumothorax)

Risk Factors
Smoking
Trauma (e.g., rib fracture, vertebral compression fracture)
Prolonged immobility
Chronic immunosuppression (e.g., corticosteroids, cancer chemotherapy)
Malnutrition, dehydration
Chronic diseases: diabetes mellitus, chronic lung disease, renal disease, cancer
URI or pneumonia

Pain Pattern
Sharp, localized
Aggravated by respiratory movements
Prefer to sit upright
Autosplinting decreasing the pain
Range of motion not reproducing symptoms (e.g., shoulder and/or trunk movements)

Associated Signs and Symptoms
Dyspnea
Persistent cough
Constitutional symptoms: fever, chills
Weak and rapid pulse with concomitant fall in blood pressure (e.g., pneumothorax)

a potential pulmonary problem. Neck or back pain that is reproduced, increased with inspiratory movements, or accompanied by dyspnea, persistent cough, cyanosis, or hemoptysis must be reevaluated by the therapist. Clients with respiratory origins of pain usually also show signs of general malaise or constitutional symptoms.

Recognizing and Reporting Renal and Urologic Red Flags

When considering the possibility of a renal or urologic cause of back pain, the PTA can keep in mind the same step-by-step approach of looking at the history, risk factors, clinical presentation, and associated signs and symptoms. For example, in anyone with back pain reported in the T9–L1 area corresponding to pain patterns from the kidney or urinary tract (see Figs. 4.7 and 4.8), ask about a history of kidney stones, urinary tract infections (UTIs), and trauma (e.g., fall, blow, lift).

Origin of Pain Patterns

As discussed in Chapter 2, there can be at least three possible explanations for visceral pain patterns, including embryologic development, multisegmental innervation, and direct pressure on the diaphragm.

All three of these mechanisms are found in the urologic system. The *embryologic* origin of urologic pain patterns begins with the testicles and ovaries. These reproductive organs begin in utero where the kidneys are in the adult and then migrate during fetal development following the pathways of the ureters. A kidney stone down the pathway of the ureter causes pain in the flank radiating to the scrotum (male) or labia (female).

Evidence of the influence of *multisegmental innervation* is observed when skin pain over the kidneys is reported. Visceral and cutaneous sensory fibers enter the spinal cord close to each other and converge on the same neurons. When visceral pain fibers are stimulated, cutaneous fibers are also stimulated. Thus visceral pain can be perceived as skin pain.

None of the components of the lower urinary tract comes in contact with the diaphragm, so the bladder and urethra are not likely to refer pain to the shoulder. Lower urinary tract impairment is more likely to refer pain to the low back, pelvic, or sacral areas. However, the upper urinary tract can impinge the diaphragm with resultant referred pain to the costovertebral area or shoulder.

Past Medical History

Kidney disorders such as acute pyelonephritis and perinephric abscess of the kidney may be confused with a back condition. Most renal and urologic conditions appear with a combination of systemic signs and symptoms accompanied by pelvic, flank, or LBP. The client may have a history of recent trauma or a past medical history of UTIs. If the therapist is not aware of this information, the PTA can alert him or her of this information.

Clinical Presentation

Acute pyelonephritis, perinephric abscess, and other kidney conditions appear with aching pain at one or several costovertebral areas, posteriorly, just lateral to the muscles at T12–L1, from acute distention of the capsule of the kidney.[117] The pain is usually dull and constant, with possible radiation to the pelvic crest or groin. The client may describe febrile chills, frequent urination, hematuria, and shoulder pain (if the diaphragm is irritated).

Nephrolithiasis (kidney stones) may appear as back pain radiating to the flank or the iliac crest (see Fig. 4.8). Kidney stones may occur in the presence of diseases associated with hypercalcemia (excess calcium in the blood) such as hyperparathyroidism, metastatic carcinoma, multiple myeloma, senile osteoporosis, specific renal tubular disease, hyperthyroidism, and Cushing disease. Other conditions associated with calculus formation are infection, urinary stasis, dehydration, and excessive ingestion or absorption of calcium.[132]

Ureteral colic, caused by passage of a kidney stone (calculus), appears as excruciating pain that radiates down the course of the ureter into the urethra or groin area. The pain is unrelieved by rest or change in position. These attacks are intermittent and may be accompanied by nausea, vomiting, sweating, and tachycardia. Localized abdominal muscle spasm may be present. The urine usually contains erythrocytes or is grossly bloody.[133]

UTI affecting the lower urinary tract is related directly to irritation of the bladder and urethra. The intensity of symptoms depends on the severity of the infection. Although LBP may be the client's chief complaint, further questioning usually elicits additional urologic symptoms. The PTA should report anytime the client describes the following:

- Urinary frequency, urgency, dysuria (burning pain on urination), or nocturia (frequency at night)
- Constitutional symptoms (fever, chills, nausea, vomiting)
- Blood in urine
- Testicular pain

The important thing to look and listen for is *change*. Many people have problems with incontinence, nocturia, or frequency. If someone has always experienced a delay before starting a flow of urine, this may be normal for him (or her).

▶▶ PTA ACTION PLAN

Points to Ponder

Many females have nocturia after childbirth, but most males do not get up at night to empty their bladders until after age 65. They may not even be aware that this has changed for them; often, the wife or partner is the one who answers the question about getting up at night. Likewise, if a male has always had a delay in starting a flow of urine, he may not be aware that the delay is now twice as long as before. Or he may not recognize that being unable to continue a flow of urine is not "normal" and, in fact, requires medical evaluation. When the PTA is aware of any incontinence issues, the therapist should be notified and a plan of care discussed that may include addressing any underlying neuromusculoskeletal causes.

Recognizing and Reporting Gastrointestinal Red Flags

Back pain of all the possible visceral origins seen in a physical therapy clinic occurs most often as a result of GI problems. Pain patterns associated with the GI system can present as sternal, shoulder, scapular, mid-back, low back, or hip pain and dysfunction.[130] If the client had *primary* symptoms of GI impairment (abdominal pain, nausea, diarrhea, or constipation), he or she would see a medical doctor.

As it is, the referred pain patterns are quite convincing that the musculoskeletal region described is the problem. Referred pain patterns for the GI system are presented in Fig. 5.7 (anterior and posterior). These are the pain patterns the PTA is more likely to hear described.

Past Medical History and Risk Factors

Paying attention to past medical history, risk factors, and clinical presentation and asking about associated signs and symptoms may reveal important red flags and clues of possible GI system involvement. The most significant and common history is one of long-term or chronic use of NSAIDs. Other significant risk factors in the history include the long-term use of immunosuppressants, past history of cancer, history of Crohn disease (also known as regional enteritis), or previous bowel obstruction.

Signs and Symptoms of Gastrointestinal Dysfunction

The most common signs and symptoms associated with the GI system are listed in Box 5.8. Back pain (as well as hip, pelvic, sacral, and lower extremity pain) with any of these

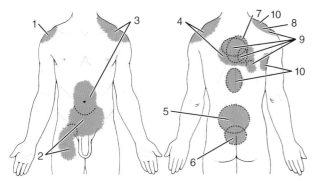

FIG. 5.7 Full-figure referred pain patterns. *1*, Liver/gallbladder/common bile duct; *2*, appendix; *3*, pancreas; *4*, pancreas; *5*, small intestine; *6*, colon; *7*, esophagus; *8*, stomach/duodenum; *9*, liver/gallbladder/common bile duct; and *10*, stomach/duodenum.

BOX 5.8 Signs and Symptoms of Gastrointestinal Dysfunction

Anterior neck pain or back pain accompanied by any of the following is a red flag:
- Esophageal pain
- Epigastric pain with radiation to the back
- Dysphagia (difficulty swallowing)
- Odynophagia (pain with swallowing)
- Early satiety; symptoms associated with meals
- Bloody diarrhea
- Fecal incontinence
- Melena (dark, tarry, sticky stools caused by oxidized blood)
- Hemorrhage (blood in the toilet)

---

accompanying features should be considered a red flag for the possibility of GI impairment.

Anterior neck (esophageal) pain may occur, usually with a burning sensation ("heartburn") or other symptoms related to eating or swallowing (e.g., dysphagia, odynophagia). Esophageal varices associated with chronic alcoholism may appear as anterior neck pain but usually occur at the xiphoid process and are attributed to heartburn.

▶▶ PTA ACTION PLAN

Recognizing Gastrointestinal Signs and Symptoms

The PTA should look and listen for other associated signs and symptoms, such as sore throat; pain that is relieved with antacids, fluids, the upright position, or avoidance of eating; and pain that is aggravated by eating, bending, or recumbency. The PTA may become aware of other unusual causes of anterior neck pain (e.g., anterior disk protrusion, eating disorders with vomiting) that should be brought to the therapist's attention.

Dysphagia (difficulty swallowing), *odynophagia* (painful swallowing), and *epigastric pain* are indicative of esophageal involvement. Certain types of drugs (e.g., antidepressants,

antihypertensives, asthma medications) can make swallowing difficult and should be considered a potential cause of dysphagia among those individuals taking these medications.

Early satiety (the client takes one or two bites of food and is no longer hungry) is another red-flag symptom of the GI system (Case Example 5.5). In general, back pain made better, worse, or altered in any way by eating is a red-flag symptom. If the change in symptom(s) occurs immediately to within 30 minutes of eating, the upper GI tract or stomach/duodenum may be a possible cause. Change in symptoms 2 to 4 hours *after* eating is more indicative of the lower GI tract (intestines/colon).

Bloody diarrhea, fecal incontinence, and *melena* are three additional signs of lower GI involvement. It is important to ask the client about the presence of specific signs that may be too embarrassing to mention (or the client may not see the connection between back pain and bowel smears on the underwear). Asking someone with back pain about bowel function can be accomplished professionally. The more experienced PTA may tell the client:

I am going to ask you a series of questions about your bowels. This may not seem like it is connected to your current problem, so just bear with me. These are important questions to make sure we have covered every possibility. If you do not know the answer to the question, pay attention over the next day or two to see how everything is working. If you notice anything unusual or different, please let me know or talk with the physical therapist when you come in next time.

▶▶ PTA ACTION PLAN

Follow-Up Questions

- When was your last bowel movement? (Look for a change of any kind in the client's normal elimination pattern. In addition, failure to have a bowel movement over a much longer period than expected for that client may be a sign of impaction/obstruction/obstipation.)
- Are you having any diarrhea?
- Is there any blood in your stool?
- Have you ever been told you have hemorrhoids or do you know that you have hemorrhoids?
- Do you have difficulty wiping yourself clean?
- Do you find smears on your underwear later after a bowel movement?
- Do you have small amounts of stool leakage?

Again, when it comes to something like bowel smears on the underpants, it is important to distinguish between pathology and poor hygiene. The key distinction is change, such as the new appearance of a problem that was not present before the onset of back pain or other symptoms. With blood in the stools a medical doctor must differentiate between internal and external bleeding.

Melena is a dark, tarry stool caused by oxidation of blood in the GI tract (usually the upper GI tract, but it can be the lower GI tract). The most common causes of abdominal bleeding are chronic use of NSAIDs (leading to ulceration), Crohn disease,

CASE EXAMPLE 5.5   Early Satiety and Weight Loss

Background: A 78-year-old female was referred to physical therapy by her orthopedic surgeon 6 weeks status post total knee replacement (TKR). Her active knee flexion was 70 degrees; passive knee flexion was only 86 degrees. There was a 15-degree extensor lag.

Her social history included the recent death of a spouse. She had taken care of her husband at home for the last 3 years after he had a severe stroke. She knew she needed a knee replacement but put it off because of her husband's poor health. Within 6 weeks of his death, she scheduled the needed operation.

During the course of her rehabilitation program, her adult daughters took turns bringing her to the clinic. There were multiple occasions that they all commented on how much weight their mother had lost.

During a specific session the physical therapist assistant (PTA) asked the client about the weight loss, she replied, "Oh, I take a bite or two and then I'm not very hungry." The PTA asked, "How long has this been going on?" The client replied that the symptom (early satiety with weight loss) had been present for the last 2 months (starting prior to the TKR).

Small Group Activity

List some questions with which the PTA could ask the client to follow-up (see Chapter 4).

The answers to the follow-up questions revealed that she did not have any other signs or symptoms associated with the gastrointestinal system. There were no reported changes in bowel function or the appearance of her stools, no blood in the stools, no back or sacral pain, no night pain that was not directly related to her knee, and no other changes in her health.

What do you see in the history, clinical presentation, and associated signs and symptoms as they are presented here that raise a red flag?

- History: age and positive social history for recent personal loss
- Clinical presentation: unremarkable; consistent with orthopedic diagnosis
- Associated signs and symptoms: early satiety with weight loss

There are really only two red flags here (age and early satiety with weight loss), but they are significant enough to warrant contact with her physician.

What is the Appropriate Action of the PTA?

The PTA should document all important information pertinent to the follow-up questions asked and the client's current status. The PTA should then notify the physical therapist (PT), if possible, while the client is still in the clinic. If immediate communication is not possible, the PTA should inform the client that he or she will follow-up with the primary PT to see what the next step will be prior to the next therapy session.

Once the PTA and PT discussed the details, the PT decided that it may be best to communicate all findings with the referring physician or health care provider.

Outcome: The orthopedic surgeon recommended referral to her primary care physician. Examination and diagnostic tests resulted in a diagnosis of esophageal cancer (early stage). The client was treated successfully for the cancer while completing her rehabilitation program.

---

or ulcerative colitis, as well as diverticulitis or diverticulosis. Anyone with a history of these problems presenting with new onset of back pain must be reevaluated by the PT.

Hemorrhage or visible blood in the toilet may be a sign of anal fissures, hemorrhoids, or colon cancer. The etiology must be determined by a medical doctor. Be aware that there is an increased incidence of rectal bleeding from anal fissures and local tissue damage associated with anal intercourse. This occurs predominantly in the male homosexual or bisexual population but can be seen in heterosexual partners who engage in anal intercourse. There are also increasing reports of adolescents engaging in oral and anal intercourse as a form of birth control.

▶▶ PTA ACTION PLAN

Communication With the Therapist

Anytime the PTA is aware of bleeding issues, immediate consultation with the PT is required. This statement may seem like it is very obvious, but many patients do not want to discuss this problem (or are too embarrassed to) with health care professionals. The PTA may also feel awkward or unsure about how to respond to comments patients might make. In general, it would be a good idea to discuss with the therapist his or her preferred approach to this type of medical history/clinical presentation.

Esophagus

Esophageal pain will occur at the level of the lesion and is usually accompanied by epigastric pain and heartburn. Severe esophagitis may refer pain to the anterior cervical or, more often, the mid-thoracic spine.

The pain pattern will most likely present in a band of pain starting anteriorly and spreading around the chest wall to the back. Rarely, pain will begin in the mid-back and radiate around to the front. Referred pain to the mid-thoracic spine occurs around T5–T6.

As with cervical pain of GI origin, there may be a history of alcoholism with esophageal varices,[134] cirrhosis, or an underlying eating disorder. If liver impairment is an underlying factor, there may be signs such as asterixis (liver flap or flapping tremor), palmar erythema, spider angiomas, and carpal (tarsal) tunnel syndrome (see discussion in Chapter 4).

Stomach and Duodenum

Long-term use of NSAIDs is the most common cause of back pain referred from the stomach or duodenum. Ulceration and bleeding into the retroperitoneal area can cause pain in the back or shoulder. The primary and referred pain patterns for pain of a stomach or duodenal source are shown in Fig. 5.8.

The referred pain to the back is at the level of the lesion, usually between T6 and T10. For the client with mid-thoracic spine pain of unknown cause or that does not fit the expected musculoskeletal presentation, listen for any patient report of associated signs and symptoms such as the following:

- Blood in the stools
- Symptoms associated with meals
- Relief of pain after eating (immediately or 2 hours later)

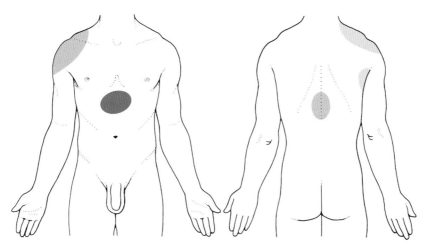

FIG. 5.8 Stomach or duodenal pain (*dark red*) may occur anteriorly in the midline of the epigastrium or upper abdomen just below the xiphoid process. There is a tendency for the stomach and duodenum to refer pain posteriorly. Referred pain (*light red*) to the back occurs at the anatomic level of the abdominal lesion (T6–10). Other patterns of referred pain (*light red*) may include the right shoulder and upper trapezius or the lateral border of the right scapula.

- Increased symptoms during a bowel movement
- Decreased symptoms after a bowel movement

The pain of peptic ulcer occasionally occurs only in the midthoracic back between T6 and T10, either at the midline or immediately to one side or the other of the spine. Posterior penetration of the retroperitoneum with blood loss and resultant-referred thoracic pain is most often caused by long-term use of NSAIDs. The therapist should be notified any time the PTA is aware of any correlation between symptoms and the timing of meals, as well as the presence of blood in the feces or relief of symptoms with antacids.

Small Intestine

Diseases of the small intestine (e.g., Crohn disease, irritable bowel syndrome, obstruction from neoplasm) usually produce midabdominal pain around the umbilicus, but the pain may be referred to the back if the stimulus is sufficiently intense or if the individual's pain threshold is low (Fig. 5.9).

For the client with LBP of unknown cause or suspicious presentation, the PTA may ask if any abdominal pain is ever present. Alternating abdominal/LBP at the same level is a red flag that requires documentation and therapist notification. Since both symptoms do not always occur together, the client may not recognize the relationship or report the symptoms to the therapist.

Look for a known history of Crohn disease (regional enteritis), irritable bowel syndrome, bowel obstruction, or cancer. Low back, sacral, or hip pain may be a new symptom of an already established disease. The client may not be aware that more than 25% of the people with GI disease also have back or joint pain.[135,136]

PICTURE THE PATIENT

Enteric-induced arthritis can be accompanied by a skin rash that comes and goes. A flat red or purple rash or raised skin lesion(s) is possible, usually preceding the joint or back pain. The PTA must ask the client if he or she has had any skin rashes in the last few weeks.

The PTA may be involved in treating joint or back pain when there is an unknown or unrecognized enteric (GI) cause. Treatment for musculoskeletal symptoms or apparent movement impairment can make a difference in the short term but does not affect the final outcome. Eventually the GI symptoms will progress; symptoms that are unrelieved by physical therapy intervention are red flags. Medical treatment of the underlying disease is essential to correcting the musculoskeletal component.

Recognizing and Reporting Hepatic Red Flags

The primary pain pattern for liver disease is directly over the liver. When a referred pain pattern occurs, the patient reports back pain. There is no complaint of anterior pain to alert the PTA to the possibility of a problem outside the scope of the PTA. Patients with the referred pain patterns depicted and described in Fig. 4.4 may require liver palpation by the PT. In addition to a painful and distended liver the client may report the following:
- Pain/nausea 1 to 3 hours after eating (gallstones)
- Pain immediately after eating (gallbladder inflammation)
- Muscle guarding/tenderness and fever/chills in the right upper quadrant (posterior)

Other signs and symptoms associated with liver impairment are discussed in detail in Chapter 4 and include the following:

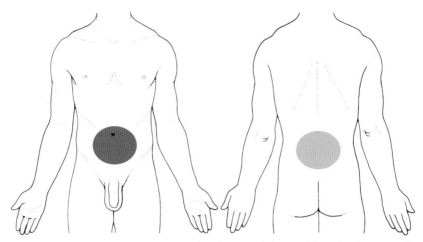

FIG. 5.9 Midabdominal pain (*dark red*) caused by disturbances of the small intestine is centered around the umbilicus (T9–11 nerve distribution) and may be referred (*light red*) to the low back area at the same anatomic level. Keep in mind the umbilicus is at the same level as the L3–4 disk space in the average adult who is not obese or who has a protruding abdomen.

- Liver flap (asterixis)
- Nail-bed changes (nail of Terry)
- Palmar erythema (liver palms)
- Spider angiomas
- Ascites, jaundice

 PTA ACTION PLAN

Reporting Signs and Symptoms of Hepatic System

Gallbladder and biliary disease may also refer pain to the interscapular or right subscapular area. The PTA should inform the therapist of any report of fever and chills, nausea and indigestion, changes in urine or stool, or signs of jaundice. The client may not associate GI symptoms with the scapular pain or discomfort. The therapist can use specific questions to rule out potential GI problems.

The Pancreas

Acute pancreatitis may appear as epigastric pain radiating to the mid-thoracic spine (Fig. 5.10). Pain from the head of the pancreas is felt to the right of the spine, whereas pain from the body and tail is perceived to the left of the spine. More rarely, pain may be referred to the upper back and midscapular areas.[22]

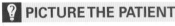 **PICTURE THE PATIENT**

There may be a history of alcohol and tobacco use. Associated symptoms, which are usually GI related, may include diarrhea, anorexia, pain after a meal, and unexplained weight loss. The pain is relieved initially by heat, which decreases muscular tension, and may be relieved by leaning forward, sitting up, or lying motionless.

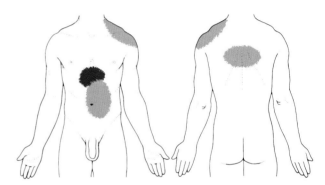

FIG. 5.10 Pancreatic pain (*dark red*) occurs in the midline or left of the epigastrium, just below the xiphoid process, but may be referred (*light red*) to the left shoulder or to the mid-thoracic spine. Posterior pain may radiate or lateralize from the spine away from the midline. Sensory nerve distribution is from T5 to T9.

PTA ACTION PLAN

Communication With the Therapist

The PTA should report to the therapist anytime a client with LBP reports a benefit from a heating pad at home or other heat modalities but then suddenly gets worse and does not improve with physical therapy intervention.

Recognizing and Reporting Red Flags of Infection

Drug abuse, immune suppression, and human immunodeficiency virus may predispose to infection. Fever in anyone taking immunosuppressants is a red-flag symptom indicating a possible underlying infection. Many people with a spinal infection do not have a fever; they are more likely to have a red-flag history or risk factors.[55]

Vertebral Osteomyelitis

Vertebral osteomyelitis is a bone infection most often affecting the first and second lumbar vertebrae, causing LBP. There are many causative factors. Osteomyelitis may occur in individuals with diabetes, intravenous drug users, alcoholics, clients taking corticosteroid drugs, clients with spinal cord injury and neurogenic bladder, and otherwise debilitated or immune-suppressed clients. Older children can be affected, although the most common peak is after the third decade of life.[137]

Vertebral osteomyelitis is increasingly being reported as a complication of health care–associated bacteremia. Methicillin-resistant *Staphylococcus aureus* (MRSA) is the most common causative organism. Osteomyelitis can also occur after surgery, open fractures, penetrating wounds, skin breakdown and ulcers, and systemic infections. It may result from a hematogenous (blood system) spread through arterial and venous routes secondary to (1) surgically implanted hardware for internal fixation of the spine, (2) pelvic inflammatory disease, or (3) GU tract infection.

▶▶ PTA ACTION PLAN

Communication With the Therapist

The therapist should be told about new onset of back pain in anyone who has been treated with vancomycin therapy for MRSA. Vancomycin therapy may give the appearance of being effective with resolution of fever and the return of white blood cell counts to normal ranges but, in fact, may be insufficient to prevent or reverse the progression of hematogenous MRSA vertebral osteomyelitis.[138,139] Medical referral is often required.

In the adult, usually two adjacent vertebrae and their intervening disk are involved, and the vertebral body(ies) may undergo destruction and collapse. Abscess formation may result, with possible neurologic involvement. The abscess can advance anteriorly to produce an abscess that can extend to the psoas muscle producing hip pain.

💡 PICTURE THE PATIENT

The most consistent clinical finding is marked local tenderness over the spinous process of the involved vertebrae with "nonspecific backache." The classic history describes pain that has been increasing in severity over a period of 1 to 3 weeks. Movement is painful, and there is marked muscular guarding and spasm of the paravertebral muscles and the hamstrings. The involved vertebrae are usually exquisitely sensitive to pressure, and pain is more severe at night. There may be no rise in temperature or a low-grade fever in adults when body temperature changes do occur.

Children are more likely to present with acute, severe complaints including high fever, intense pain, and localized manifestations such as edema, erythema, and tenderness. Acute hematogenous osteomyelitis seen in children usually originates in the metaphysis of a long bone. Precipitating trauma is often present in the history, and well-localized, acute bone pain of 1 day to several days' duration is the primary symptom. The pain is most commonly severe enough to limit or restrict the use of the involved extremity, and fever and malaise consistent with sepsis are usual.[140]

▶▶ PTA ACTION PLAN

What to Watch for

Clinical signs and symptoms of vertebral osteomyelitis can include the following:
* Pain and local tenderness over the involved spinous process(es); possible swelling, redness, and warmth in the affected area
* Night pain
* Stiff back with difficulty bearing weight, moving, walking
* Paravertebral muscle guarding or spasm
* Pain with straight leg raise (SLR)
* Hip pain if infection spreads to the psoas muscle
* May be constitutional symptoms (fever, malaise)
* Recent history of bacterial infection (e.g., pharyngitis, otitis media in children)

Disk Space Infection

Disk space infection is a form of subacute osteomyelitis involving the vertebral end-plates and the disk in both children and adults. The lower thoracic and lumbar spines are the most common sites of infection.

Symptoms associated with postoperative disk space infection occur 2 to 8 weeks after diskectomy. Diskitis of an infectious type occurs following bacteremia resulting from UTI, with or without instrumentation (e.g., catheterization or cystoscopy). Low-grade viral or bacterial infection (e.g., gastroenteritis, upper respiratory infection, UTI) is most often implicated in young children with diskitis (4 years old and younger).[53] The PTA can ask the parent, guardian, or caretaker of any young child with back pain if there has been a recent history of sore throat, cold, ear infection, or other upper respiratory illness. A positive response (if unknown to the therapist) must be reported immediately.

💡 PICTURE THE PATIENT

Adults with disk space infection often complain of LBP localized around the disk area. The pain can range from mild to "excruciating" and sometimes described as "knife like." Such severe pain is accompanied by restricted movement and constant pain, present both day and night. The pain is usually made worse by activity, but unlike most other causes of back pain, it is not relieved by rest.

If the condition becomes chronic, pain may radiate into the abdomen, pelvis, and lower extremities. The affected individual may have localized tenderness over the involved disk space, paraspinal muscle spasm, and restricted lumbar motion. SLR may be positive, and fever is common (Case Example 5.6).

Children present with a history of increasingly severe localized back pain often accompanied by a limp or refusal to walk. There may be an increased lumbar lordosis. Pain may occur in the flank, abdomen, or hip. Symptoms may get worse with a passive straight leg position or other hip motion.

CASE EXAMPLE 5.6   Septic Diskitis

A 72-year-old male with leg myalgia and stabbing back pain of 2 weeks' duration was referred to physical therapy for evaluation by a rural nurse practitioner.

Initial Evaluation Information

Past Medical History: The client reported a prostatectomy 22 years ago with no further problems. He was not aware of any other associated signs and symptoms but reported a recurring dermatitis that was being treated by his nurse practitioner. There were no skin lesions associated with the dermatitis present at the time of the physical therapist (PT) evaluation.

Clinical Presentation: The examination revealed spasm of the thoracolumbosacral paraspinal muscles bilaterally. The client reported extreme sensitivity to palpation of the spinous processes at L3 and L4; tap test reproduced painful symptoms. Spinal accessory motions could not be tested because of the client's state of acute pain and immobility.

Hip flexion and extension reproduced the symptoms and produced additional radiating flank pain. A straight leg raise (SLR) caused severe back pain with each leg at 30 degrees on both sides. A neurologic examination was otherwise within normal limits. Vital signs were not taken during the initial evaluation. A physical therapy plan of care was developed and the client was set up with another session for the very next day.

Upon the client's return to the clinic for his second treatment session, he reported to the physical therapist assistant (PTA) that he has an increase in pain and discomfort. The PTA assessed the vital signs: blood pressure of 180/100 mm Hg; heart rate of 100 bpm; temperature of 101°F.

What are the Red Flags in this Case?

- Age
- Recurring dermatitis
- Positive tap test
- Bilateral SLR
- Vital signs

The PTA documented the observations and immediately reported the details of the client's complaints of pain and vital sign information to the PT.

Result: The therapist contacted the nurse practitioner by telephone to report the findings, especially the vital signs and results of the SLR. It was determined that the client needed a medical evaluation, and he was referred to a physician's center in the nearest available city. A summary of findings from the PT was sent with the client along with a request for a copy of the physician's report.

The client returned to the PT's clinic with a copy of the physician's report with the following diagnosis: *Clostridium perfringens* septic diskitis (made on the basis of blood culture). The prescribed treatment was intravenous antibiotic therapy for 6 weeks, progressive mobilization, and a spinal brace to be provided and fitted by the PT. The client's back pain subsided gradually over the next 2 weeks. He was followed up at intervals until he was weaned from the brace and resumed normal activities.

Note: Septic diskitis may occur following various invasive procedures, or it may be related to occult infections, urinary tract infections, septicemia, and dermatitis. Contact dermatitis was the most likely underlying cause in this case.

Bacterial Endocarditis

Bacterial endocarditis often presents initially with musculoskeletal symptoms, including arthralgia, arthritis, LBP, and myalgias. Half of these clients will have only musculoskeletal symptoms, without other signs of endocarditis.[76,109,141]

The early onset of joint pain and myalgia is more likely if the client is older and has had a previously diagnosed heart murmur or prosthetic valve (risk factors). Other risk factors include injection drug use, previous cardiac surgery, recent dental work, and recent history of invasive diagnostic procedures (e.g., shunts, catheters).[142]

Almost one-third of clients with bacterial endocarditis have LBP. In many persons, LBP is the principal musculoskeletal symptom reported. Back pain is accompanied by decreased ROM and spinal tenderness. Pain may affect only one side, and it may be limited to the paraspinal muscles.[83,137]

🔖 PICTURE THE PATIENT

Endocarditis-induced LBP may be very similar to the pain pattern associated with a herniated lumbar disk; it radiates to the leg and may be accentuated by raising the leg, coughing, or sneezing. The key difference is that neurologic deficits are usually absent in clients with bacterial endocarditis.

REFERENCES

1. Waterman BR, Belmont PJ, Schoenfeld AJ: Low back pain in the United States: incidence and risk factors for presentation in the emergency setting, *Spine* 12:63–70, 2012.
2. Deyo RA, Von Korff M, Duhrkoop D: Opioids for low back pain, *BMJ* 350:g6380, 2015.
3. Maas ET, Juch JNS, Groeneweg JG, et al: Cost-effectiveness of minimal interventional procedures for chronic mechanical low back pain: design of four randomized controlled trials with an economic evaluation, *BMC Musculoskelet Disorders* 13:260, 2012.
4. Jarvik J, Deyo R: Diagnostic evaluation of low back pain with emphasis on imaging, *Ann Intern Med* 137:586–597, 2002.
5. Spitzer WO: Quebec task force on spinal disorders: scientific approach to the assessment and management of activity-related spinal disorders: a monograph for clinicians, *Spine* 12(Suppl 1): 51–59, 1987.
6. Sembrano JN, Polly DW: How often is low back pain not coming from the back? *Spine* 34:E27–E32, 2009.
7. Bernard TN Jr, Kirkaldy-Willis WH: Recognizing specific characteristics of nonspecific low back pain, *Clin Orthop* 217:266–280, 1987.
8. Shaw JA: The role of the sacroiliac joint as a cause of low back pain and dysfunction. In Vleeming A, Mooney V, Snijders C, editors: *The First Interdisciplinary World Congress on low back pain and its relation to the sacroiliac joint*, Rotterdam, 1992, Economic Cooperation Organization, pp 67–80.
9. Depalma MJ: What is the source of chronic low back pain and does age play a role? *Pain Med* 12(2):224–233, 2011.
10. Vora AJ: Functional anatomy and pathophysiology of axial low back pain: discs, posterior elements, sacroiliac joint, and associated pain generators, *Phys Med Rehabil Clin North Am* 21(4):679–709, 2010.
11. Vanelderen P: Sacroiliac joint pain, *Pain Pract* 10(5):470–478, 2010.
12. Cohen SP, Chen Y, Neufeld NJ: Sacroiliac joint pain: a comprehensive review of epidemiology, diagnosis and treatment, *Expert Rev Neurother* 13(1):99–116, 2013.

13. Kim DH, Hilibrand AS: Rheumatoid arthritis in the cervical spine, *J Am Acad Orthop Surg* 13(7):463–474, 2005.

14. Magarelli N: MR imaging of atlantoaxial joint in early rheumatoid arthritis, *Radiol Med* 115(7):1111–1120, 2010.

15. Krauss WE: Rheumatoid arthritis of the craniovertebral junction, *Neurosurgery* 66(3 Suppl):83–95, 2010.

16. McDonnell M, Lucas P: Cervical spondylosis, stenosis, and rheumatoid arthritis, *Med Health R I* 95(4):105–109, 2012.

17. Guzman J: A new conceptual model of neck pain, *Spine* 33(4S):S14–S23, 2008.

18. Boissonnault WG, Koopmeiners MB: Medical history profile: orthopaedic physical therapy outpatients, *J Orthop Sports Phys Ther* 20:2–10, 1994.

19. Boissonault WG: Prevalence of comorbid conditions, surgeries, and medication use in a physical therapy outpatient population: a multi-centered study, *J Orthop Sports Phys Ther* 29:506–519, 1999; discussion 520–525.

20. Boissonnault WG, Meek PD: Risk factors for antiinflammatory drug or aspirin induced gastrointestinal complications in individuals receiving outpatient physical therapy services, *J Orthop Sports Phys Ther* 32:510–517, 2002.

21. Biederman RE: Pharmacology in rehabilitation: non-steroidal antiinflammatory agents, *J Orthop Sports Phys Ther* 35:356–367, 2005.

22. Goldman L, Schafer AI: *Goldman's Cecil medicine*, ed 24, Philadelphia, 2012, Saunders.

23. Fillit HM: *Brocklehurst's textbook of geriatric medicine*, ed 7, Philadelphia, 2010, Saunders.

24. Daniels JM: Evaluation of low back pain in athletes, *Sports Health* 3(4):336–345, 2011.

25. Witkin LR: Abscess after a laparoscopic appendectomy presenting as low back pain in a professional athlete, *Sports Health* 3(1):41–45, 2011.

26. Cosar M: The major complications of transpedicular vertebroplasty, *J Neurosurg Spine* 11(5):607–613, 2009.

27. Johnson BA: Epidurography and therapeutic epidural injections: technical considerations and experience with 5334 cases, *Am J Neuroradiol* 20:697–705, 1999.

28. Davenport TE: Subcutaneous abscess in a patient referred to physical therapy following spinal epidural injection for lumbar radiculopathy, *J Orthop Sports Phys Ther* 38(5):287, 2008.

29. Ganske CM, Horning KK: Levofloxacin-induced tendinopathy of the hip, *Ann Pharmacother* 46(5):e13, 2012.

30. Kaleagasioglu F, Olcay E: Fluoroquinolone-induced tendinopathy: etiology and preventive measures, *Tohoku J Exp Med* 226(4):251–258, 2012.

31. Tsai WC, Yang YM: Fluoroquinolone-associated tendinopathy, *Chang Gung Med J* 34(5):461–467, 2011.

32. van den Bosch MAAJ: Evidence against the use of lumbar spine radiography for low back pain, *Clin Radiol* 59:69–76, 2004.

33. Bogduk N, McQuirk B: *Medical management of acute and chronic low back pain: an evidence based approach*, Amsterdam, 2002, Elsevier.

34. Burton AK: Psychosocial predictors of outcome in acute and subchronic low back trouble, *Spine* 20(6):722–728, 1995.

35. McCarthy CJ: The reliability of the clinical tests and questions recommended in International Guidelines for Low Back Pain, *Spine* 32(6):921–926, 2007.

36. Moore JE: Chronic low back pain and psychosocial issues, *Phys Med Rehabil Clin North Am* 21(4):801–815, 2010.

37. Kendall NAS, Linton SJ, Main CJ: *Guide to assessing psychosocial yellow flags in acute low back pain: risk factors for long-term disability and work loss*, Wellington, 1998, Accident Rehabilitation and Compensation Insurance Corporation of New Zealand and the National Health Committee.

38. Pincus T: A systematic review of psychological factors as predictors of chronicity/disability in prospective cohorts of low back pain, *Spine* 27(5):E109–E120, 2002.

39. George SZ, Fritz JM, Childs JD: Investigation of elevated fear-avoidance beliefs for patients with low back pain: a secondary analysis involving patients enrolled in physical therapy clinical trials, *J Orthop Sports Phys Ther* 38(2):50–58, 2008.

40. Burns SA: A treatment-based classification approach to examination and intervention of lumbar disorders, *Sports Health* 3(4):363–372, 2011.

41. Waljee AK, Rogers MA, Lin P, et al: Short term use of oral corticosteroids and related harms among adults in the United States: population based cohort study, *BMJ* 357:j1415, 2017.

42. Henschke N: Prevalence of and screening for serious spinal pathology in patients presenting to primary care settings with acute low back pain, *Arthritis Rheum* 60(10):3072–3080, 2009.

43. Henschke N: A systematic review identifies five "red flags" to screen for vertebral fracture in patients with low back pain, *J Clin Epidemiol* 61:110–118, 2008.

44. National Osteoporosis Foundation: *Learn about osteoporosis: risk factors*, 2012. http://www.nof.org. Accessed January 5, 2013.

45. Sizer PS, Brismee JM, Cook C: Medical screening for red flags in the diagnosis and management of musculoskeletal spine pain, *Pain Pract* 7(1):53–71, 2007.

46. Deyo RA, Diehl AK: Cancer as a cause of back pain: frequency, clinical presentation, and diagnostic strategies, *J Gen Intern Med* 3(3):230–238, 1988.

47. Sanpera I: Bone scan as a screening tool in children and adolescents with back pain, *J Pediatr Orthop* 26(2):221–225, 2006.

48. Feldman DS: The use of bone scan to investigate back pain in children and adolescents, *J Pediatr Orthop* 20:790–795, 2000.

49. Borenstein DG, Balague F: Low back pain in adolescent and geriatric populations, *Rheum Dis Clin North Am* 47(2):149–163, 2021.

50. Bento TP, Cornelio GP, De Oliveira P, et al: Low back pain in adolescents and association with sociodemographic factors, electronic devices, physical activity and mental health, *J Pediatr (Rio J)* 96(6):717–724, 2020.

51. Bhatia N: Diagnostic modalities for the evaluation of pediatric back pain: a prospective study, *J Pediatr Orthop* 28(2):230–233, 2008.

52. Leroux J: Early diagnosis of thoracolumbar spine fractures in children. A prospective study, *Orthop Traumatol Surg Res* 99(1):60–65, 2013.

53. Achar S, Yamanaka J: Back pain in children and adolescents, *Am Fam Physician* 102(1):19–28, 2020 Jul 1.

54. Kliegman RM: *Nelson's textbook of pediatrics*, ed 19, Philadelphia, 2011, WB Saunders.

55. Waddell G: *The back pain revolution*, ed 2, Edinburgh, 2004, Churchill Livingstone.

56. León-Díaz A, González-Rabelino G, Alonso-Cerviño M: Analysis of the etiologies of headaches in a pediatric emergency service, *Rev Neurol* 39(3):217–221, 2004.

57. Helweg-Larsen J, Astradsson A, Richhall H, et al: Pyogenic brain abscess, a 15 year survey, *BMC Infect Dis* 12:332, 2012.

58. Petersen SM: Articular and muscular impairments in cervicogenic headache, *J Orthop Sports Phys Ther* 33(1):21–30, 2003.

59. Huber J, Lisi´nski P, Polowczyk A: Reinvestigation of the dysfunction in neck and shoulder girdle muscles as the reason

of cervicogenic headache among office workers, *Disabil Rehabil* 35(10):793–802, 2013.

60. Ryan LM, Warden DL: Post concussion syndrome, *Int Rev Psychiatry* 15(4):310–316, 2003.

61. Seiffert TD, Evans RW: Posttraumatic headache: a review, *Curr Pain Headache Rep* 14(4):292–298, 2010.

62. Silberstein SD, Olesen J, Bousser MG, et al: The international classification of headache disorders, ed 2 (ICHD-II)— revision of criteria for 8.2 medication overuse headache, *Cephalalgia* 25(6):460–465, 2005.

63. Agostoni E: Headache in cerebral venous thrombosis, *Neurol Sci* 25(suppl 3):S206–S210, 2004.

64. Agostoni E, Aliprandi A: Alterations in the cerebral venous circulation as a cause of headache, *Neurol Sci* 30(suppl 1): S7–S10, 2009.

65. Lucas S: Characterization of headache after traumatic brain injury, *Cephalalgia* 32(8):600–606, 2012.

66. Gerber MR, Fried LE, Pineles SL, et al: Posttraumatic stress disorder and intimate partner violence in a women's headache center, *Women Health* 52(5):454–471, 2012.

67. Jacobson SA, Folstein MF: Psychiatric perspectives on headache and facial pain, *Otolaryngol Clin North Am* 36(6):1187–1200, 2003.

68. Farmer K: Psychologic factors in childhood headaches, *Semin Pediatr Neurol* 17(2):93–99, 2010.

69. Hering-Hanit R, Gadoth N: Caffeine-induced headache in children and adolescents, *Cephalalgia* 23(5):332–335, 2003.

70. Chang PY, Kuo YB, Wu TL, et al: Association and prognostic value of serum inflammation markers in patients with leukoplakia and oral cavity cancer, *Clin Chem Lab Med* 15:1–10, 2012.

71. Lian IB, Tseng YT, Su CC, Tsai KY: Progression of precancerous lesions to oral cancer: results based on the Taiwan National Health Insurance Database, *Oral Oncol* 49(5):427–430, 2013.

72. Neville BW, Day TA: Oral cancer and precancerous lesions, *CA Cancer J Clin* 52(4):195–215, 2002.

73. Purdy RA, Kirby S: Headaches and brain tumors, *Neurol Clin* 22(1):39–53, 2004.

74. Kirby S: Headache and brain tumours, *Cephalalgia* 30(4): 387–388, 2010.

75. Valentinis L: Headache attributed to intracranial tumours: a prospective cohort study, *Cephalalgia* 30(4):389–398, 2010.

76. Gorski JM, Schwartz LH: Shoulder impingement presenting as neck pain, *J Bone Joint Surg* 85A(4):635–638, 2003.

77. Firestein GS: *Kelley's textbook of rheumatology*, ed 9, Philadelphia, 2013, Saunders.

78. Lee L, Elliott R: Cervical spondylotic myelopathy in a patient presenting with low back pain, *J Orthop Sports Phys Ther* 38(12):798, 2008.

79. Kawakita E, Kasai Y, Uchida A: Low back pain and cervical spondylotic myelopathy, *J Orthop Surg (Hong Kong)* 17(2): 187–189, 2009.

80. Manchikanti L, Kaye AD, Soin A, et al: Comprehensive evidence-based guidelines for facet joint interventions in the management of chronic spinal pain: American Society of Interventional Pain Physicians (ASIPP) guidelines facet joint interventions 2020 guidelines, *Pain Physician* 23(3S):S1–S127, 2020.

81. Fruth SJ: Differential diagnosis and treatment in a patient with posterior upper thoracic pain, *Phys Ther* 86(2):154–268, 2006.

82. Dutton M: *Dutton's orthopaedic examination evaluation and intervention*, ed 3, New York, 2012, McGraw-Hill Medical.

83. Leslie KO, Wick MR: *Leslie & Wick: practical pulmonary pathology*, ed 2, Philadelphia, 2011, Saunders.

84. Bonow RO: *Braunwald's heart disease: a textbook of medicine*, ed 9, Philadelphia, 2011, Saunders.

85. Feldman M: *Sleisenger and Fordtran's gastrointestinal and liver disease*, ed 9, Philadelphia, 2010, Saunders.

86. Hartvigsen J, Christensen K, Frederiksen H: Back pain remains a common symptom in old age. A population-based study of 4,486 Danish twins aged 70-102, *Eur Spine J* 12(5):528–534, 2003.

87. Mason RJ: *Murray and Nadel's textbook of respiratory medicine*, ed 5, Philadelphia, 2010, Saunders.

88. Braun J, Inman R: Clinical significance of inflammatory back pain for diagnosis and screening of patients with axial spondyloarthritis, *Ann Rheum Dis* 69(7):1264–1268, 2010.

89. Ozgen S: Lumbar disc herniation in adolescence, *Pediatr Neurosurg* 43:77–81, 2007.

90. O'Neill CW, Kurgansky ME, Derby R, et al: Disc stimulation and patterns of referred pain, *Spine* 27(24):2776–2781, 2002.

91. Giamberardino MA, Costantini R, Affaitati G, et al: Viscero-visceral hyperalgesia: characterization in different clinical models, *Pain* 151(2):307–322, 2010.

92. Koes BW: Diagnosis and treatment of sciatica, *BMJ* 334: 1313–1317, 2007.

93. Crowell MS, Gill NW: Medical screening and evacuation: cauda equina syndrome in a combat zone, *J Orthop Sports Phys Ther* 39(7):541–549, 2009.

94. O'Laughlin SJ, Kokosinski E: Cauda equina syndrome in a pregnant woman referred to physical therapy for low back pain, *J Orthop Sports Phys Ther* 38(11):721, 2008.

95. Kauppila LI: Atherosclerosis and disc degeneration/low-back pain—a systemic review, *Eur J Endovasc Surg* 37(6):661–670, 2009.

96. Qaseem A, Forciea MA, McLean RM: Treatment of low bone density or osteoporosis to prevent fractures in men and women: a clinical practice guideline update from the American College of Physicians, *Ann Intern Med* 166(11):818–839, 2017.

97. Ebeling PR, Nguyen HH, ALeksova J, et al: Secondary osteoporosis, *Endocr Rev* 43(2):240–313, 2022.

98. Kiebzak G, Beinart G, Perser K, et al: Under treatment of osteoporosis in men with hip fracture, *Arch Intern Med* 162(19):2217–2222, 2002.

99. Ebeling PR: Osteoporosis in men, *N Engl J Med* 358(14): 1474–1482, 2008.

100. Ebeling PR: Androgens and osteoporosis, *Curr Opin Endocrinol Diabetes Obes* 17(3):284–292, 2010.

101. Blain H: Osteoporosis in men: epidemiology, physiopathology, diagnosis, prevention, and treatment, *Rev Med Interne* 25(suppl 5): S552–S559, 2005.

102. Lee HM, Park SY, Lee SH, et al: Comparative analysis of clinical outcomes in patients with osteoporotic vertebral compression fractures: conservative treatment versus balloon kyphoplasty, *Spine J* 12(11):998–1005, 2012.

103. Badke MB, Boissonnault WG: Changes in disability following physical therapy intervention for patients with low back pain: dependence on symptom duration, *Arch Phys Med Rehab* 87(6):749–756, 2006.

104. Whooley MA: Case-finding instruments for depression. Two questions are as good as many, *J Gen Intern Med* 12:439–445, 1997.

105. Haggman S: Screening for symptoms of depression by physical therapists managing low back pain, *Phys Ther* 84:1157–1165, 2004.

106. Slipman C: Epidemiology of spine tumors presenting to musculoskeletal physiatrists, *Arch Phys Med Rehabil* 84: 492–495, 2003.

107. Rose PS, Buchowski JM: Metastatic disease in the thoracic and lumbar spine: evaluation and management, *J Am Acad Orthop Surg* 19(1):37–48, 2011.

108. Henschke N: Screening for malignancy in low back pain patients: a systematic review, *Eur Spine J* 16(10):1673–1679, 2007.

109. Briggs HK: The physical therapist's management of a patient with low back pain following an atypical response to treatment: a case report, *J Orthop Sports Phys Ther* 41(1):A16, 2011.

110. Cleveland Clinic: *Current clinical medicine*, ed 2, Philadelphia, 2010, Saunders.

111. Mazanec DJ, Segal AM, Sinks PB: Identification of malignancy in patients with back pain: red flags, *Arthritis Rheum* 36(suppl): S251–S258, 1993.

112. van Tulder M, Becker A, Bekkering T, et al: Chapter 3: European guidelines for the management of acute nonspecific low back pain in primary care, *Euro Spine J* 15(Suppl 2):S169–S191, 2006.

113. Skoffer B: Low back pain in 15- to 16-year-old children in relation to school furniture and carrying of the school bag, *Spine* 32(24):E713–E717, 2007.

114. Neuschwander TB: The effect of backpacks on the lumbar spine in children, *Spine* 35(1):83–88, 2009.

115. Patchell RA: Direct decompressive surgical resection in the treatment of spinal cord compression caused by metastatic cancer: a randomized trial, *Lancet* 366(9486):643–648, 2005.

116. Abeloff MD: *Abeloff's clinical oncology*, ed 4, Philadelphia, 2008, Churchill Livingstone.

117. Wein AJ: *Campbell-Walsh urology*, ed 10, Philadelphia, 2011, Saunders.

118. Wong DA, Fornasier VL, MacNab I: Spinal metastases: the obvious, the occult, and the imposters, *Spine* 15(1):1–4, 1990.

119. Ross MD, Bayer E: Cancer as a cause of low back pain in a patient seen in a direct access physical therapy setting, *J Orthop Sports Phys Ther* 35(10):651–658, 2005.

120. Goldberger AL: *Clinical electrocardiography: a simplified approach*, ed 8, Philadelphia, 2012, Saunders.

121. Marx JA: *Rosen's emergency medicine*, ed 7, St Louis, 2009, Mosby.

122. Cosford PA, Leng GC: Screening for abdominal aortic aneurysm, *Cochrane Database Syst Rev* 18(2):CD002945, 2007.

123. Fleming C, Whitlock EP, Beil TL, et al: Screening for abdominal aortic aneurysm: a best evidence systematic review for the U.S. Preventive Services Task Force, *Ann Intern Med* 142(3):203–211, 2005.

124. Lederle FA: Smokers' relative risk for aortic aneurysm compared with other smoking-related diseases: a systematic review, *J Vasc Surg* 38:329–334, 2003.

125. Dua MM, Dalman RL: Identifying aortic aneurysm risk factors in postmenopausal women, *Womens Health* 5(1):33–37, 2009.

126. Lederle FA: Abdominal aortic aneurysm events in the women's health initiative: cohort study, *BMJ* 337:1724–1734, 2008.

127. Mechelli F, Preboski Z, Boissonnault W: Differential diagnosis of a patient referred to physical therapy with low back pain: abdominal aortic aneurysm, *J Orthop Sports Phys Ther* 38(9):551–557, 2008.

128. Adam A: *Grainger & Allison's diagnostic radiology*, ed 5, Philadelphia, 2008, Churchill Livingstone.

129. Owens DK: Screening for abdominal aortic aneurysm. US Preventive Services Task Force Recommendation Statement, *JAMA* 322(22):2211–2218, 2019.

130. Jarvis C: *Physical examination and health assessment*, ed 6, St. Louis, 2011, Mosby.

131. Crapo JD, Karlinsky JB, King TE: *Baum's textbook of pulmonary diseases*, ed 7, Philadelphia, 2003, Lippincott, Williams & Wilkins.

132. McDermott MT: *Endocrine secrets*, ed 5, St. Louis, 2009, Mosby.

133. Taal MW: *Brenner & Rector's the kidney*, ed 9, Philadelphia, 2011, Saunders.

134. Harward MP: *Medical secrets*, ed 5, St. Louis, 2011, Mosby.

135. Barkhodari A, Lee KE, Shen M, Shen B, Yao Q: Inflammatory bowel disease: focus on enteropathic arthritis and therapy, *Rheumatol Immunol Res* 3(2):69–76, 2022.

136. Gran JT, Husby G: Joint manifestations in gastrointestinal diseases, *Digest Dis* 10:295–312, 1992.

137. Mandell GL: *Mandell, Douglas, and Bennett's principles and practice of infectious diseases*, ed 7, Philadelphia, 2009, Churchill Livingstone.

138. Gelfand MS, Cleveland KO: Vancomycin therapy and the progression of methicillin-resistant *Staphylococcus aureus* vertebral osteomyelitis, *South Med J* 97(6):593–597, 2004.

139. Van Hal SJ: Emergence of daptomycin resistance following vancomycin-unresponsive Staphylococcus aureus bacteraemia in a daptomycin-naive patient—a review of the literature, *Eur J Clin Microbiol Infect Dis* 30(5):603–610, 2011.

140. Long SS: *Principles and practice of pediatric infectious diseases*, ed 4, Philadelphia, 2012, Saunders.

141. Tamura K: Clinical characteristics of infective endocarditis with vertebral osteomyelitis, *J Infect Chemother* 16(4):260–265, 2010.

142. Daroff RB: *Bradley's neurology in clinical practice*, ed 6, Philadelphia, 2012, Saunders.

6

Recognizing and Reporting Red Flags in the Upper Extremity

Systemic and viscerogenic problems can effectively masquerade as shoulder and arm pain and bypass detection. For example, systemic diseases and medical conditions affecting the neck, breast, and any organs in the chest or abdomen can present clinically as shoulder pain (Table 6.1).[1,2]

💡 PICTURE THE PATIENT

Peptic ulcers, heart disease, ectopic pregnancy, and myocardial ischemia are only a few examples of systemic diseases that can cause shoulder pain and movement dysfunction. Each disorder listed can present clinically as a shoulder problem before ever demonstrating systemic signs and symptoms.

Only until progression of the disease creates a clearer picture of the true underlying problem might the physical therapist assistant (PTA) observe something suspicious requiring further evaluation by the physical therapist (PT).

This chapter takes a look at each system that can refer pain or symptoms to the shoulder. This will include vascular, pulmonary, renal, gastrointestinal (GI), and gynecologic causes of shoulder and upper extremity pain and dysfunction (Fig. 6.1). Knowing the key red flags for cancer, vascular disease, pulmonary, GI, and gynecologic causes of shoulder pain and/or dysfunction will help the PTA quickly recognize the need for reevaluation.

There are no new guidelines presented in the remaining two chapters that have not been discussed in the previous chapters. The PTA must remain alert to yellow (caution) or red (warning) flags in the history and clinical presentation and while asking about associated signs and symptoms. At the same time, the PTA must keep in mind that many neuromuscular and musculoskeletal conditions in the neck, cervical spine, axilla, thorax, thoracic spine, and chest wall can refer pain to the shoulder and arm. For this reason, the PT's examination usually includes assessment above and below the involved joint for referred musculoskeletal pain.

⟫ PTA ACTION PLAN
Clinical Scenario

Because clinical signs and symptoms affecting the shoulder and upper extremity can come from musculoskeletal, neuromuscular, and visceral or systemic sources, the PTA must be prepared to recognize a clinical presentation that requires documentation and communication with the PT (or physician if the therapist is not available immediately) (Case Example 6.1).

💡 PICTURE THE PATIENT

When symptoms seem out of proportion to the injury or persist beyond the expected time of healing, reevaluation by the PT may be needed.[5] Likewise, pain that is unrelieved by rest or change in position or pain/symptoms that do not fit the expected mechanical or neuromuscular (NMS) system pattern should serve as red-flag warnings. A past medical history of cancer warrants close observation.

RECOGNIZING AND REPORTING RED FLAGS IN THE SHOULDER

Past Medical History

It is important for the PTA to review and thoroughly understand the prior medical history provided in the initial evaluation to safely and accurately observe the patient's tolerance to physical therapy interventions provided on a daily basis. Other times, the PTA will acquire important medical information from the patient, family members, or medical staff that was not discussed during the evaluation process; this information should be followed up with appropriate communication to the supervising PT.

While reviewing the various potential systemic causes of shoulder symptomatology listed in Table 6.1, think about the most common risk factors and red-flag histories the PTA might see with each of these conditions. For example, a history of any kind of cancer is always a red flag. Breast and lung cancer are the two most common types of cancer to metastasize to the shoulder.

Heart disease can cause shoulder pain, but it usually occurs in an age-specific population.[2,6,7] Anyone over 50 years old, postmenopausal females, and anyone with a positive first-generation family history is at increased risk for symptomatic heart disease. Younger individuals and anyone having a heart attack for the first time may be more likely to demonstrate atypical symptoms such as shoulder pain without chest pain.[8,9]

Hypertension, diabetes, and hyperlipidemia are other red-flag histories associated with cardiac-related shoulder pain. A history of angina,[10] heart attack, angiography, stent or pacemaker placement,[11-13] coronary artery bypass graft (CABG), or other cardiac procedure is also a yellow (caution) flag.

TABLE 6.1 Systemic and Medical Conditions as Causes of Shoulder and Upper Extremity Symptoms

	Neck	Chest/Trunk/Back	Abdomen
Cancer	Metastases (leukemia, Hodgkin lymphoma) Cervical cord tumors Bone tumors	Metastases to nodes in axilla or mediastinum Metastases to lungs from: • Bone • Breast • Kidney • Colorectal • Pancreas • Uterus Bone metastases to thoracic spine: • Breast • Lung • Thyroid Breast cancer Lung cancer	Pancreatic cancer Spinal metastases: • Kidney • Testicle • Prostate
Cardiovascular/ vascular	TOS	Angina/MI Acute coronary syndrome ICU/s/p CABG Pacemaker (complications) Bacterial endocarditis Pericarditis Thoracic aortic aneurysm Empyema and lung abscess Collagen vascular disease	Dissecting aortic aneurysm
Pulmonary	Pulmonary tuberculosis	Pulmonary embolism Pulmonary tuberculosis Spontaneous pneumothorax Pancoast tumor Pneumonia	
Renal/urologic			Kidney stones Obstruction, inflammation, or infection of upper urinary tract
Gastrointestinal/ hepatic		Hiatal hernia	Peptic/duodenal ulcer (perforated) Ruptured spleen Liver disease Gallbladder disease Pancreatic disease
Infection		Septic arthritis Necrotizing fasciitis Mononucleosis Osteomyelitis/transverse myelitis Syphilis/gonorrhea Herpes zoster (shingles) Pneumonia Cellulitis (skin anywhere in neck, chest, arm, hand)	Subphrenic abscess
Gynecologic			Ectopic pregnancy (rupture) Endometriosis (cysts)
Other	Cervical central cord lesion Trauma: Cervical fractures or ligamentous instability; whiplash	Mastodynia (breast) Diabetes mellitus (adhesive capsulitis) Sickle cell anemia Hemophilia	Diaphragmatic hernia Anterior spinal surgery (postoperative hemorrhage)

ICU/s/p CABG, Intensive care unit status post coronary artery bypass graft; *MI,* myocardial infarction; *TOS,* thoracic outlet syndrome.

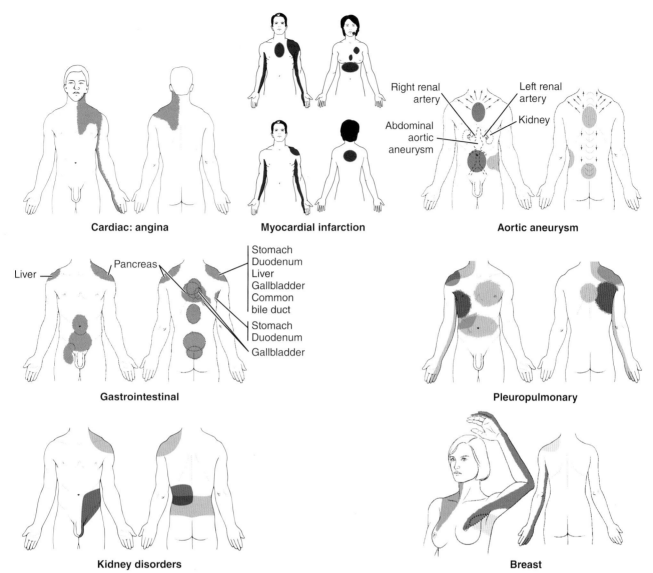

Cardiac: angina

Myocardial infarction

Right renal artery

Left renal artery

Kidney

Abdominal aortic aneurysm

Aortic aneurysm

Liver

Pancreas

Stomach
Duodenum
Liver
Gallbladder
Common
bile duct
Stomach
Duodenum
Gallbladder

Gastrointestinal

Pleuropulmonary

Kidney disorders

Breast

FIG. 6.1 Composite picture of referred shoulder and upper extremity pain patterns.

CASE EXAMPLE 6.1   Initial Evaluation of a Professional Golfer

Referral: A 38-year-old male, professional golfer presented to physical therapy with a diagnosis of shoulder impingement syndrome, with partial thickness tears of the supraspinatus tendon.

Prior to the physical therapy intervention, x-rays taken were reported as negative for fracture or tumor. Magnetic resonance imaging (MRI) was reported as positive for bursitis and supraspinatus tendinitis with some partial tears. The shoulder specialist also provided the client with one corticosteroid injection, which gave him some relief of his shoulder pain.

Past Medical History: Past medical history and review of systems were negative for any systemic issues. He was on no medication at the time of evaluation.

Clinical Presentation: Functional deficits were reported as pain with the take-away phase of the golf swing and with the adduction motion of the shoulder in follow-through. He also reported a loss of distance associated with his drive by 20 to 30 yards. He had trouble sleeping and reported pain would wake him up if his head were turned into left rotation. He also had pain when turning his head to the left (e.g., when driving a car).

Upper Quarter Screen

Shoulder Range of Motion (ROM)

Active ROM:

Left		Right
160 degrees	Flexion (Flex)	170 degrees
165 degrees	Abduction (Abd)	170 degrees
50 degrees	Internal rotation (IR)	55 degrees
55 degrees	External rotation (ER)	85 degrees

Passive ROM:

Left		Right
170 degrees	Flex	175 degrees
170 degrees	Abd	175 degrees
55 degrees	IR	60 degrees
60 degrees	ER	75 degrees

Continued

CASE EXAMPLE 6.1 Initial Evaluation of a Professional Golfer—cont'd

Isometric Muscle Testing of Rotator Cuff

Abd	Painful/strong
Abd with IR	Painful/strong
IR	Painless/strong
ER	Painless/strong

Special Tests

Hawkins/Kennedy +

Neer +

Speed +

ER lag test −

IR lag test −

Cervical ROM

Flexion 40 degrees	
Extension (ext) 20 degrees	Report of left scapular pain
Left side bend 20 degrees	Report of left scapular pain
Right side bend 25 degrees	No report of pain
Left rotation 45 degrees	Report of left scapular pain
Right rotation 70 degrees	No report of pain
Quadrant position	Right and left: Reproduced left posterior scapular pain with radicular pain to the thumb and second finger area
Quadrant position	Right and left: Reproduced left posterior scapular pain with radicular pain to the thumb and second finger area

Deep Tendon Reflexes

Left		Right
2+	Biceps	2+
0	Triceps	2+
2+	Brachioradialis	2+

Strength

Left		Right
5/5	Shoulder flex	5/5
4/5	Shoulder abd	5/5
5/5	Elbow flex	5/5
2/5	Elbow ext	5/5
3/5	Wrist ext	5/5
5/5	Wrist flex	5/5
5/5	Thumb ext	5/5
5/5	Finger abd	5/5

He did have intact sensation to light touch and proprioceptive sense. Strength testing on the Cybex weight-lifting machines showed he was able to do 10 triceps extensions on the right with four plates while he was only able to do one repetition on the left with one plate.

Result: With the data obtained in the examination the patient was determined to have an impingement syndrome as described by Neer, with involvement of the bursa and rotator cuff tendons.[3] Cyriax muscle testing revealed some musculotendon involvement with the strong/painful tests.[4]

The cervical findings required consultation with the referring physician. A provisional medical diagnosis was made of cervical radiculopathy with a C5–C6 herniated disk. The client was referred to a neurosurgeon for evaluation. An MRI confirmed the diagnosis and the client underwent an anterior cervical fusion with diskectomy.

Summary: This case example helps the physical therapist assistant (PTA) to understand the clinical decision-making a physical therapist uses while completing a thorough examination process, even if a physician specialist refers a client for physical therapy services. The therapist must "clear" or examine the joints above and below the region thought to be the cause of the dysfunction. The major reason for the symptoms or a secondary diagnosis may be missed if the screening step is left out because of a lack of time or the assumption that someone else checked out the client. A basic understanding of the evaluation process will allow the PTA to more accurately report important information back to the therapist when needed.

(From Voshell S: *Case report presented in fulfillment of DPT 910*, Chester, 2005, Institute for Physical Therapy Education, Widener University, used with permission.)

The presence of even one previously undetected or new yellow flag should alert the PTA of the potential need for further screening by the PT. Knowledge of past medical history of pathologic conditions, illnesses, and diseases helps all health care professionals safely monitor and treat individual clients.

- Recent (past 1–3 months) myocardial infarction (MI) (complex regional pain syndrome [CRPS]; formerly reflex sympathetic dystrophy)
- Recent implantation of pacemaker[11–13]
- Cancer, especially breast or lung cancer (metastasis)
- Recent history of pneumonia, recurrent upper respiratory infection (URI), or influenza (diaphragmatic pleurisy)

►► PTA ACTION PLAN

Ask Yourself

Is there a history of the following:
- Rheumatic disease
- Diabetes mellitus (adhesive capsulitis)
- "Frozen" shoulder of unknown cause in anyone with coronary artery disease, recent history of hospitalization in the critical care unit or intensive care unit (ICU) following CABG

Risk Factors

Identifying risk factors is an important part of disease prevention. The PTA can have an active role in prevention through follow-up questions and education. The past medical history just discussed is often a red flag as well as a risk factor. Recognizing risk factors may guide the PTA in notifying the PT of potential red flags sooner than otherwise would seem necessary. Notifying the PT of potentially important risk factors may result in the PT generating a medical referral early on in the disease process. Educating clients about their risk factors is a key element in risk factor reduction.

▶▶ PTA ACTION PLAN

Shoulder Pain Associated With Tuberculosis

Who is most likely to develop tuberculosis (TB)?

Although less common in the United States compared with other less-developed countries, pulmonary TB is still a possible cause of shoulder pain and/or frozen shoulder[14,15]; therefore the PTA monitoring individuals with unknown or questionable cause of shoulder pain will want to keep in mind potential risk factors for TB.[16–18]

The PTA should be aware of the following risk factors:

Health care workers

Homeless population

Prison inmates

Immunocompromised individuals (e.g., transplant recipients, long-term use of immunosuppressants, anyone treated for long-term rheumatoid arthritis [RA], anyone undergoing chemotherapy)

Older adult (over 65 years)

Immigrants from areas where TB is endemic

Injection drug users

Malnourished (e.g., eating disorders, alcoholism, drug users, cachexia)

For patients with TB, there will usually be other associated signs and symptoms such as fever, sweats, and cough. Whenever working with a client who has shoulder pain of unknown origin or an unusual clinical presentation, vital signs may provide key information previously undetected. For example, recognizing the effect of increased respiratory movements on shoulder symptoms could be an important finding for the PTA to report (Case Example 6.2).

Clinical Presentation

Shoulder pain of a systemic or visceral source can be difficult to recognize because any pain that is felt in the shoulder often affects the joint as though the pain were originating in the joint.[3] Shoulder pain with any of the components listed in this chapter may be a manifestation of systemic visceral illness. This is true even if shoulder movements make the pain worse or if there are objective findings at the shoulder. It is especially important for the PTA to be knowledgeable in observing these pain patterns and effectively communicate observations to the PT.

Many visceral diseases present as unilateral shoulder pain (Table 6.2). As the table indicates, esophageal, pericardial (or other myocardial diseases), aortic dissection, and diaphragmatic irritation from thoracic or abdominal diseases (e.g., upper GI, renal, hepatic/biliary) can appear as unilateral pain. This presentation corresponds with information presented in Fig. 2.4 regarding direct pressure from the viscera in contact with the respiratory diaphragm, which can refer pain to the ipsilateral shoulder.

Adhesive capsulitis, a condition in which both active and passive glenohumeral motions are restricted, can be associated with diabetes mellitus, hyperthyroidism,[21,22] ischemic heart disease, infection, and lung diseases (e.g., TB, emphysema, chronic bronchitis, Pancoast tumors).[14,17,18,23–26]

Shoulder pain (unilateral or bilateral) progressing to adhesive capsulitis can occur 6 to 9 months after CABG. Similarly, anyone immobile in the ICU or coronary care unit can experience loss of shoulder motion, resulting in adhesive capsulitis (Case Example 6.3). Clients with pacemakers who have

CASE EXAMPLE 6.2 Homeless Male With Tuberculosis

Referral: A 36-year-old male was referred to physical therapy as an inpatient for a short-term hospitalization. He was a homeless male brought to the hospital by the police and admitted with an extensive medical problem list, including the following:

Malnutrition

Alcoholism

Depression

Hepatitis A

Broken wrist

Shoulder pain

Dehydration

There was no past medical history of cancer. The client was a smoker when he could get cigarettes. He expresses that he would like to support a one-pack/day habit.

Medical service requested an evaluation of the client's shoulder pain. X-rays were not taken because the male had full active range of motion (ROM), no history of trauma, and no insurance to cover additional testing.

Clinical Presentation: During the initial evaluation the therapist was unable to reproduce the shoulder pain with palpation, position, or provocation testing. There was no sign of rotator cuff dysfunction, adhesive capsulitis, tendinitis, or trigger points in the upper quadrant. There was a noticeable stiffening of the neck with very limited cervical ROM in all planes and directions. Supraclavicular lymph nodes were palpable, tender, and moveable on both sides.

During the second therapy session with the physical therapist assistant (PTA), the following observations were documented. Vital signs were unremarkable,

but the client was perspiring heavily despite being in threadbare clothing and at rest. He reported getting the "sweats" everyday around this same time.

The PTA asked the client to take a deep breath and cough. He went into a paroxysm of coughing, which he said caused his shoulder to start aching. The cough was productive, but the client swallowed the sputum.

PTA Action Plan: The PTA contacted the charge nurse to request an immediate assessment of the patient. Auscultation of lung sounds by the nurse revealed rales (crackles) in the right upper lung lobe.

Based on the information received from the evaluation documentation from the physical therapist and the appropriate observational skills applied during this session, the PTA was able to report the following concerns to the nurse:

- Constitutional symptoms of sweats and fatigue (although fatigue could be caused by his extreme malnutrition)
- Pulmonary impairment with reproduction of symptoms with coughing
- Suspicious (aberrant) lymph nodes (bilateral)
- Cervical spine involvement with no apparent cause or recognizable musculoskeletal pattern

Result: The charge nurse followed up with a consult with the on-call physician, which resulted in a medical evaluation and x-ray. The client was diagnosed with pulmonary tuberculosis, which was confirmed by a skin test. Shoulder and neck pain and dysfunction were attributed to a pulmonary source and not considered appropriate for physical therapy intervention.

The client was sent to a halfway house where he could receive adequate nutrition and medical services to treat his tuberculosis.

TABLE 6.2   Location of Shoulder Pain

Systemic Origin	Right Shoulder Location	Systemic Origin	Left Shoulder Location

Peptic ulcer	Lateral border, right scapula	Internal bleeding:
		    Spleen (trauma, rupture)
		    Postoperative laparoscopy
			Left shoulder (Kehr sign)

Myocardial ischemia	Right shoulder, down arm	Myocardial ischemia	Left pectoral/left shoulder
		Thoracic aortic aneurysm	Left shoulder (or between shoulder blades)
Hepatic/biliary:		Pancreas	Left shoulder
Acute cholecystitis	Right shoulder; between scapulae; right subscapular area		
Gallbladder	Right upper trapezius, right shoulder	Infectious mononucleosis (hepatomegaly, splenomegaly)	Left shoulder/left upper trapezius
Liver disease (hepatitis, cirrhosis, metastatic tumors, abscess)	Right shoulder, right subscapular		
Pulmonary: Pleurisy Pneumothorax Pancoast tumor Pneumonia	Ipsilateral shoulder; upper trapezius	Pulmonary: Pleurisy Pneumothorax Pancoast tumor Pneumonia	Ipsilateral shoulder; upper trapezius
Kidney	Ipsilateral shoulder	Kidney	Ipsilateral shoulder
Gynecologic: Endometriosis	Reported in right shoulder[19,20]; possible in either shoulder, depending on location of cysts	Gynecologic: Ectopic pregnancy	Ipsilateral shoulder

CASE EXAMPLE 6.3   Pleural Effusion With Fibrosis, Late Complication of Coronary Artery Bypass Graft

A 53-year-old male was referred to physical therapy by his primary care physician for left shoulder pain. He is currently working with a physical therapist assistant (PTA) in a cardiac rehab program.

Past Medical History: The client had a recent (6 months ago) history of cardiac bypass surgery (i.e., coronary artery bypass graft [CABG]). Hypertension is currently being controlled with medications. He has a 60-pack/year history (smoking three cigarettes/day for 20 years), but he quit smoking 10 years ago after having a heart attack.

Subjective Information: The patient reports, "I am 50 pounds overweight and I need to go on a diet."

Clinical Presentation: The client presented with good posture and alignment. Shoulder range of motion was equal and symmetric bilaterally, but the client reported pain when the left arm was raised over 90 degrees of flexion or abduction. His position of preference was left side-lying. The pain could be reduced in this position from a rated level of 6 to a 2 on a scale from 0 (no pain) to 10 (worst pain).

Scapulohumeral motion on the left was altered compared with the right. Medial and lateral rotations were within normal limits (WNL) with the upper arm against the chest. Lateral rotation reproduced painful symptoms when performed with the shoulder in 90 degrees of abduction.

Neurologic screen was negative.

Vital Signs:

Blood pressure:	122/68 mm Hg
Resting pulse:	60 bpm
Body temperature:	98.6°F

Lung Sounds:

Diminished basilar (lower lobes) breath sounds on the left compared with the right.

Decreased chest wall excursion on the left; increased shoulder pain with deep inspiration

Dyspnea was not observed at rest

When asked if there were any symptoms of any kind anywhere else in the body, the client reported ongoing but intermittent chest pain and shortness of breath for the last 3 months. The client had not reported these "new" symptoms to the physical therapist (PT) during the initial evaluation.

What are the Red Flags (If Any)? Which Red Flags Need to be Reported to the PT?

Shoulder problems are not uncommon following CABG, but the number and type of red flags present caught the PTA's attention. The client was not in any apparent physiologic distress and vital signs were WNL (although he was on antihypertensive medications).

PTA Action Plan: The PTA discussed these red flags with the supervising PT, and a decision was made to report these findings to the physician. The physician requested immediate follow-up with the client, who was seen the next day.

Result: The client was diagnosed with pleural effusion causing pleural fibrosis, a rare long-term complication of cardiac bypass surgery. The physician noted that the left lower lobe was adhered to the chest wall.

Pleural effusion is a common complication of cardiac surgery and is associated with other postoperative complications. Pleural effusion complications can occur more often in females and individuals with associated cardiac or vascular comorbidities.[27-30]

The client was treated medically but also continued in physical therapy to restore full and normal motion of the shoulder complex. The physician also asked the therapist to review the client's cardiac rehab program and modify it accordingly because of the pulmonary complications.

complications and revisions that result in prolonged shoulder immobilization can also develop CRPS and/or adhesive capsulitis.[31]

It is not uncommon for the older adult to attribute "overdoing it" to the appearance of physical pain or NMS dysfunction. Any adult over age 65 years presenting with new shoulder pain and/or dysfunction or shoulder symptoms that have not been evaluated will need to be screened by the PT for systemic or viscerogenic origin of symptoms, even when there is a known (or attributed) cause or injury.

▶▶ PTA ACTION PLAN

Follow-Up Questions

Whether the client presents with an unknown etiology of injury or impairment or with an assigned cause, it is important to keep these questions in mind:
- Is it really insidious (no known cause)?
- Is it really caused by [whatever the client told you]?

The client may wrongly attribute onset of symptoms to an activity. The alert PTA may recognize a true causative factor. Any information obtained by asking the following questions should be given to the supervising PT through appropriate face-to-face or phone call communication. A written note or recorded information in the client's chart is not recommended due to the uncertainty in the PT actually seeing it in a timely matter.
- Since the beginning of your shoulder problem, have you had any unusual perspiration for no apparent reason, sweats, or fever?
- Have you sustained any injuries in the last week during a sports activity, car accident, etc.? (e.g., ruptured spleen associated with pain in the left shoulder: positive Kehr sign)
- Has the client had a laparoscopy in the last 24 to 48 hours? (left shoulder pain: positive Kehr sign)[32]

Anytime a surgical procedure is performed, the PT should be notified as a reevaluation of the patient will need to be completed prior to the PTA continuing with general daily therapeutic interventions.
- Have you been in a fight or been assaulted?
- Have you ever been pulled by the arm, pushed against the wall, or thrown by the arm?

If the answer is positive and the history relates to the current episode of symptoms, the PT may need to conduct a more complete screening interview related to domestic violence and assault.
- Do you have any symptoms of any kind anywhere else in your body that you have not mentioned to the PT?

As previously stated, shoulder pain can be referred from the neck, back, chest, abdomen, and elbow (Fig. 6.2). During orthopedic assessment the therapist always checks "above and below" the impaired level for a possible source of referred pain. With this guideline in mind the therapist knows to look for potential musculoskeletal or neuromuscular causes from the cervical and thoracic spine[33] and elbow. It is important that the therapist alert the PTA for any important red flags or clinical signs to watch for based on findings from the orthopedic assessment.

Associated Signs and Symptoms

One of the most basic clues in recognizing a possible viscerogenic or systemic cause of shoulder pain is to notice if the patient has shoulder pain accompanied by any of the following features:
- Pleuritic component (chest pain, cough, wheeze, shortness of breath, sputum production)
- Exacerbation by recumbency

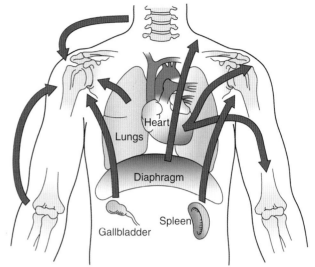

FIG. 6.2 Musculoskeletal and systemic structures referring pain to the shoulder.

- Recent history of laparoscopic procedure (risk factor)[34-37]
- Coincident diaphoresis (cardiac)
- Associated GI signs and symptoms
- Exacerbation by exertion unrelated to shoulder movement (cardiac)
- Associated urologic signs and symptoms

Shoulder pain with any of these conditions present should be approached as a manifestation of systemic visceral illness until proven otherwise. This is true even if the pain is exacerbated by shoulder movement or if there are objective findings at the shoulder.[38] These findings will direct the PTA to communicate with the PT immediately.

▶▶ PTA ACTION PLAN

Points to Ponder

Shoulder dysfunction can look like a true neuromuscular or musculoskeletal problem and still be viscerogenic or systemic in origin.

RECOGNIZING AND REPORTING PULMONARY RED FLAGS

Extensive disease may occur in the lung without pain until the process extends to the parietal pleura. Pleural irritation then results in sharp, localized pain that is aggravated by any respiratory movement.

❓ PICTURE THE PATIENT

Clients usually note that the pain is alleviated by lying on the affected side, which diminishes the movement of that side of the chest (called autosplinting[39]), whereas shoulder pain of musculoskeletal origin is usually aggravated by lying on the symptomatic shoulder.

Shoulder symptoms made worse by lying supine may be a yellow flag for pulmonary involvement. Lying down increases the venous return from the lower extremities. A compromised cardiopulmonary system may not be able to accommodate the increase in fluid volume. Referred shoulder pain from the taxed and overworked pulmonary system may result. Look for tachypnea, dyspnea, wheezing, hyperventilation, or other noticeable changes and report these as well.

At the same time, recumbency or the supine position causes a slight shift of the abdominal contents upward toward the head. This shift may put pressure on the diaphragm, which in turn presses up against the lower lung lobes. The combination of increased venous return and diaphragmatic pressure may be enough to reproduce the musculoskeletal symptoms.

Pneumonia in the older adult may appear as shoulder pain when the affected lung presses on the diaphragm; usually there are accompanying pulmonary symptoms, but in older adults, confusion (or increased confusion) may be the only other associated sign.

Any time the PTA becomes aware of a pleuritic component such as a persistent or productive cough and/or chest pain, documentation in the medical record and notification of the therapist are required.

▶▶ PTA ACTION PLAN

Reviewing Pulmonary Clinical Presentation

The PTA should be alert to the following list of pulmonary clinical presentations. Observations should be documented immediately in the medical chart and reported verbally to the supervising PT if they are new or previously unknown or unreported.

- Presence of a pleuritic component such as a persistent, dry, hacking, or productive cough; blood-tinged sputum; or chest pain; musculoskeletal symptoms are aggravated by respiratory movements.
- Exacerbation by recumbency despite proper positioning of the arm in neutral alignment (diaphragmatic or pulmonary component).
- Presence of associated signs and symptoms (e.g., tachypnea, dyspnea, wheezing, hyperventilation).
- Shoulder pain of unknown cause in older adults with accompanying signs of confusion or increased confusion (pneumonia).
- Shoulder pain aggravated by the supine position may be an indication of mediastinal or pleural involvement; shoulder or back pain alleviated by lying on the painful side may indicate autosplinting (pleural).
- Watch for the exacerbation of symptoms by recumbency even with proper positioning of the arm; lying down in the supine position can put the shoulder in a position of slight extension. This can put pressure on soft tissue structures in and around the shoulder, causing pain in the presence of a true neuromuscular or musculoskeletal problem.
- For this reason, when assessing the effect of recumbency, make sure the shoulder is in a neutral position. You may have to support the upper arm with a towel roll under the elbow and/or put a pillow on the client's abdomen to give the forearms a place to rest.
- Pain is relieved or made better by side-lying on the involved side (autosplinting).
- Pressure on the ribcage prevents respiratory movement on that side, thereby reducing symptoms induced by respiratory movements. This is quite the opposite of a musculoskeletal or neuromuscular cause of shoulder pain; the client often cannot lie on the involved side without increased pain.

In the older adult, listen for a self-report or family report of unknown cause of shoulder pain/dysfunction and/or any signs of confusion (confusion or increased confusion is a common first symptom of pneumonia in the older adult).

▶▶ PTA ACTION PLAN

Follow-Up Questions (Pulmonary)

Not all questions need to be presented; however, based on the patient's report at each session, the history, and any changes in clinical presentation from the initial evaluation documented by the PT, the PTA may see the need to ask some follow-up questions. If the client answers positively to any of the following questions, the PTA should provide an accurate verbal summary to the primary PT.

- Ask about the presence of pleuritic component. Does the patient have any of the following:
  - Persistent cough (dry or productive)
  - Blood-tinged sputum; rust, green, or yellow phlegm
  - Chest pain
  - Musculoskeletal symptoms are aggravated by respiratory movements. Ask the client to take a deep breath; does this reproduce or increase the pain/symptoms?
- Have you been treated recently for a lung problem (or think you have any lung or respiratory problems)?
- Do you currently have a cough?
  - *If yes*, is this a smoker's cough?
  - *If no*, how long has this been present?
  - Is this a productive cough (can you bring up sputum)? Is the sputum yellow, green, black, or tinged with blood?
  - Does coughing bring on your shoulder pain (or make it worse)?
- Do you ever have shortness of breath, have trouble catching your breath, or feel breathless?
- Does your shoulder pain increase when you cough, laugh, or take a deep breath?
- Do you have any chest pain?
- What effect does lying down or resting have on your shoulder pain? (In the supine or recumbent position a pulmonary problem may be made worse, whereas a musculoskeletal problem may be relieved; on the other hand, pulmonary pain may be relieved when the client lies on the affected side, which diminishes the movement of that side of the chest.)
- Remember to ask our final question: Are there any symptoms of any kind anywhere else in your body that I should report to your PT?

RECOGNIZING AND REPORTING CARDIOVASCULAR RED FLAGS

Shoulder symptoms from a cardiac cause get worse when the client increases activity that does not necessarily involve the arm or shoulder. For example, walking up stairs or riding a stationary bicycle can bring on cardiac-induced shoulder pain. In cases like this, ask about the presence of nausea, unexplained sweating, jaw pain or toothache, back pain, or chest discomfort or pressure.

Angina or Myocardial Infarction

Angina and/or MI can appear as arm and shoulder pain that can be masquerading as arthritis or other musculoskeletal pathologic conditions. Shoulder pain associated with MI is unaffected by position, breathing, or movement. Because of the well-known association between shoulder pain and angina, cardiac-related shoulder pain may be medically diagnosed without ruling out other causes, such as adhesive capsulitis or supraspinatus tendinitis, when, in fact, the client may have both a cardiac and a musculoskeletal problem.

PICTURE THE PATIENT

Shoulder pain that starts 3 to 5 minutes after the start of activity is a cardiovascular red flag. This includes shoulder pain with isolated lower extremity motion (e.g., shoulder pain starts after the client climbs a flight of stairs, guides a self-propelled lawn mower, or rides a stationary bicycle). If the client has known angina and takes nitroglycerin, ask about the influence of the nitroglycerin on shoulder pain.

» PTA ACTION PLAN

The clinical scenarios presented in Case Example 6.4 and Case Example 6.5 will help the reader problem solve through the appropriate PTA action plan individually or in a small group.

Clinical Signs and Symptoms
Bacterial Endocarditis

The most common musculoskeletal symptom in clients with bacterial endocarditis is arthralgia, generally in the proximal joints. The shoulder is affected most often, followed by (in declining incidence) the knee, hip, wrist, ankle, metatarsophalangeal and metacarpophalangeal joints, and by acromioclavicular involvement.

Most clients with endocarditis-related arthralgias have only one or two painful joints, although some may have pain in several joints.[40] Painful symptoms begin suddenly in one or two joints, accompanied by warmth, tenderness, and redness. As a rule, morning stiffness is not as prevalent in clients with endocarditis as in those with RA or polymyalgia rheumatica.

Pericarditis

The inflammatory process accompanying pericarditis may result in an accumulation of fluid in the pericardial sac, preventing the heart from expanding fully. The subsequent chest pain of pericarditis (Fig. 6.3) closely mimics that of a MI because it is substernal, is associated with cough, and may radiate to the shoulder.[41]

 PICTURE THE PATIENT

Pericarditis pain is sharp and relieved by leaning over when seated. Irritation of the diaphragm can cause shoulder pain. The chest and shoulder pain associated with pericarditis may be relieved by kneeling with hands on the floor, leaning forward, or sitting upright. Pericardial pain is often made worse by deep breathing, swallowing, or belching.

Aortic Aneurysm

Aortic aneurysm appears as sudden, severe chest pain with a tearing sensation (see Fig. 5.5), and the pain may extend to the neck, shoulders, lower back, or abdomen but rarely to the joints and arms, which distinguishes it from MI.

Shoulder pain by itself is not associated with aortic aneurysm; shoulder pain with aneurysm is more likely to occur when the primary pain pattern radiates up and over the trapezius and upper arm(s) (Fig. 6.4).[42] The client may report a bounding or throbbing pulse (heartbeat) in the abdomen. Such a report would require an immediate recheck by the PT or contact with the medical doctor if the PT is not immediately available.

Deep Venous Thrombosis of the Upper Extremity

Deep venous thrombosis (DVT) of the upper extremity is not as common as in the lower extremity, but incidence may be on the rise as a result of the increasing use of peripherally inserted central catheters (PICC lines) or central venous catheters (CVC).[43-46] Thrombosis affects the subclavian vein, axillary vein, or both most often, with less common sites being the internal jugular and brachial veins.[47]

CASE EXAMPLE 6.4   Strange Case of the Flu

Referral: A 53-year-old butcher at the local grocery store stopped by the physical therapy clinic located in the same shopping complex with a complaint of unusual shoulder pain. He had been seen at this same clinic several years ago for shoulder bursitis and tendinitis from repetitive overuse (cutting and wrapping meat).

Clinical Presentation: His clinical presentation for this new episode of care was exactly as it had been during the last episode of shoulder impairment. The therapist reinstituted a program of soft tissue mobilization and stretching, joint mobilization, and exercises to improve postural alignment. Modalities were used during the first two sessions to help gain pain control.

At the third appointment the client mentioned feeling "dizzy and sweaty" all day. His shoulder pain was described as a constant, deep ache that had increased in intensity from a 6 to a 10 on a 0-to-10 scale. He attributed these symptoms to having the flu.

PTA Action Plan: At this point the physical therapist assistant (PTA) discussed with the therapist the following red flags:
- Age
- Recent history (past 3 weeks) of middle ear infection on the same side as the involved shoulder

- Constant, intense pain (escalating over time)
- Constitutional symptoms (dizziness, perspiration)
- Symptoms unrelieved by physical therapy treatment

Result: The therapist suggested the client get a medical checkup before continuing with physical therapy. Even though the clinical presentation supported shoulder impairment, enough red flags and soft signs of systemic distress existed to warrant further evaluation.

It turns out the client was having myocardial ischemia masquerading as shoulder pain, the flu, and an ear infection. He had an angioplasty with complete resolution of all his symptoms and even reported feeling energetic for the first time in years.

Is there Anything Else The PTA Could Have Done to Gather Further Pertinent Information for the PT?
This is a good example of how shoulder pain and dysfunction can exactly mimic a true musculoskeletal problem—even to the extent of reproducing symptoms from a previous condition.

This case highlights the fact that PTAs must be careful to fully assess clients with each episode of care.

CASE EXAMPLE 6.5   Angina Versus Shoulder Pathology

A 54-year-old male was referred to physical therapy for preprosthetic training after a left transtibial (TT) amputation.

Past Medical History

A right TT amputation was performed 4 years ago

Coronary artery disease with coronary artery bypass graft, myocardial infarction (heart attack), and angina

Peripheral vascular disease

Long-standing diabetes mellitus (insulin dependent × 47 years)

Gastroesophageal reflux disease

Clinical Presentation: During the third session the client reported to the physical therapist assistant (PTA) substernal chest pain and left upper extremity pain with activity. Typical anginal pain pattern was described as substernal chest pain. The pain occurs with exertion and is relieved by rest.

Critical Thinking for Small Group Discussion

Review concepts in the text and apply them by listing the appropriate follow-up questions the PTA should ask the patient to gather information to report back to the physical therapist (PT).

As a result of the follow-up questions by the PTA, the patient who reported arm pain has never been a part of his usual anginal pain pattern. He reports that his arm pain began 10 months ago with intermittent pain starting in the left shoulder and radiating down the anterior-medial aspect of the arm, halfway between the shoulder and the elbow.

The pain is made worse by raising his left arm overhead, pushing his own wheelchair, and using a walker. He was not sure if the shoulder pain was caused by repetitive motions needed for mobility or by his angina. The shoulder pain is relieved by avoiding painful motions. He has not received any treatment for the shoulder problem.

Neurologic screening included deep tendon reflex testing, manual muscle testing, and light touch. All results were negative.

Vital Signs

Heart rate:	88 bpm
Blood pressure:	120/66 mm Hg (position and extremity, not recorded)
Respirations:	Within normal limits

Vital Signs (after transfer and pregait activities)

Heart rate:	92 bpm
Blood pressure:	152/76 mm Hg
Respirations:	"Minimal shortness of breath" recorded

Special Tests (performed by the PT)

Yergason's sign:	Positive
Apprehension test:	Positive
Relocation test:	Positive
Speed's test:	Positive

Palpation of the biceps and supraspinatus tendons increased the client's shoulder pain.

Active Range of Motion (AROM): Left Shoulder

Flexion:	100 degrees
Abduction:	70 degrees
Internal/external rotation:	60 degrees

There is a capsular pattern in the left glenohumeral joint with limitations in rotation and adduction.

Manual Muscle Test (gross)

Bilateral upper extremity:	4/5 (throughout available AROM)

PTA Action Plan

Based on the above observations, the PTA will request further evaluation of the shoulder by the PT.

Result: Further testing performed by the PT revealed an untreated biceps and supraspinatus tendinitis. This tendinitis combined with adhesive capsulitis most likely accounted for the left shoulder pain. This assessment was based on the decreased left glenohumeral AROM and decreased joint mobility.

With objective clinical findings to support a musculoskeletal dysfunction, medical referral was not required. There were no indications that the shoulder pain was a signal of a change in the client's anginal pattern.

Left shoulder impairments were limiting factors in his mobility and rehabilitation process. Shoulder intervention to alleviate pain and to improve upper extremity strength was included in the plan of care. The desired outcome was to improve transfer and gait activities.

The observations made by the PTA resulted in the modification of the plan of care by the PT. These modifications brought about resolution of left shoulder pain within the first week of the new treatment plan.

The client gained independence with bed mobility and supine-to-sit transfers. The client continued to make improvements in ambulation, ROM, and functional mobility.

Physical therapy intervention for the shoulder impairments had a significant impact on the outcomes of this client's rehab program. By differentiating and treating the shoulder movement dysfunction, the intervention enabled the client to progress faster in the transfer and gait training program than he would had his left shoulder pain been attributed to angina.

(From Smith ML: Differentiating angina and shoulder pathology pain, *Phys Ther Case Rep* 1(4):210–212, 1998.)

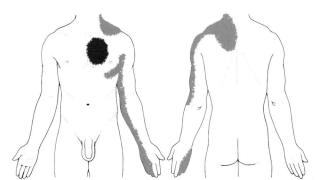

FIG. 6.3 Substernal pain associated with pericarditis (*dark red*) may radiate anteriorly (*light red*) to the costal margins, neck, upper back, upper trapezius muscle, and left supraclavicular area or down the left arm.

CVCs are frequently used in people with hematologic/oncologic disorders to administer drugs,[48] stem cell infusions, blood products, parenteral alimentation, and blood sampling. Other risk factors include blood clotting disorders,[49] clavicle fracture,[50,51] insertion of pacemaker wires, and arthroscopy of the shoulder or reconstructive shoulder arthroplasty.[52–55]

▶ PTA ACTION PLAN

Communication With the Physical Therapist

The therapist should be notified of pain and pitting edema or swelling of the entire (usually upper) limb and/or an area of the limb that is 2 cm or more larger than the surrounding area, which indicates swelling and requires further investigation.

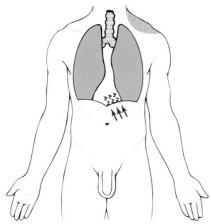

FIG. 6.4 Irritation of the peritoneal (*outside*) or pleural (*inside*) surface of the *central* area of the diaphragm can refer sharp pain to the upper trapezius muscle, neck, and supraclavicular fossa. The pain pattern is ipsilateral to the area of irritation. Irritation to the *peripheral* portion of the diaphragm can refer sharp pain to the ipsilateral costal margins and lumbar region (*not shown*).

Other red-flag symptoms that require reporting include redness or warmth of the arm, dilated veins, or low-grade fever, possibly accompanied by chills and malaise. Be aware of bruising or discoloration of the area or proximal to the area on the arm with the thrombosis.[56] Swelling can contribute to decreased neck or shoulder motion. Severe thromboses can cause superior vena cava syndrome; symptoms include edema of the face and arm, vertigo, and dyspnea.[57,58]

🔎 PICTURE THE PATIENT

The following are indications of upper extremity DVTs:
- Numbness or heaviness of the extremity
- Itching, burning, or coldness of the extremity
- Swelling, discoloration, warmth, or redness of the extremity; pitting edema
- Limited range of motion (ROM) of neck or shoulder
- Low-grade fever, chills, or malaise
- (For individuals with a PICC line [in addition to any of the signs and symptoms listed above]): Pain or tenderness at or above the insertion site

▶ PTA ACTION PLAN

Reviewing Cardiovascular Clinical Presentation

The PTA should be alert to the following list of cardiovascular clinical presentations. Observations should be immediately documented in the medical chart and verbally reported to the supervising PT if these signs and symptoms are new or previously unknown or unreported.
- Exacerbation by exertion unrelated to shoulder movement (e.g., using only the lower extremities to climb stairs or ride a stationary bicycle).
- Unexplained profuse sweating when the shoulder pain occurs.
- Shoulder pain relieved by leaning forward, kneeling with hands on the floor, or sitting upright (pericarditis).
- Shoulder pain accompanied by dyspnea, temporomandibular joint pain, toothache, belching, nausea, or pressure behind the sternum (angina).
- Shoulder pain relieved by nitroglycerin (males) or antacids/acid-relieving drugs (females) (angina).
- Difference of 10 mm Hg or more at rest in blood pressure in the affected arm compared with the uninvolved or a symptomatic arm (dissecting aortic aneurysm, vascular component of thoracic outlet syndrome).

- Excessive, unexplained coincident diaphoresis (i.e., the client breaks out in a cold sweat just before or during an episode of shoulder pain; this may occur at rest but is more likely with mild physical activity).
- Bilateral shoulder pain that comes on after using the arms overhead for 3 to 5 minutes.
- Remember to correlate any of the clinical presentations listed above with the client's past medical history.

▶ PTA ACTION PLAN

Follow-Up Questions

If the client answers "yes" to any of the following questions, the PTA should provide an accurate verbal summary to the primary PT.
- Have you recently (ever) had a heart attack? (referred pain)
  Note: This should be asked only if the patient had not reported this to the PT during the initial evaluation.
- Do you ever notice sweating, nausea, or chest pain when the pain in your shoulder occurs?
- Have you noticed your shoulder pain increasing with exertion that does not necessarily cause you to use your shoulder (e.g., climbing stairs, stationary bicycle)?
- Do(es) your mouth, jaw, or teeth ever hurt when your shoulder is bothering you? (angina)
- [For the client with known angina]: Does your shoulder pain go away when you take nitroglycerin? (Ask about the effect of taking antacids/acid-relieving drugs for females.)

RECOGNIZING AND REPORTING UROLOGIC RED FLAGS

The anatomic position of the kidneys (and ureters) is in front of and on both sides of the vertebral column at the level of T11 to L3. The right kidney is usually lower than the left.[59] Because of its location in the posterior upper abdominal cavity in the retroperitoneal space, touching the diaphragm, the upper urinary tract can refer pain to the (ipsilateral) shoulder on the same side as the involved kidney.

Renal pain is aching and dull in nature but can occasionally be a severe, boring type of pain. The distention or stretching of the renal capsule, pelvis, or collecting system from intrarenal fluid accumulation (e.g., inflammatory edema, inflamed or bleeding cysts, and bleeding or neoplastic growths) accounts for the constant, dull, and aching quality of reported pain.

🔎 PICTURE THE PATIENT

Ischemia of renal tissue caused by blockage of blood flow to the kidneys can produce either a constant dull or sharp pain. True renal pain is seldom affected by change in position or movements of the shoulder or spine.

If the diaphragm becomes irritated because of pressure from a renal lesion, ipsilateral shoulder pain can be the only symptom or may occur in conjunction with other pain and red-flag signs and symptoms. For example, generalized abdominal pain may develop, accompanied by nausea, vomiting, and impaired intestinal motility (progressing to intestinal paralysis) when pain is acute and severe. Nerve fibers from the renal plexus are also in direct communication with the spermatic plexus; because of this close relationship, testicular pain may also accompany renal pain in males.[60,61]

>> PTA ACTION PLAN
Communication With the Physical Therapist

Elevation in temperature or changes in color, odor, or amount of urine (flow, frequency, nocturia) presenting with shoulder pain should be brought to the attention of the supervising PT. Shoulder pain that is not affected by movement requires a closer look.

The presence of constitutional symptoms, constant pain (even if dull), and failure to change the symptoms with a position change are also indications that the therapist may need to conduct a more thorough screening examination. A past medical history of cancer is always an important risk factor requiring careful assessment. This is true even when patients/clients have a known or traumatic cause for their symptoms.

Flank pain combined with unexplained weight loss, fever, pain, and hematuria are red flags requiring further evaluation by the PT, who may also report these to the physician. The presence of any amount of blood in the urine always requires referral to a physician for further diagnostic evaluation because this is a primary symptom of urinary tract neoplasm.

>> PTA ACTION PLAN
Reviewing Urologic Clinical Presentation

The PTA should be alert to the following list of urologic clinical presentations. Observations should be immediately documented in the medical chart and verbally reported to the supervising PT if they are new or previously unknown or unreported.
- Shoulder pain accompanied by elevation in temperature or changes in color, odor, or amount of urine (flow, frequency, nocturia); pain is not affected by movement.
- Shoulder pain accompanied by or alternating with flank pain, abdominal pain, or pelvic pain (or, in males, testicular pain).

>> PTA ACTION PLAN
Follow-Up Question

If the client answers "yes" to any of the following questions, the PTA should provide an accurate verbal summary to the primary PT (if this is new information).
- Have you had any recent kidney infections, tumors, or kidney stones? (pressure from kidney on diaphragm referred to shoulder)

RECOGNIZING AND REPORTING GASTROINTESTINAL RED FLAGS

Upper abdominal or GI problems with diaphragmatic irritation can refer pain to the ipsilateral shoulder on the same side as the affected diaphragm (i.e., irritation of the left side of the diaphragm can cause left shoulder pain and vice versa). Perforated gastric or duodenal ulcers, gallbladder disease, and hiatal hernia are the most likely GI causes of shoulder pain seen in a physical therapy clinic or rehab facility.

? PICTURE THE PATIENT

Usually there are associated signs and symptoms, such as nausea, vomiting, anorexia, melena, or early satiety, but the client may not connect the shoulder pain with GI disorders.

History of previous ulcer, especially in association with the use of nonsteroidal antiinflammatory drugs (NSAIDs), is a red flag. With a true musculoskeletal problem, peak NSAID dosage (usually 2–4 hours after ingestion; variable with each drug) should reduce or alleviate painful shoulder symptoms. Shoulder pain that worsens 2 to 4 hours after taking the NSAID can be suggestive of GI bleeding and is considered a yellow (caution) flag. Any pain increase instead of decrease may be a symptom of GI bleeding.

>> PTA ACTION PLAN
Reviewing Gastrointestinal Red Flags

The PTA can ask about the effect of eating on shoulder pain. If eating makes shoulder pain better or worse (anywhere from 30 minutes to 2 hours after eating), there may be a GI problem. The client may not be aware of the link between these two events until the PTA asks. If the client is not sure, repeat the question at a future appointment. Ask again if the client has noticed any unusual symptoms or connection between eating and shoulder pain.

The PTA should be alert to the following list of GI clinical presentations. Observations should be immediately documented in the medical chart and verbally reported to the supervising PT if they are new or previously unknown or unreported.
- Coincident nausea, vomiting, dysphagia; presence of other GI complaints such as anorexia, early satiety, epigastric pain or discomfort and fullness, melena
- Shoulder pain relieved by belching or antacids and made worse by eating
- History of previous ulcer, especially in association with the use of NSAIDs
- History of chronic (>6 months) NSAID use and history of previous ulcer, especially in association with NSAID use. This is the most common cause of medication-induced shoulder pain in all ages, but especially adults over 65 years.
- History of other GI diseases that can refer pain to the shoulder, such as:
  - Gallbladder
  - Acute pancreatitis
  - Reflex esophagitis

It is important to know that true NMS shoulder pain is not relieved or made worse by eating. If a peptic ulcer in the upper GI tract is causing referred pain to the shoulder, there is often a history of NSAID use. This client will have that red-flag history along with shoulder pain that gets better after eating. Other GI symptoms may also be present, such as nausea, loss of appetite, or melena from oxidized blood in the upper GI tract.

>> PTA ACTION PLAN
Follow-Up Questions

If the client answers "yes" to any of the following questions, the PTA should provide an accurate verbal summary to the primary PT.

Again, pay attention to the prior medical history included in the PT's initial evaluation before asking any of the following questions.

- Have you ever had an ulcer?
  - *If yes*, when? Do you still have any pain from your ulcer?
  - Have you noticed any association between when you eat and when your symptoms increase or decrease?
- Does eating relieve your pain? (ulcer)
  - How soon is the pain relieved after eating?
- Does eating aggravate your pain? (gastric ulcer, gallbladder inflammation)
- Does your pain occur 1 to 3 hours after eating or between meals? (duodenal or pyloric ulcers, gallstones)
- [For the client taking NSAIDs]: Does your shoulder pain increase 2 to 4 hours after taking your NSAIDs? (If the client does not know, ask him or her to pay attention for the next few days to the response of shoulder symptoms after taking the medication.)
- Have you ever had gallstones?
- Do you have a feeling of fullness after only one or two bites of food? (early satiety: stomach and duodenum or gallbladder)
- Have you had any nausea, vomiting, difficulty in swallowing, loss of appetite, or heartburn since the shoulder started bothering you?

RECOGNIZING AND REPORTING LIVER AND BILIARY RED FLAGS

As with many of the organ systems in the human body, the hepatic and biliary organs (liver, gallbladder, and common bile duct) can develop diseases that mimic primary musculoskeletal lesions.

The musculoskeletal symptoms associated with hepatic and biliary pathologic conditions are generally confined to the mid-back, scapular, and right shoulder regions (see Fig. 4.4). These musculoskeletal symptoms can occur alone (as the only presenting symptom) or in combination with other systemic signs and symptoms. In most cases of shoulder pain referred from visceral processes, shoulder motion is not compromised and local tenderness is not a prominent feature.

Individuals who have avoided medical treatment may have shoulder pain caused by hepatic and biliary diseases that has created biomechanical changes in muscular contractions and shoulder movement. These changes eventually create pain of a biomechanical nature.[62]

Liver dysfunction resulting in increased serum ammonia and urea levels can result in impaired peripheral nerve function, causing what appears to be carpal tunnel syndrome (CTS). Many potential causes of CTS exist, both musculoskeletal and systemic (see Box 4.5). The presence of *bilateral* CTS can be a red-flag warning of hepatic involvement.[63] Because this is a system-wide event, peripheral nerves on both sides and in hands and feet may be involved.

The client with shoulder pain (GI bleed) and symptoms of CTS (liver impairment) may demonstrate other signs of liver impairment, such as the following:
- Liver flap (asterixis) (see Fig. 3.5)
- Liver palms (palmar erythema) (see Fig. 3.4)
- Nail-bed changes (white nails of Terry) (see Fig. 3.3)
- Spider angiomas (over the abdomen) (see Figs. 3.6 and 3.7)

Flapping tremors or *liver flap* (asterixis) is described as the inability to maintain wrist extension with forward flexion of the upper extremities. It is tested by asking the client to actively hyperextend the wrist and hand with the rest of the arm supported on a firm surface or with the arms held out in front of the body. The test is positive if quick, irregular extensions and flexions of the wrist and fingers occur. Asterixis may also be observed when releasing the pressure in the arm cuff during blood pressure readings.

Palmar erythema (warm redness of the skin over the palms, also called *liver palms*), caused by an extensive collection of arteriovenous anastomoses, is especially evident on the hypothenar and thenar eminences and pulps of the finger. The person may complain of throbbing, tingling palms. The soles of the feet may be similarly affected. Throbbing and tingling may be associated with these anastomoses.

Spider angiomas (arterial spider, spider telangiectasias, vascular spider), branched dilations of the superficial capillaries resembling a spider in appearance, may be vascular manifestations of increased estrogen levels (hyperestrogenism). Spider angiomas and palmar erythema both occur in the presence of liver impairment as a result of increased estrogen levels normally detoxified by the liver.

RECOGNIZING AND REPORTING RED FLAGS OF INFECTION

The most likely infectious causes of shoulder pain in a physical therapy clinic include infectious (septic) arthritis, herpes zoster (shingles), pneumonia, cellulitis, osteomyelitis, and infectious mononucleosis (mono). Immunosuppression for any reason puts people of all ages at risk for infection.

▶▶ PTA ACTION PLAN

Points to Ponder

Postoperative infection of any kind may not appear with any clinical signs/symptoms for weeks or months, especially in a client who is on corticosteroids or immunocompromised.

▶▶ PTA ACTION PLAN

The clinical scenario presented in Case Example 6.6 is an excellent example of the PTA exhibiting strong observation skills and taking action early on in the treatment schedule.

Septic arthritis of the acromioclavicular joint or hand can present as insidious onset of shoulder pain. Likewise, septic arthritis of the sternoclavicular joint can present as chest pain. Usually, there is local tenderness at the affected joint. A possible history of intravenous drug use, diabetes, trauma (puncture wound, surgery, human or animal bite), and infection is usually present. Punching someone in the mouth (hand coming in contact with teeth, resulting in a puncture wound) has been reported as a potential cause of septic arthritis. With infection of this type, there may or may not be constitutional symptoms.[64,65]

Herpes Zoster (shingles): see Chapter 3.

CASE EXAMPLE 6.6 Osteomyelitis

The following information was provided to the physical therapist assistant (PTA) via the initial evaluation made by the physical therapist (PT).

Referral: S.C., an active 62-year-old cardiac nurse, was referred by her orthopedic surgeon for "PT [for] possible rotator cuff tear (RCT), three times a week for 4 weeks." S.C. reported an "open" magnetic resonance imaging (MRI) was negative for RCT and plain films were also negative. She noted that laboratory testing was not done.

Past Medical History

Medications: Current medications included Motrin 800 mg tid for pain; Decadron 0.75 mg qid for atypical dermatitis and asthma (45-year use of corticosteroids); Avapro 75 mg qid to control hypertension; HydroDIURIL 25 mg qid to counteract fluid retention from corticosteroids; and Chlor-Trimeton 12 mg qid to suppress the high level of blood histamine resulting from the long-term comorbid condition of atypical dermatitis and asthma.

Social History: The client consumes one glass of wine per day, quit smoking 20 years ago, and has never done illicit drugs.

Clinical Presentation

Pain Pattern: The client presented with primary complaints of severe and limiting pain of nearly 4 weeks' duration with any active movement at her left shoulder and at rest. Her pain was rated on the visual analog scale as 7/10 at rest and 9/10 to 10/10 with motion at glenohumeral (GH) joint. Pain onset was gradual over a 3-day period; she was not aware of injury or trauma.

She reported an inability to (1) use her left upper extremity (UE); (2) lie on or bear weight on left side; (3) perform activities of daily living; (4) sleep uninterrupted due to pain, awakening four or five times nightly; or (5) participate in regular weekly yoga classes.

Vital Signs: Temperature: 98.6°F (37°C); blood pressure: 120/98 mm Hg. S.C. reported that her medication combination of Decadron and Chlor-Trimeton had been implicated in the past by her physician as acting to suppress low-grade fevers.

Observation: Slight puffiness but minimal swelling observed in the left supraclavicular area. S.C. holds left UE at her side with the elbow flexed to 90 degrees and the shoulder held in internal rotation.

Standing Posture: Forward head position with increased cervical spine lordosis and thoracic spine kyphosis, with an inability to attain neutral or reverse either spinal curve.

Palpation revealed exquisite tenderness at distal clavicle and both anterior and posterior aspects of proximal humerus.

Cervical spine screen: Spurling compression, distraction, and quadrant testing were all negative; deep tendon reflexes at C5, C6, and C7 were symmetrically increased bilaterally; dermatomal testing was within normal limits; myotomes could not be reliably tested because of pain.

Special tests at the shoulder could not be performed or were unreliable because of pain limitation.

Range of Motion (ROM): Left GH joint active ROM (AROM) and passive ROM (PROM) were severely limited. AROM: Unable to actively perform flexion or abduction at left shoulder. PROM left shoulder (measured in supine with arm at side and elbow flexed to 90 degrees):

Flexion:	35 degrees
Abduction:	35 degrees
Internal rotation:	50 degrees
External rotation:	−10 degrees

All ranges were pain limited with an "empty" end feel.

Evaluation/Assessment: S.C.'s signs, symptoms, and examination findings were consistent with those of a severe, full-thickness RCT, including severity of pain and functional loss with empty end feel at GH joint ROM. However, the inability to obtain results of special test results at the shoulder limited the certainty of the RCT diagnosis.

PTA Observations

Over the course of four therapy sessions, the PTA became concerned about the patient's severe loss of motion with empty end feel, constancy and severity of pain, inability to relieve pain or obtain a comfortable position, bony tenderness, and insidious onset of the condition. Additional risk factors included long-term use of corticosteroids to treat atypical dermatitis with asthma.

Based on the objective findings, including swelling and bone tenderness, along with the severity and unrelenting nature of her pain, the PTA determined the need for further evaluation by the PT.

Outcomes: The client made very little progress after the prescribed physical therapy intervention. The severity of pain and functional loss remained unchanged. Numerous attempts were made by the client and the therapist to discuss this case with the referring physician. The client eventually referred herself to a second physician.

Result: The PTA's early observations and report of the unusual signs and symptoms resulted in a diagnosis with osteomyelitis as a result of a repeat MRI and a triple-phase bone scan, and laboratory test results of elevated levels of erythrocyte sedimentation rate and C-reactive protein values. A surgical biopsy confirmed the diagnosis. She underwent three different surgical procedures culminating in a total shoulder arthroplasty along with repair of the full-thickness RCT.

(From West PR: *Case report presented in fulfillment of DPT 910,* Chester, 2005, Institute for Physical Therapy Education, Widener University, used with permission.)

Pneumonia is usually preceded by a URI, frequently viral. Signs and symptoms of pneumonia include sudden and sharp pleuritic chest pain aggravated by chest movement and accompanied by a hacking, productive cough with rust-colored or green purulent sputum. Other symptoms include dyspnea, tachypnea accompanied by decreased chest excursion on the affected side, cyanosis, headache, fatigue, fever and chills, and generalized aches and myalgias.

Older adults with bronchopneumonia have fewer symptoms than younger people, and many remain afebrile because of the changes in temperature regulation as part of the normal aging process.[66,67] Associated changes in gas exchange (hypoxia and hypercapnia) may result in altered mental status (e.g., confusion) or loss of balance and may lead to falls.

Cellulitis, an acute spreading inflammation of the skin and subcutaneous tissues, usually results from infection of burns, wounds, or other breaks in the skin, although in some cases no entry site is noted.[68] Recurrent episodes of cellulitis may occur in extremities in which lymphatic drainage has been impaired (e.g., postaxillary node dissection, site of saphenous vein harvest) or chronic fungal infections serve as a reservoir.[69]

The skin is painful and swollen with accompanying erythema. Systemic symptoms such as fever and chills are often associated with the skin infection. Cellulitis can rapidly spread or involve bacteremia or lymphangitis. Lymphangitis is readily recognized by the presence of red, tender, linear streaks directed toward enlarged, tender regional lymph nodes. It is accompanied by systemic symptoms such as chills, fever, malaise, and headache.

Osteomyelitis (bone or bone marrow infection) is caused most commonly by *Staphylococcus aureus*. Hematogenous spread from a wound, abscess, or systemic infection (e.g., fracture, TB, urinary tract infection, URI, finger felons) occurs most often. Osteomyelitis of the spine is associated with injection drug use.

 PICTURE THE PATIENT

Onset of clinical signs and symptoms is usually gradual in adults but may be more sudden in children with high fever, chills, and inability to bear weight through the affected joint. In all ages, there is marked tenderness over the site of the infection when the affected bone is superficial (e.g., spinous process, distal femur, proximal tibia). The most reliable way to recognize infection is the presence of both local and systemic symptoms.

Mononucleosis is a viral infection that affects the respiratory tract, liver, and spleen. Splenomegaly with subsequent rupture is a rare but serious cause of left shoulder pain (Kehr sign).[70] Left upper abdominal pain usually occurs, and, in many cases, trauma to the enlarged spleen (e.g., sports injury) is the precipitating cause in an athlete with an unknown or undiagnosed case of mono.

 PICTURE THE PATIENT

The virus can be present 4 to 10 weeks before any symptoms develop, so the person may not know mono is present. Acute symptoms can include sore throat, headache, fatigue, lymphadenopathy, fever, myalgias, and, occasionally, skin rash. Enlarged tonsils can cause noisy or difficulty breathing.

RECOGNIZING AND REPORTING RED FLAGS OF CANCER

A past medical history of cancer anywhere in the body with new onset of back or shoulder pain (or impairment) is a red-flag finding requiring close observation for any change in clinical presentation. Brachial plexus radiculopathy can occur in either or both arms with cancer metastasized to the lymphatics. Invasion of the upper humerus and glenoid area by secondary malignant deposits affects the joint and the adjacent muscles.

▶▶ **PTA ACTION PLAN**

The clinical scenarios presented in Case Example 6.7 and Case Example 6.8 will provide the reader the opportunity to develop a unique action plan based on small group discussion.

Primary Bone Neoplasm

Bone cancer occurs chiefly in young people, in whom a cause-less limitation of movement of the shoulder leads the physician to order x-rays. If the tumor originates from the shaft of the humerus, the first symptoms may be a feeling of "pins and needles" in the hand, associated with fixation of the biceps and triceps muscles and leading to limitation of movement at the elbow.

▶▶ **PTA ACTION PLAN**

The clinical scenario presented in Case Example 6.9 will help the reader begin to develop a mental checklist of red flags and a routine of proper communication with the PT.

Pulmonary (Secondary) Neoplasm

Occasionally, shoulder pain is referred from metastatic lung cancer. The affected individual is unable to lift the arm beyond the horizontal position. Muscles respond with spasm that limits joint movement.

 PICTURE THE PATIENT

If the neoplasm interferes with the diaphragm, diaphragmatic pain (C3–5–phrenic nerve) is often felt at the shoulder at each breath (at the deltoid area).[71] Although the lung is insensitive, large tumors invading the chest wall set up local pain and cause spasm of the pectoralis major muscle, with consequent shoulder pain and/or limitation of elevation of the arm.[72] If the neoplasm encroaches on the ribs, stretching the muscle attached to the ribs leads to spasm of the pectoralis major. By contrast, the scapula is mobile, and a full range of passive movement is present at the shoulder joint.

CASE EXAMPLE 6.7   **Upper Extremity Radiculopathy**

A 72-year-old female was referred to physical therapy by her neurologist with a diagnosis of "nerve entrapment" for a postural exercise program and home traction. She was experiencing symptoms of left shoulder pain with numbness and tingling in the ulnar nerve distribution. She had a moderate forward head posture with slumped shoulders and loss of height from known osteoporosis.

Past Medical History: Her past medical history was significant for right breast cancer treated with a radical mastectomy and chemotherapy 20 years ago. She had a second cancer (uterine) 10 years ago that was considered separate from her previous breast cancer.

Clinical Presentation: The physical therapy examination was consistent with the physician's diagnosis of nerve entrapment in a classic presentation. There were significant postural components to account for the development of symptoms. The physical therapist assistant (PTA) observed and palpated several large masses in the axillary and supraclavicular fossa on both the right and left sides. There was no local warmth, redness, or tenderness associated with these lesions.

Critical Thinking for Small Group Discussion
Review concepts in the text and apply them by listing the appropriate follow-up questions the PTA should ask the patient to gather information to report back to the physical therapist (PT).

Result: Given the significant past medical history for cancer, her age, presence of progressive night pain, and palpable masses, the PTA consulted with the PT. When the PT asked the patient if the physician had seen or felt the masses, the client responded with a definite "no."

The therapist returned the client to the physician with a brief (one-page) written report summarizing the findings.

Further medical testing was performed, and a medical diagnosis of lymphoma was made.

CASE EXAMPLE 6.8   Shoulder and Leg Pain

Referral: A 33-year-old female came to a physical therapy clinic located inside a large health club. She reported right shoulder and right lower leg pain that is keeping her from exercising. She could walk but had an antalgic gait resulting from pain on weightbearing.

She linked these symptoms with heavy household chores. She could think of no other trauma or injury. She was screened for the possibility of domestic violence with negative results.

Past Medical History: There was no past history of disease, illness, trauma, or surgery. There were no other symptoms reported (e.g., no fever, nausea, fatigue, bowel or bladder changes, sleep disturbance).

Clinical Presentation: During the treatment session with the physical therapist assistant (PTA), the right shoulder and right leg were visibly and palpably swollen. Any and all (global) motions of either the arm or the leg were painful. The skin was tender to light touch in a wide band of distribution around the painful sites. No redness or skin changes of any kind were noted.

Pain prevented strength training exercises today. Functionally, she was able to climb stairs and walk, but these and other activities (e.g., exercising, biking, household chores) were limited by pain.

Critical Thinking for Small Group Discussion
What further information should the PTA gather prior to reporting back to the physical therapist?

Result: X-rays of the right shoulder showed complete destruction of the right humeral head consistent with a diagnosis of metastatic disease. X-rays of the right leg showed two lytic lesions. There was no sign of fracture or dislocation. Computed tomography scans showed destructive lytic lesions in the ribs and ilium.

Additional testing was performed, including lab values, bone biopsy, mammography, and pelvic ultrasonography. The client was diagnosed with bone tumors resulting from hyperparathyroidism.

A large adenoma was found and removed from the left inferior parathyroid gland. Medical treatment resulted in decreased pain and increased motion and function over a period of 3 to 4 months. Physical therapy intervention was prescribed for residual muscle weakness.

(From Insler H: Shoulder and leg pain in a 33-year-old woman, *J Musculoskelet Med* 14(6):36–37, 1997.)

CASE EXAMPLE 6.9   Osteosarcoma

A 24-year-old male presented to a sports medicine clinic with a complaint of left shoulder pain that had been present off and on for the last 4 months. There was no reported history of injury or trauma despite active play on the regional soccer team.

Past Medical History: It was diagnosed as "tendinitis" with the suggestion to see a physical therapist (PT) of the family's choice. No x-rays or other diagnostic imaging was performed to date. The client could not remember if any laboratory work (blood or urinalysis) had been done.

Subject Information: The client reports to the physical therapist assistant (PTA) that his arm feels "heavy" and has become more difficult to move in the last week. The only other symptom present was intermittent tingling in the left hand.

Current Level of Function: The PTA noted moderate loss of active motion in shoulder flexion, abduction, and external rotation with an empty end feel and pain during passive range of motion. There was no pain with palpation or isometric resistance of the rotator cuff tendons. Gross strength of the upper extremity was 4/5 for all motions.

There was a palpable firm, soft, but fixed mass along the lateral proximal humerus. The client reported it was "tender" when the PTA applied moderate pressure. The client was not previously aware of this lump.

Upper extremity pulses, deep tendon reflexes, and sensation were all intact. There were no observed skin changes or palpable temperature changes.

Critical Thinking for Individual or Small Group Activity: Make a list of the red flags presented by this client and describe the most appropriate way for the PTA to communicate this information to the supervising PT.

Result: The PTA brought the red flags to the PT's attention. As a result of the follow-up examination with the PT, the physician was notified of possible changes in the patient status. The family was advised by the doctor's office staff to bring him to the clinic as a walk-in the same day. X-rays showed an irregular bony mass of the humeral head and surrounding soft tissues. The biopsy confirmed a diagnosis of osteogenic sarcoma. The cancer had already metastasized to the lungs and liver.

PANCOAST TUMOR

Pancoast tumors of the lung apex usually do not cause symptoms while confined to the lungs. Shoulder pain occurs if they extend into the surrounding structures, infiltrating the chest wall into the axilla. Occasionally, brachial plexus involvement (eighth cervical and first thoracic nerve) presents with radiculopathy.[73,74]

? PICTURE THE PATIENT

This nerve involvement produces sharp pain in the axilla, shoulder, and subscapular area on the affected side, with eventual atrophy of the upper extremity muscles. Bone pain is aching, exacerbated at night, and a cause of restlessness and musculoskeletal movement.[75]

Usually, general associated systemic signs and symptoms are present (e.g., sore throat, fever, hoarseness, unexplained weight loss, productive cough with blood in the sputum). These features are not found in any regional musculoskeletal disorder, including such disorders of the shoulder.

▶ PTA ACTION PLAN

Reviewing Cancer-Related Red Flags

The PTA should be alert to the following list of clinical presentations. Observations should be immediately documented in the medical chart and verbally reported to the supervising PT if they are new or previously unknown or unreported.

- Pectoralis major muscle spasm with no known cause; limited active shoulder flexion but with full passive shoulder motions and mobile scapula (tumor).
- Presence of localized warmth felt over the scapular area (tumor).
- Marked limitation of movement at the shoulder joint.
- Severe muscular weakness and pain with resisted movements.
- Previous history of cancer (any kind, but especially breast or lung cancer).
- Pectoralis major muscle spasm with no known cause, but full passive ROM and a mobile scapula; no relief from symptoms or change in movement pattern after trigger point therapy.
- Shoulder flexion and abduction limited to 90 degrees with empty end feel.
- Presence of localized warmth over scapular area; look for other trophic changes (e.g., increased hair growth, dry or flaking skin, unusual sweating, hot or cold skin temperature).

> ## ▶▶ PTA ACTION PLAN

Follow-Up Questions

Pain that is associated with any of the scenarios previously discussed and the client answers positively to the questions below should result in early verbal communication with the primary PT.

- Does your pain ever wake you at night from a sound sleep?
  - Can you find any way to relieve the pain and get back to sleep?
  - If yes, how? (cancer pain is usually intense and constant; nothing relieves it or, if relief is obtained in any way, pain gets progressively worse over time.)

RECOGNIZING AND REPORTING GYNECOLOGIC RED FLAGS

Shoulder pain as a result of gynecologic conditions is uncommon, but still very possible. Occasionally a client may present with breast pain as the primary complaint, but most often the description is of shoulder or arm, neck, or upper back pain.

Many breast conditions (e.g., tumors, infections, myalgias, implants, lymph disease, trauma) can refer pain to the shoulder either alone or in conjunction with chest and/or breast pain.[76-78] Shoulder pain or dysfunction in the presence of any of these conditions as part of the client's current or past medical history raises a red flag.

When asked if the client has any symptoms anywhere else in the body, breast pain may be mentioned. This new report of breast pain should be documented and the supervising PT notified.

> ## ▶▶ PTA ACTION PLAN

Reviewing Gynecologic Red Flags

The PTA should be alert to the following list of gynecologic clinical presentations. Observations should be documented immediately in the medical chart and reported verbally to the supervising PT if they are new or previously unknown or unreported.

- Shoulder pain preceded or accompanied by one-sided lower abdominal or pelvic pain in a sexually active female of reproductive age may be a symptom of ectopic pregnancy; there may be irregular bleeding or spotting after a light or late menstrual period.
- Shoulder (and/or abdominal or chest) pain with reports of lightheadedness, dizziness, or fainting in a sexually active female of reproductive age (ectopic pregnancy).[79-81]
- Presence of endometrial cysts and/or scar tissue impinging diaphragm, nerve plexus, or the shoulder itself.
- Remember that males can have breast diseases, although not as often as females. Red-flag clinical presentation and associated signs and symptoms of breast disease referred to the shoulder may include the following:
  - Jarring or squeezing the breast refers pain to the shoulder.
  - Resisted shoulder motions do not reproduce shoulder pain but do cause breast pain or discomfort.
  - Obvious change in breast tissue (e.g., lump[s], dimpling or peau d'orange, distended veins, nipple discharge or ulceration, erythema, change in size or shape of the breast).
  - Suspicious or aberrant axillary or supraclavicular lymph nodes.

> ## ▶▶ PTA ACTION PLAN

Follow-Up Questions

If the client answers "yes" to any of the following questions, the PTA should provide an accurate and concise verbal report to the PT.

- Have you ever had a breast implant, mastectomy, or other breast surgery? (altered lymph drainage, scar tissue)
- Have you ever had a tubal or ectopic pregnancy?
- [For a female of childbearing age of unknown cause associated with missed menses]: Do you have shoulder pain? (rupture of ectopic pregnancy)
- Have you ever been diagnosed with endometriosis[19] (possible cause of shoulder pain)?
- Have you missed your last period? (ectopic pregnancy, endometriosis; blood in the peritoneum irritates the diaphragm, causing referred pain)
- Are you having any spotting or irregular bleeding?
- Have you had any spontaneous or induced abortions recently? (blood in peritoneum that irritates the diaphragm)
- Have you recently had a baby? (excessive muscle tension during birth)
- *If yes:* Are you breastfeeding with the infant supported on pillows?
- Do you have a breast discharge, or have you had mastitis?

REFERENCES

1. Walsh RM, Sadowski GE: Systemic disease mimicking musculoskeletal dysfunction: a case report involving referred shoulder pain, *J Orthop Sports Phys Ther* 31(12):696–701, 2001.
2. Lollino N: Non-orthopaedic causes of shoulder pain: what the shoulder expert must remember, *Musculoskelet Surg* 96(Suppl 1): S63–S68, 2012.
3. Cyriax J: *Textbook of orthopaedic medicine*, ed 8, Baltimore, 1982, Williams & Wilkins.
4. Prasarn ML, Ouellette EA: Acute compartment syndrome of the upper extremity, *J Am Acad Orthop Surg* 19(1):49–58, 2011.
5. Neer CS: Anterior acromioplasty for the chronic impingement syndrome in the shoulder: a preliminary report, *J Bone Joint Surg* 54(1):41–50, 1972.
6. Berg J, Björck L, Dudas K, et al: Symptoms of a first acute myocardial infarction in men and women, *Gend Med* 6(3):454–462, 2009.
7. Lovlien M, Johansson I, Hole T, Schei B: Early warning signs of an acute myocardial infarction and their influence on symptoms during the acute phase, with comparisons by gender, *Gend Med* 6(3):444–453, 2009.
8. Hwang SY, Park EH, Shin ES, Jeong MH: Comparison of factors associated with atypical symptoms in younger and older patients with acute coronary syndromes, *J Korean Med Sci* 24(5): 789–794, 2009.
9. Hwang SY, Ahn YG, Jeong MH: Atypical symptom cluster predicts a higher mortality in patients with first-time acute myocardial infarction, *Korean Circ J* 42(1):16–22, 2012.
10. Smith ML: Differentiating angina and shoulder pathology pain, *Phys Ther Case Rep* 1(4):210–212, 1998.
11. Delos D, Rodeo SA: Venous thrombosis after arthroscopic shoulder surgery: pacemaker leads as a possible cause, *HSS J* 7(3):282–285, 2011.
12. Ahrens PM, Siddiqui NA, Rakhit RD: Pacemaker placement and shoulder surgery: is there a risk? *Ann R Coll Surg Engl* 94(1): 39–42, 2012.
13. Lelakowski J, Domagala TB, Cies´la-Dul M, et al: Association between selected risk factors and the incidence of venous

obstruction after pacemaker implantation: demographic and clinical factors, *Kardiol Pol* 69(10):1033–1040, 2011.

14. Li JQ, Tang KL, Xu HT, et al: Glenohumeral joint tuberculosis that mimics frozen shoulder: a retrospective analysis, *J Shoulder Elbow Surg* 21(9):1207–1212, 2012.

15. Longo UG, Marinozzi A, Cazzato L, et al: Tuberculosis of the shoulder, *J Shoulder Elbow Surg* 20(4):e19–e21, 2011.

16. Ogawa K: Advanced shoulder joint tuberculosis treated with debridement and closed continuous irrigation and suction, *Am J Orthop* 39(2):E15–E18, 2010.

17. Ba-Fall K: Shoulder pain revealing tuberculosis of the humerus, *Rev Pneumonol* 65(1):13–15, 2009.

18. Nagaraj C, Singh S, Singh B, et al: Tuberculosis of the shoulder joint with impingement syndrome as initial presentation, *J Microbiol Immunol Infect* 41(3):275–278, 2008.

19. Unterscheider J: Shoulder pain and diaphragmatic endometriosis, *Eur J Obstet Gynecol Reprod Biol* 153(1):109–110, 2010.

20. Seoud AA, Saleh MM, Yassin AH: Endometriosis: a possible cause of right shoulder pain, *Clin Exp Obstet Gynecol* 37(1):19–20, 2010.

21. Wohlgethan JR: Frozen shoulder in hyperthyroidism, *Arthritis Rheum* 30(8):936–939, 1987.

22. Roy A: *Adhesive capsulitis in physical medicine and rehabilitation*, eMedicine Specialties. http://emedicine.medscape.com/article/326828-overview. Accessed July 16, 2023, updated October 15, 2009.

23. Lebiedz-Odrobina D: Rheumatic manifestations of diabetes mellitus, *Rheum Dis Clin North Am* 36(4):681–699, 2010.

24. Garcilazo C: Shoulder manifestations of diabetes mellitus, *Curr Diabetes Rev* 6(5):334–340, 2010.

25. Saha NC: Painful shoulder in patients with chronic bronchitis and emphysema, *Am Rev Respir Dis* 94:455–456, 1966.

26. Deng PB, Luo YY, Hu CP, Zhou LH: [Misdiagnosis of pancoast cancer: analysis of 26 cases], *Zhonghua Jie He He Hu Xi Za Zhi* 34(9):663–665, 2011.

27. Labidi M: Pleural effusions following cardiac surgery: prevalence, risk factors, and clinical features, *Chest* 136(6):1604–1611, 2009.

28. Ashikhmina EA, Schaff HV, Sinak LJ, et al: Pericardial effusion after cardiac surgery: risk factors, patient profiles, and contemporary management, *Ann Thorac Surg* 89(1):112–118, 2010.

29. Ahmed WA: Survival after isolated coronary artery bypass grafting in patients with severe left ventricular dysfunction, *Ann Thorac Surg* 87(4):1106–1112, 2009.

30. Jensen L, Yang L: Risk factors for postoperative pulmonary complications in coronary artery bypass graft surgery patients, *Eur J Cardiovasc Nurs* 6(3):241–246, 2007.

31. Okada M, Suzuki K, Hidaka T, et al: Complex regional pain syndrome type I induced by pacemaker implantation, with a good response to steroids and neurotrophin, *Intern Med* 41:498–501, 2002.

32. Söyüncü S, Bektaş F, Cete Y: Traditional Kehr's sign: left shoulder pain related to splenic abscess, *Ulus Travma Acil Cerrahi Derg* 18(1):87–88, 2012.

33. Giles LGF, Singer KP: *The clinical anatomy and management of thoracic spine pain*, Oxford, 2000, Butterworth Heinemann.

34. Leff D, Nortley M, Melly L, Bhutiani RP: Ruptured spleen following laparoscopic cholecystectomy, *JSLS* 11(1):157–160, 2007.

35. Kandil TS: Shoulder pain following laparoscopic cholecystectomy: factors affecting the incidence and severity, *J Laparoendosc Adv Surg Tech A* 20(8):677–682, 2010.

36. Chang SH: An evaluation of perioperative pregabalin for prevention and attenuation of postoperative shoulder pain after laparoscopic cholecystectomy, *Anesth Analg* 109(4):1284–1286, 2009.

37. Yasir M, Mehta KS, Banday VH, et al: Evaluation of post operative shoulder tip pain in low pressure versus standard pressure pneumoperitoneum during laparoscopic cholecystectomy, *Surgeon* 10(2):71–74, 2012.

38. Hadler NM: The patient with low back pain, *Hosp Pract* 22(10A):17–18, 1987. 20, 22, October 30

39. Crapo JD, Karlinsky JB, King TE: *Baum's textbook of pulmonary diseases*, ed 7, Philadelphia, 2003, Lippincott, Williams & Wilkins.

40. Cabell CH, Abrutyn E, Karchmer AW: Cardiology patient page. Bacterial endocarditis: the disease, treatment, and prevention, *Circulation* 107(20):e185–e187, 2003.

41. Hooper AJ, Celenza A: A descriptive analysis of patients with an emergency department diagnosis of acute pericarditis, *Emerg Med J* 30(12):1003–1008, 2013.

42. Philip S, Missov E, Gilon D: Head and neck pain in patients presenting with acute aortic dissection, *Aorta (Stamford)* 6(6):130–138, 2018.

43. Tran H: Deep venous thromboses in patients with hematological malignancies after peripherally inserted central venous catheters, *Leuk Lymphoma* 51(8):1473–1477, 2010.

44. Jones MA: Characterizing resolution of catheter-associated upper extremity deep venous thrombosis, *J Vasc Surg* 51(1):108–113, 2010.

45. Grant JD, Stevens SM, Woller SC, et al: Diagnosis and management of upper extremity deep-vein thrombosis in adults, *Thromb Haemost* 108(6):1097, 2012.

46. Liem TK: Peripherally inserted central catheter usage patterns and associated symptomatic upper extremity venous thrombosis, *J Vasc Surg* 55(3):761–767, 2012.

47. Shah MK: Upper extremity deep vein thrombosis, *South Med J* 96(7):669–672, 2003.

48. Aw A, Carrier M, Koczerginski J, et al: Incidence and predictive factors of symptomatic thrombosis related to peripherally inserted central catheters in chemotherapy patients, *Thromb Res* 130(3):323–326, 2012.

49. Linneman B: Hereditary and acquired thrombophilia in patients with upper extremity deep-vein thrombosis, *Thromb Haemost* 100(3):440–446, 2008.

50. Jones RE: Upper limb deep vein thrombosis: a potentially fatal complication of clavicle fracture, *Ann R Coll Surg Engl* 92(5):W36–W38, 2010.

51. Peivandi MT, Nazemian Z: Clavicular fracture and upper-extremity deep venous thrombosis, *Orthopedics* 34(3):227, 2011.

52. Garofalo R: Deep vein thromboembolism after arthroscopy of the shoulder: two care reports and review of the literature, *BMC Musculoskelet Disord* 11:65, 2010.

53. Willis AA: Deep vein thrombosis after reconstructive shoulder arthroplasty: a prospective observational study, *J Shoulder Elbow Surg* 18(1):100–106, 2009.

54. Bents RT: Axillary artery thrombosis after humeral resurfacing arthroplasty, *Am J Orthop (Belle Mead NJ)* 40(7):E135–E137, 2011.

55. Ojike NI: Venous thromboembolism in shoulder surgery: a systematic review, *Acta Orthop Belg* 77(3):281–289, 2011.

56. Lancaster SL, Owens A, Bryant AS, et al: Upper-extremity deep vein thrombosis, *Am J Nurs* 110(5):48–52, 2010.

57. Gaitini D: Prevalence of upper extremity deep venous thrombosis diagnosed by color Doppler duplex sonography in cancer patients with central venous catheters, *J Ultrasound Med* 25(10):1297–1303, 2006.

58. Shaheen K: Superior vena cava syndrome, *Cleve Clin J Med* 79(6):410–412, 2012.

59. Netter FH: *Atlas of human anatomy*, ed 5, Philadelphia, 2010, WB Saunders.
60. Delavierre D: Symptomatic approach to referred chronic pelvic and perineal pain and posterior ramus syndrome, *Prog Urol* 20(12):990–994, 2010.
61. Maynard JW: Testicular pain followed by microscopic hematuria, a renal mass, palpable purpura, polyarthritis, and hematochezia, *J Clin Rheumatol* 16(8):388–391, 2010.
62. Rose SJ, Rothstein JM: Muscle mutability: general concepts and adaptations to altered patterns of use, *Phys Ther* 62:1773, 1982.
63. Goodman CC, Asavasopon S, Godges JJ: Screening for gastrointestinal, hepatic/biliary, and renal/urologic disease, j*J Hand Ther* 23(2):140–156, 2010. quiz 157
64. Yung E: Screening for head, neck, and shoulder pathology in patients with upper extremity signs and symptoms, *J Hand Ther* 23:173–185, 2010.
65. McKay P: Osteomyelitis and septic arthritis of the hand and wrist, *Curr Ortho Pract* 21(6):542–550, 2010.
66. Norman DC: Fever in the elderly, *Clin Infect Dis* 31(1):148–151, 2000.
67. Norman DC: Fever of unknown origin in older persons, *Infect Dis Clin North Am* 21(4):937–945, 2007.
68. Bisno AL, Stevens DL: Streptococcus pyogenes. In Mandell GL, Bennett JE, Dolin R, editors: *Principles and practice of infectious diseases* ed 7, Philadelphia, 2009, Elsevier Churchill Livingstone. Ch. 198
69. Semel JD, Goldin H: Association of athlete's foot with cellulitis of the lower extremities: diagnostic value of bacterial cultures of ipsilateral interdigital space samples, *Clin Infect Dis* 23:1162–1164, 1996.
70. Bonsignore A: Occult rupture of the spleen in a patient with infectious mononucleosis, *G Chir* 31(3):86–90, 2010.
71. Schumpelick V: Surgical embryology and anatomy of the diaphragm with surgical applications, *Surg Clin North Am* 80(1):213–239, 2000.
72. Tateishi U: Chest wall tumors: radiologic findings and pathologic correlation, *Radiographics* 23:1491–1508, 2003.
73. Vargo MM, Flood KM: Pancoast tumor presenting as cervical radiculopathy, *Arch Phys Med Rehabil* 71(8):606–609, 1990 Jul.
74. Gu R, Kang MY, Gao ZL, et al: Differential diagnosis of cervical radiculopathy and superior pulmonary sulcus tumor, *Chin Med J (Engl)* 125(15):2755–2757, 2012.
75. Cailliet R: *Shoulder pain*, ed 3, Philadelphia, 1991, FA Davis.
76. Chaniotis SA: Clinical reasoning for a patient with neck and upper extremity symptoms: a case requiring referral, *J Bodyw Mov Ther* 16(3):359–363, 2012.
77. Jeong HJ, Sim YJ, Hwang KH, Kim GC: Causes of shoulder pain in women with breast cancer-related lymphedema: a pilot study, *Yonsei Med J* 52(4):661–667, 2011.
78. Kloth JK, Egermann M, Weber MA: [Symptomatic bilateral soft tissue tumor of the breast wall], *Radiologe* 51(5):388–391, 2011.
79. Bildik F, Demircan A, Keles A, et al: Heterotopic pregnancy presenting with acute left chest pain, *Am J Emerg Med* 26(7):835.e1–835.e2, 2008.
80. Biolchini F, Giunta A, Bigi L, et al: Emergency laparoscopic splenectomy for haemoperitoneum because of ruptured primary splenic pregnancy: a case report and review of literature, *ANZ J Surg* 80(1–2):55–57, 2010.
81. Julania S, Tai R: Heterotopic simultaneous splenic and intrauterine pregnancy after spontaneous conception and review of literature, *J Obstet Gynaecol Res* 39(1):367–370, 2013.
82. Smith ML: Differentiating angina and shoulder pathology pain, *Phys Ther Case Rep* 1(4):210–212, 1998.

7

Recognizing and Reporting Red Flags in the Lower Extremity

Lower extremity pain or dysfunction can be caused by a wide variety of medical conditions; presentation of symptoms is equally wide ranging. For example, vascular conditions (e.g., arterial insufficiency, abdominal aneurysm), infectious or inflammatory conditions, gastrointestinal (GI) disease, and gynecologic and male reproductive systems may cause symptoms in the lower extremity,[1] including the pelvis, buttock, hip, groin, thigh, and knee.

Cancer may present as primary hip, groin, or leg pain or symptoms. Primary cancer can metastasize to the low back, pelvis, and sacrum, thus referring pain to the hip and groin. Primary cancer may also metastasize to the hip, causing hip or groin pain and symptoms.

Pain may be referred to the lower extremity from other locations such as the scrotum, kidneys, abdominal wall, abdomen, peritoneum, or retroperitoneal region. Lower extremity pain may be referred through conditions that affect nearby anatomic structures, such as the spine, spinal nerve roots or peripheral nerves, and overlying soft tissue structures (e.g., hernia, bursitis, fasciitis).

The physical therapist assistant (PTA) should be aware of two important points: (1) understanding that not all pain present in the lower extremity originates in the soft tissues of the leg, and (2) recognizing and reporting to the physical therapist (PT) any red-flag signs and symptoms that might require reevaluation or further assessment.

Recognition of red-flag signs and symptoms of systemic or viscerogenic problems can direct the client toward the necessary medical attention early in the disease process. In many cases, early detection and treatment may result in improved outcomes.

PAST MEDICAL HISTORY

Some of the more common histories associated with lower extremity, hip, or groin pain of a visceral nature are listed in Box 7.1. A previous history of cancer such as prostate cancer (males), any reproductive cancers (females), bone cancer, or breast cancer is a red flag because these cancers may be associated with metastases to the lower quadrant (femur, pelvis, and/or hip).[2–5] Medical treatment for cancer can also result in side effects (e.g., osteoporosis, fractures) that can cause pain and impairments of the lower quadrant.[6]

Past history of joint replacement (especially hip arthroplasty) combined with recent infection of any kind and new onset of hip, groin, or knee pain should be discussed with the therapist. The PTA should keep in mind that postoperatively, orthopedic pins may migrate, referring pain from the hip to the back, tibia, or ankle. Loose components, improper implant

size, muscular imbalance, and infection that occur any time after joint arthroplasty may cause lower extremity pain or symptoms (Case Example 7.1).

There have been reports of hip, groin, and/or pelvic pain and/or mass associated with wear debris from hip arthroplasty. Polyethylene wear debris can also cause deep vein thrombosis, lower extremity edema, ureteral or bladder compression, or sciatic neuropathy.[7]

RISK FACTORS

Each condition, illness, or disease that can cause referred pain to the buttock, hip, thigh, groin, or other areas of the lower extremity has its own unique risk factors. Many of the items listed as past medical history are risk factors. For example, femoral artery catheterization used to monitor ongoing hemodynamic status (arterial line; status post burn injuries, and/or individuals in the intensive care unit) or used for individuals with poor upper extremity intravenous access can cause retroperitoneal hematoma formation or septic arthritis and subsequent hip pain.

Other known risk factors for systemically induced problems affecting the lower quadrant have been discussed either in this chapter or elsewhere in the text as appropriate. For example, arterial insufficiency can be a cause of low back, hip, buttock, or leg pain. Likewise, known risk factors for bone cancer or metastases as a cause of hip, groin, or lower extremity pain are also presented.

▶▶ PTA ACTION PLAN

PTA Awareness of Risk Factors and Red Flags to Report

Awareness of red-flag risk factors for various problems can help the PTA alert the therapist early on when additional red-flag signs and symptoms exist. Many risk factors for disease are modifiable. Exercise often plays a key role in prevention and treatment of pathologic conditions. Recognizing red flags in the history and clinical presentation and knowing when to refer versus when to treat are topics the PTA can discuss with the therapist.

Points to Ponder

If no neuromuscular or musculoskeletal cause of the client's symptoms can be identified, the PTA and therapist can discuss the following:

- Are there any red flags suggestive of a viscerogenic cause of pain or symptoms? (See Box 5.1; the lack of diagnostic testing or imaging studies may be an additional red flag.[8])
- What kind of pain patterns do we expect to see with viscerogenic causes?
- Are any associated signs and symptoms suggestive of a particular organ system?

BOX 7.1   Red-Flag Histories Associated With the Lower Extremity

Previous history of cancer

Previous history of renal or urologic disease such as kidney stones and urinary tract infections

Trauma/assault (fall, blow, lifting)

Femoral artery catheterization

History of infectious or inflammatory condition

- Crohn disease (regional enteritis) or ulcerative colitis
- Diverticulitis
- Pelvic inflammatory disease
- Reactive arthritis
- Appendicitis

History of gynecologic condition(s):

- Recent pregnancy, childbirth, or abortion
- Multiple births (multiparity)
- Other gynecologic conditions

History of alcoholism (e.g., hip osteonecrosis)

Long-term use of immunosuppressants (e.g., Crohn disease, sarcoidosis, cancer treatment, organ transplant, autoimmune disorders)

History of heart disease (e.g., arterial insufficiency, peripheral vascular disease)

Receiving anticoagulation therapy (risk factor for hemarthrosis)

History of acquired immunodeficiency syndrome–related tuberculosis

History of hematologic disease (e.g., sickle cell anemia, hemophilia)

CASE EXAMPLE 7.1   Screening After Total Hip Replacement

A 74-year-old retired homemaker had a total hip replacement (THR) 2 days ago. She remains as an inpatient with complications related to congestive heart failure. She has a previous medical history of gallbladder removal 20 years ago, total hysterectomy 30 years ago, and surgically induced menopause with subsequent onset of hypertension.

Her medications include intravenous furosemide (Lasix), digoxin, and potassium replacement.

During the initial physical therapy intervention the client reported muscle cramping and headache but was able to complete the entire exercise protocol. Blood pressure was 100/76 mm Hg (measured in the right arm while lying in bed). Systolic measurement dropped to 90 mm Hg when the client moved from supine to standing. Pulse rate was 56 bpm with a pattern of irregular beats. Pulse rate did not change with postural change. Platelet count was 98,000 cells/mm³ when it was measured yesterday.

What Areas Should the *PTA* be Prepared to Assess when Working With this Patient?
Neuromusculoskeletal

- Assess orthopedic complications such as signs of infection, increased skin temperature, localized swelling, and pain.
- Observe patient's adherence to hip precautions; note surgical technique and approach used, type of implant, and location of incision.
- Be aware that orthostatic hypotension can cause dizziness, loss of balance, or falls—a very dangerous situation with a recent THR.
- This can be compounded by osteoporosis, if present as a result of surgical menopause.

Systemic

- Monitor all vital signs.
- Observe for bruising, joint bleeds, and deep venous thrombosis; follow precautions and exercise guidelines.[1]
- Watch for signs and symptoms of cardiovascular/pulmonary impairments such as the following:
  - Fatigue and muscle weakness
  - Tachycardia
  - Fluid migration from the legs to the lungs during the supine position
  - Dyspnea, orthopnea,* spasmodic cough

- Peripheral edema
- Check nail beds for signs of decreased perfusion

Observe for side effects of medications or drug interactions:

- Diuresis from Lasix (loop diuretic) can result in potassium depletion and lead to increased sensitivity of myocardium to digoxin (digitalis); monitor serum electrolytes, and observe for signs/symptoms of potassium imbalance; observe for urinary frequency and headache.
- Common adverse effects of Lasix include:
  - Dehydration; muscle cramping, fatigue, weakness, headache, paresthesias, nausea, confusion, orthostatic hypotension, blurred vision, rash
- Digoxin: Headache, drowsiness, other central nervous system disturbance, bradycardia, arrhythmia, gastrointestinal upset, blurred vision, halos.

What Signs and Symptoms Should the *PTA* Report to the Medical Staff?

Nurses will be closely monitoring the patient's signs and symptoms. Read the medical record to stay up with what the other practitioners know or have observed about the patient. Read the physician's notes to see whether medical intervention has been ordered.

Report anything observed but not already recorded in the chart, such as muscle cramping, headache, irregular heartbeat with bradycardia, low pulse, and orthostatic hypotension.

Bradycardia is one of the first signs of digitalis toxicity. In some hospitals a pulse less than 60 bpm in an adult would indicate that the next dose of digoxin should be withheld and the physician contacted. The protocol may be different from institution to institution.

The PTA is advised to report the following:

- Irregular heartbeat with bradycardia (a possible sign of digoxin/digitalis toxicity).
- Muscle cramping (adverse effect of Lasix) and headache (possible adverse effect of digoxin).
- Charting of vital signs; her blood pressure was not too unusual and pulse rate did not change with position change (probably because of medications), so she does not have medically defined orthostatic hypotension.
- Monitor vital signs throughout intervention; record the time it takes for vital signs to return to normal after exercise or treatment for your own documentation of measurable outcomes.

* Ask if the patient must use pillows and sit up or have the head of the bed elevated; often described as "one-pillow orthopnea" or "two-pillow orthopnea."

Hip and Buttock

There are many different causes of hip or buttock pain (Box 7.2) as a result of regional neuromuscular or musculoskeletal disorders. The PTA must be aware that disorders affecting the organs within the pelvic and abdominal cavities can also refer pain to the hip region, mimicking a musculoskeletal lesion. A careful history and physical examination by the PT usually differentiate these entities from true hip disease, but sometimes the picture does not become clear enough to recognize a problem outside the scope of a PT's practice until much later (e.g., during subsequent treatment sessions with the PTA).[9]

BOX 7.2   Causes of Hip Pain

Systemic/Medical Conditions

Cancer

Metastasis

Bone tumors[†]
  Osteoid osteoma
  Chondrosarcoma
  Giant cell tumor
  Ewing sarcoma

Vascular

Arterial insufficiency

Abdominal aortic aneurysm

Avascular necrosis

Urogenital

Kidney (renal) impairment; kidney stones

Urinary tract infection

Testicular cancer

Infectious/Inflammatory Conditions

Abdominal or peritoneal inflammation (psoas abscess; see Box 7.6)

Ankylosing spondylitis

Appendicitis

Ischial rectal abscess[†]

Crohn disease; ulcerative colitis

Diverticulitis

Osteomyelitis (upper femur)[†]

Pelvic inflammatory disease

Reactive arthritis

Inflammatory arthritis (rheumatoid arthritis, systemic lupus erythematosus, seronegative arthropathies, gout)

Septic hip or sacroiliac arthritis[†]

Septic hip bursitis[†]

Tuberculosis

Metabolic Disease

Osteomalacia, osteoporosis

Gaucher disease

Paget disease

Ochronosis

Hemochromatosis

Other

Sickle cell crisis

Hemophilia

Ectopic pregnancy

Femoral artery catheterization

Neuromusculoskeletal*

Lumbar spine, sacroiliac joint, sacral, or knee pathology

Osteoarthritis

Synovitis

Femoral, inguinal, or sports hernia/athletic pubalgia

Femoroacetabular impingement

Bursitis (trochanteric, iliopectineal, iliopsoas, ischial)

Fasciitis, myofascial pain

Muscle impairment (weakness, loss of flexibility, hypertonus, hypotonus sprain/
  strain/tear/avulsion); snapping hip syndrome

Tendinopathy (tendinitis, tendinosis)

Piriformis syndrome

Stress reactions/fractures

Occult fracture of the femoral neck

Peripheral nerve injury or entrapment; meralgia paresthetica

Total hip arthroplasty
  • Infection
  • Implant loosening
  • Intraoperative blood vessel injury
  • Bone loss; subsidence

Acetabular labral or cartilage lesions

Developmental hip dysplasia; hip dislocation

Legg-Calvé-Perthes disease

Slipped capital femoral epiphysis

Osteitis pubis (pubic pain radiates to anterior hip)

* This is not an exhaustive, all-inclusive list, but rather, it includes the most commonly encountered adult neuromuscular or musculoskeletal causes of hip pain.
† Most common causes of the sign of the buttock.

PAIN PATTERN

True hip pain, whether from a neuromusculoskeletal or systemic cause (see Box 7.2), is usually felt posteriorly deep within the buttock or anteriorly in the groin, sometimes with radiating pain down the anterior thigh. Pain perceived on the outer (lateral) side or posterior aspect of the hip is usually not caused by an intraarticular problem, but more likely results from a trigger point (TrP), bursitis, knee, sacroiliac (SI), or back problem.

With true hip joint disease, pain will occur with active or passive motion of the hip joint; this pain increases with weightbearing.[10] Often, an antalgic gait pattern is observed as the individual leans away from the affected hip and shortens the swing phase to avoid weightbearing.

When the underlying problem is related to soft tissue (e.g., abductor weakness) rather than to the joint as the source of symptoms, the client may lean toward the affected side to compensate for the downward rotation of the pelvis.[11] With soft tissue involvement of the bursa or tendons (e.g., gluteus medius, gluteus minimus), pain may radiate from the buttock, greater trochanter, and/or lateral thigh down the leg to the level of insertion of the iliotibial tract on the proximal tibia.[12–14]

Pain with medial rotation and decreased hip medial range of motion is associated with hip osteoarthritis.[15] Cyriax's "Sign of the Buttock" (Box 7.3) can help the therapist differentiate between hip and lumbar spine disease.[16–18] The presence of any of these signs may be an indication of osteomyelitis, neoplasm (upper femur, ilium), fracture (sacrum), abscess, or other infection and should be reported to the PT.[17]

BOX 7.3   Sign of the Buttock

James Cyriax, MD, was the first to write about the "Sign of the Buttock," which is actually made up of seven signs that indicate serious disease posterior to the axis of flexion and extension of the hip. These signs of neural tension deficit suggest severe central nervous system compromise, requiring medical referral. When positive, this test may help the therapist to identify serious extracapsular hip or pelvic disease.

- Primary sign of the buttock: Passive hip flexion more limited and more painful than the straight leg raise
- Limited (and painful) straight leg raise
- Trunk flexion limited to the same extent as hip flexion
- Painful weakness of hip extension
- Noncapsular pattern of restriction (hip); the capsular pattern is marked limitation of hip medial rotation first, then hip flexion with some limitation of abduction and little or no limitation of adduction and lateral rotation
- Swelling (and tenderness) in the buttocks region
- Empty end feel with hip flexion

(From Cyriax J: *Textbook of orthopaedic medicine: diagnosis of soft tissue lesions*, ed 8, Philadelphia, 1983, WB Saunders.)

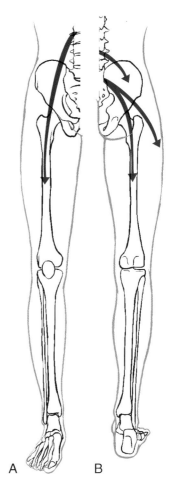

FIG. 7.2 Pain referred *to* the hip *from* other structures and anatomic locations. (A) Hip pain referred from the upper lumbar vertebrae can radiate into the anterior aspect of the thigh. (B) Hip pain from the lower lumbar vertebrae and sacrum is usually felt in the gluteal region, with radiation down the back or outer aspect of the thigh.

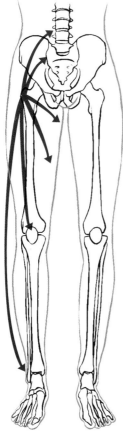

FIG. 7.1 Pain referred *from* the hip *to* other structures and anatomic locations. Pain from a pathologic condition of the hip can be referred to the low back, sacroiliac or sacral area, groin, anterior thigh, knee, or ankle.

NEUROMUSCULOSKELETAL PRESENTATION

Identifying the hip as the source of a client's symptoms can be difficult because pain originating in the hip may not localize to the hip but rather may present as low back, buttock, groin, SI, anterior thigh, or even knee or ankle pain (Fig. 7.1).

On the other hand, regional pain from the low back, SI, sacrum, or knee can be referred to the hip. SI pain that localizes to the base of the spine may be accompanied by radicular pain extending across the buttock and down the leg. It can also cross the lateral hip area. In addition, SI joint dysfunction can cause groin pain and, with referred pain to the hip, may be accompanied by an ipsilateral decrease in hip joint internal rotation of 15 degrees or more, thereby confusing the clinical picture even further.[19,20]

Overlying soft tissue structure disorders such as femoral hernia, bursitis, or fasciitis; muscle impairments such as weakness, loss of flexibility, hypertonus or hypotonus, strain, sprain, or tears; and peripheral nerve injury or entrapment, including meralgia paresthetica, can also cause localized hip (and/or groin) pain.

Hip pain referred from the upper lumbar vertebrae can radiate into the anterior aspect of the thigh, whereas hip pain from the lower lumbar vertebrae and sacrum is usually felt in the gluteal region, with radiation down the back or outer aspect of the thigh (Fig. 7.2).

The client with pain following total hip arthroplasty caused by component instability may report hip or groin pain with activity, pain at rest, or both.[21] The client reports a dull aching pain in the thigh with no history of systemic illness or recent trauma. Often, the pain is localized to the site of the prosthetic stem tip. The client points to a specific spot along the anterolateral thigh. Pain on initiation of activity that resolves with continued activity can be a red flag of a loose prosthesis.

PTA ACTION PLAN

Recognizing and Reporting Red Flags Associated With Hip Implants

Clinically, a history of "start-up" pain may indicate a loose component. After 5 or 10 steps the groin pain subsides. Pain may increase again after a moderate amount of walking. Groin or thigh pain is most common with micromotion at the bone-prosthesis interface or other loose component, periosteal irritation, or a standard-length femoral stem.[22–24] Persistent pain that is not relieved with rest and continues through the night should be reported to the therapist.[22,25]

SYSTEMIC PRESENTATION

Red-flag patterns of restricted hip motion include limited hip extension, adduction, and lateral rotation and may be a sign of a serious underlying disease—something other than the typical joint problems seen in association with osteoarthritis (Case Example 7.2). An empty end feel can be an indicator of potentially serious disease such as infection or neoplasm and should be reported to the therapist immediately. Empty end feel is described as limiting pain before the end range of motion is reached but with no resistance perceived by the examiner.[17]

The presence of GI symptoms (e.g., nausea, vomiting, diarrhea, constipation, abdominal bloating or cramping) or urologic symptoms (e.g., urinary frequency, nocturia, dysuria, or flank pain) along with hip pain should be documented and discussed with the therapist.

Negative radiographs of the hip may not rule out bone lesions. When intervention by the PT and PTA does not yield relief of symptoms (or only temporary relief), further imaging studies may be needed. A careful review of risk factors and clinical presentation will guide this decision.[26]

Groin

The PTA may provide treatment for a client with an isolated groin problem, especially in the sports populations; more often, however, the individual has low back, pelvic, hip, knee, or SI problems with a secondary complaint of groin pain. Possible systemic and/or visceral causes of groin pain are wide ranging, whether appearing as an isolated symptom or in combination with pelvic, hip, low back, or thigh pain (Box 7.4).

Palpating the groin area is usually necessary in making a differential diagnosis, thus the PTA should immediately report the

---

CASE EXAMPLE 7.2   Noncapsular Hip Pattern

A 46-year-old male long-distance runner developed sudden onset of right hip pain. He was given a diagnosis of trochanteric bursitis (now called greater trochanteric pain syndrome [GTPS]) by an orthopedic physician and was referred to physical therapy.

Initial Evaluation: Objective Findings
- For tenderness on palpation over the greater trochanter
- Trigger points of the hip and low back region
- Noncapsular pattern of restriction of the hip (capsular pattern in the hip is flexion, abduction, and medial rotation); client was limited in extension and lateral rotation
- Heel strike test

The major criteria for a medical diagnosis of trochanteric bursitis (or GTPS) consist of marked tenderness to deep palpation of the greater trochanter and relief of pain after peritrochanteric injection with a local anesthetic and corticosteroid.

The absence of greater trochanter tenderness and the presence of a noncapsular pattern of restriction of the hip were not consistent with the given diagnosis. Local injection was not administered.

During the second therapy session the physical therapist (PT) performed the initial assessment of the patient prior to the physical therapist assistant (PTA) performing the general treatment session that included modalities for pain control and gentle therapeutic exercise/stretching. During the treatment session the PTA followed through with asking a few questions that were discussed earlier with the PT.

Gastrointestinal: Are you having any nausea, vomiting, or abdominal pain? Changes in bowel function? Blood in the stool? (Client answered "no" to all questions.)

Vascular: Any throbbing pain? Presence of varicose veins? Trophic changes? History of heart disease? (Client answered "no" to all questions.)

Infectious: Any history of inflammatory bowel conditions such as Crohn disease, ulcerative colitis, or diverticulitis? Ever have appendicitis? Any recent skin rashes in the legs? (Client answered "no" to all questions.)

Cancerous: Previous history of cancer? Bone pain at night? Night sweats? (Client answered "yes" to all questions.)

The *PTA* Determines That the Red Flags Included the Following:
- Age.
- Past history of prostate cancer at age 44 with current symptoms of night pain and night sweats.
- Positive heel strike test.
- Noncapsular hip pattern.
- Inconsistent symptoms with diagnosis.

The PTA immediately reported the results of the questioning and concerns of the red flags to the primary PT.

The results of the physical therapy examination and PTA follow-up work/communication with the PT warranted further medical evaluation, and the client was instructed to return to the physician with a recommendation for imaging studies. Magnetic resonance imaging results indicated a nondisplaced, complete fracture of the femoral neck from prostate cancer that had metastasized to the bone.

(From Jones DL, Erhard RE: Differential diagnosis with serious pathology: a case report, *Phys Ther* 76:S89–S90, 1996.)

BOX 7.4   Causes of Groin Pain

Systemic/Medical Conditions

Cancer
- Spinal cord tumors
- Osteoid osteoma
- Hodgkin disease/lymphoma
- Leukemia
- Testicular
- Prostate
- Soft tissue masses

Osteoporosis

Fluid in peritoneal cavity
- Ascites (cirrhosis)
- Congestive heart failure
- Cancer
- Hyperaldosteronism

Hemophilia
- Gastrointestinal bleeding

Abdominal aortic aneurysm, peripheral arterial aneurysm

Gynecologic conditions
- Cancer (uterine/ovarian masses)
- Uterine fibroids
- Ovarian cyst
- Endometriosis (causing pubalgia)
- Ectopic pregnancy (not common)
- Sexually transmitted infection
- Pelvic inflammatory disease

Infection, usually intraabdominal or intraperitoneal infection (see Box 7.6)

Urologic
- Prostate impairment (prostatitis, benign prostatic hyperplasia, prostate cancer)
- Epididymitis; testicular torsion
- Urethritis/urinary tract infection
- Upper urinary tract problems affecting the kidneys or ureters (inflammation, infection, obstruction)

- Hydrocele/varicocele

Gastrointestinal
- Diverticulitis
- Inflammatory bowel disease

Seronegative spondyloarthropathy

Neuromusculoskeletal

Musculotendinous strain (adductors, hamstrings, iliopsoas, abdominals, tensor fascia lata, gluteus medius)[27]

Internal oblique avulsion

Nerve compression or entrapment (ilioinguinal, obturator, lateral femoral cutaneous, sciatic nerves)

Stress reaction, stress fracture, avulsion fracture, or complete bone fracture (femoral neck, pubic ramus)

Bursitis (iliopectineal)

Pubalgia*

Osteitis pubis

Apophysitis (young athletes)

Trauma (physical, sexual, birth)

Sports, inguinal, or femoral hernia

Hip joint impairment
- Subluxation, dislocation, dysplasia
- Avascular necrosis (osteonecrosis)
- Total hip arthroplasty (loosening, infection, bone loss, subsidence)
- Slipped capital femoral epiphysis
- Legg-Perthes disease
- Labral tear with or without femoroacetabular impingement
- Arthritis, arthrosis

Sacroiliac joint impairment

Lumbar spine impairment (spinal stenosis, disk disease)

Trigger points

Thoracic disc disease (lower thoracic spine)

*Pubalgia is really a description of painful symptoms of the groin that can be caused by a wide range of muscular, tendinous, osseous, and even visceral structures. This condition may be labeled osteitis pubis when there is articular involvement such as arthritis, articular instability, or other articular lesions involving the pubic symphysis.[27]

---

need for a palpation examination. This can be a sensitive issue, and the therapist is advised to have a third person in the examination area. That third person may be the PTA but should be the same gender as the client.

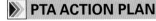 **PTA ACTION PLAN**

The PTA as a Third-Person Observer

If you are asked to fulfill this role but are not the same gender as the individual being evaluated, take the time to ask the therapist for a (private) moment to request someone else.

Neuromusculoskeletal Presentation

Neuromuscular or musculoskeletal causes of groin pain are within the scope of the physical therapy practice (Case Example 7.3).[28,29] Intraarticular pathology of the hip can manifest as groin pain owing to the innervation of the hip capsule. Extraarticular hip conditions radiate to the lateral or posterior aspects of the hip.[30]

Groin pain is a common complaint in sports that involve kicking and rapid change of direction (e.g., soccer, hockey). The most common musculoskeletal cause of groin pain is strain of the adductor muscles, most often involving the adductor longus. The history includes a specific trauma, repetitive motion, or injury, which occurs primarily at the junction of the muscle fibers and the extended tendon of origin. Acutely, this injury causes unilateral or bilateral pain during or after activity, with local palpation of the adductor longus origin, and during passive stretching or active contraction; eccentric activation may be even more painful.[31,32] Acute injury may be followed in several days by ecchymosis.

Chronic groin or inguinal pain in the active athletic, sports, or military groups is often referred to as *athletic pubalgia*. Athletic pubalgia is sometimes used interchangeably to describe a *sports* or *athletic hernia*, which is a tear in the muscles of the inner thigh, lower abdomen, and/or the fascia.[33] The term *sports hernia* may be a bit misleading because experts in this area do not consider this condition the same as a true inguinal or femoral hernia.[34]

CASE EXAMPLE 7.3 Groin Pain—Musculoskeletal Cause

A 44-year-old male patient came to physical therapy with a 7-year history of right groin pain. X-rays, bone scan, and arthrogram of the hip were negative. At the time of initial examination the client was taking morphine for pain that was described as constant, severe, and sharp, and that was rated 8 out of 10 on the Numeric Rating Scale. Sitting and driving made the symptoms worse, and he was unable to work as a mechanic because prolonged squatting was required. Lying supine relieved the pain.

Physical examination revealed extreme hip medial rotation associated with active hip flexion, abduction, and knee extension; each of these movements reproduced his symptoms. Passive range of motion of the right hip was painful and was limited to 95 degrees of flexion and 0 degrees of lateral rotation.

Visual inspection during movement and palpation of the greater trochanter indicated that the proximal femur had medially rotated and moved anteriorly during hip flexion. The client was able to moderate his symptoms by avoiding hip medial rotation during hip and knee movements.

Red Flags: Age (over 40); constant, intense pain

Further Screening Performed by the PT Revealed: The length of time that symptoms have been present without accompanying signs and symptoms of a urologic or gastrointestinal nature (7 years) is not typical of systemic origin of musculoskeletal symptoms.

The fact that no aggravating and relieving factors are known further rules out a viscerogenic cause of pain.

Communication Between the PT and PTA: The physical therapist assistant (PTA) initiated discussion with the physical therapist (PT) regarding appropriate follow-up questions to ask this client throughout the physical therapy process. The PT confirmed that it was appropriate for the PTA to ask the following questions: Have you ever had prostate problems? Have you ever been told you have a hernia or do you have one now? (If yes, an immediate report to the PT is required.) Have you recently had kidney stones or bladder or kidney infection? Have you had changes in urination recently?

Result: The client was treated for femoral anterior glide with medial rotation (movement impairment diagnosis).[28] Training to teach the client to modify hip medial rotation during sustained postures and functional activities was a key component of the intervention. Exercises were given to strengthen the right iliopsoas muscle, hip lateral rotator muscles, and posterior gluteus medius muscle.

The client was pain free and off pain medications 2 months later, after six treatment sessions. He was able to return to full-time work.

Comment: Knowledge of red-flag signs and symptoms, risk factors for various systemic conditions and illnesses, associated signs and symptoms of viscerogenic pain, and typical clinical presentations for neuromuscular and musculoskeletal problems can guide the PTA in quickly sizing up a situation and accurately reporting to the PT when warranted.

In this case the PTA should be aware that only a few follow-up questions are in order. The need for any additional special tests depends on the client's answers to screening questions and will be immediately reported to the PT. The PTA will also need to be aware that the client's failure to progress with intervention is a red flag that indicates the need for reevaluation by the PT.

(From Bloom NJ, Sahrmann SA: Groin pain caused by movement system impairments: a case report. In *Poster presented at: combined sections meeting*, New Orleans, 2004, used with permission.)

Symptoms associated with athletic pubalgia are often described as deep groin or lower abdominal pain with exertion (usually unilateral). A localized sharp burning sensation may occur in the lower abdomen and/or inguinal region. Symptoms are relieved with rest but aggravated by activity, especially sport-related activities. As the condition progresses, symptoms may radiate to the adductor region, testes (male), and labia (female).[35,36]

Labral tears of the acetabulum can also cause groin pain. There may be a history of trauma but acetabular labral tears can occur without trauma. The clinical presentation can vary and include night pain, activity-related pain, positive Trendelenburg sign, and positive impingement sign (pain reproduced with hip flexion, adduction, and internal rotation). In young, active individuals with a primary complaint of groin pain with or without a history of trauma, the diagnosis of a labral tear should be suspected and investigated further.[37]

Femoroacetabular impingement presents as groin pain in young adults. Onset is gradual and progressive with intermittent groin pain after prolonged walking, prolonged sitting, or athletic activities that stress the hip. The impingement test (performed by the PT) is always positive. Referral for a medical orthopedic examination and imaging studies may be warranted.[38]

Another common problem in the young athlete or long-distance runner is osteitis pubis. Repetitive stress of the adductor group can cause inflammation at the musculotendinous attachment on the pubic bone, contributing to sclerosis and bony changes.[39]

Osteitis pubis with inflammation and sclerosis of the pubic symphysis can cause both acute and chronic groin pain. Individuals affected most often include competitive sports athletes involved in running, leaping and landing with force, repetitive kicking motions, or training on concrete, uneven, or other hard surfaces. Osteitis pubis can also occur as a result of leg length differences, faulty foot and body mechanics, muscular imbalances, and pregnancy. Tenderness on palpation of the pubic symphysis helps identify this condition.[31] Onset of midline pain that radiates to the groin is typical. Pain is reproduced by palpation of the pubis (anterior), passive hip abduction, and resisted hip adduction. Articular lesions involving the pubis symphysis can also lead to pubalgia.[27]

Insertional injuries of the upper attachment of the rectus abdominis muscle over the anteroinferior pubis (just lateral to the pubic symphysis) can lead to tendinopathy presenting as pubalgia. Without magnetic resonance imaging, insertional abdominis pathology cannot be differentiated from adductor pathology because the abdominis pubic attachment and the thigh adductor tendon blend to form one unit.[27]

Older adults are more likely to experience hip, buttock, or groin pain associated with arthritis, lumbar stenosis, insufficiency fractures, or hip arthroplasty. Arthritis is characterized by radiating pain to the knee, but not below, with decreased hip range of motion. Gait disturbances may be seen as arthritis progresses.[23,40] Insufficiency fracture of the pubic rami can also cause hip/groin pain, resulting in a reluctance to bear weight on the affected side along with an antalgic gait.[41]

PTA ACTION PLAN

Confirming the Need for Special Tests and Palpation

Accurate documentation and verbal communication of the red flags discussed previously will be the responsibility of the PTA. The PTA should always report the observed red-flag signs and symptoms of neuromuscular or musculoskeletal causes of groin pain to the PT. The PT will then be responsible for confirming the need for follow-up special testing or palpation assessments.

? PICTURE THE PATIENT

Hip and groin pain resulting from lumbar stenosis can manifest as low back pain that radiates to the lower extremities. The pain begins and gets worse with ambulation. Standing and walking may also increase symptoms when the lumbar spine assumes a more lordotic position and the ligamentum flavus folds in on itself, pinching the foramina closed. The client who has stenosis bends forward or sits to avoid painful symptoms. Clients who have a total hip arthroplasty for hip pain may have continued groin and buttock pain, resulting from sciatica or lumbar spinal stenosis.[23,40]

Systemic Presentation

The clinical presentation of groin pain from a systemic source does not vary from musculoskeletally induced groin pain. Red flags include the client's age (e.g., atherosclerotically induced vascular problems in the older adult), past medical history (e.g., previous history of cancer, liver disease, hemophilia), and gender (e.g., ectopic pregnancy, prostate or testicular problems).

 PTA ACTION PLAN

Follow-Up Questions

Asking about the presence of other symptoms may help the PTA recognize and report red flags that could be associated with any one of the systemic causes listed in Box 7.4.

Thigh

Anterior thigh pain is more common than posterior thigh pain (Box 7.5), but the latter may occur, with ruptured abdominal aortic aneurysm (AAA). Local anterior or posterior thigh pain of systemic origin generally occurs as a deep aching generated by soft tissue irritation or bone involvement.

? PICTURE THE PATIENT

Radicular pain is usually a sharp, stabbing pain that projects in dermatomal distributions caused by compression of the dorsal nerve roots.

Neuromusculoskeletal Presentation

The lower lumbar vertebrae and sacrum can refer pain to the gluteal and hip region, with pain radiating down the posterior or posterolateral thigh. Pain down the lateral aspect of the thigh to the knee may also be caused by inflammation of the tensor fascia lata with iliotibial band syndrome.

BOX 7.5   Causes of Thigh Pain

Systemic/Medical Conditions

Retroperitoneal or intraabdominal tumor or abscess (see Box 7.6)
Kidney stones (nephrolithiasis, ureteral or renal colic)
Peripheral neuropathy (bilateral, symmetric)
- Diabetes mellitus
- Neoplasm
- Chronic alcohol use

Thrombosis (femoral artery, great saphenous vein)
Bone tumor (primary or metastases)
Bone fracture associated with long-term bisphosphonates (rare; under investigation)*

Neuromusculoskeletal

Musculotendinous strains (e.g., adductor, abductor, quadriceps)
Iliopectineal bursitis (anterior and medial thigh pain); trochanteric bursitis/greater trochanteric pain syndrome (lateral thigh)
Peripheral neuropathy (unilateral, asymmetric)
Contusions (collisions with balls, hockey pucks, the ground, other athletes)
Nerve compression (e.g., meralgia paresthetica from compression of the lateral femoral cutaneous nerve)
Myositis ossificans (injury with contusion and hematoma formation)
Femoral shaft or subtrochanteric stress reaction or fracture; insufficiency fracture/stress reaction
Hip disease (osteoarthritis, labral tear)
Total hip arthroplasty (loose component, polyethylene wear debris, undersized/oversized femoral stem, periosteal irritation)
Sacroiliac joint dysfunction
Upper lumbar spine dysfunction; spondylolisthesis, herniated disk, previous surgery
Trigger points
Inguinal hernia

*Reports of thigh pain and weakness in affected thigh for weeks to months before a low-energy fracture occurs. Thighbone fractures in women taking bisphosphonate drugs, *Harv Womens Health Watch* 17(7):6–7, 2010; Abrahamsen B: Subtrochanteric and diaphyseal femur fractures in patients treated with alendronate: a register-based national cohort study, *J Bone Miner Res* 24(6):1095–1102, 2009.

BOX 7.6   Causes of Psoas Abscess

Diverticulitis
Crohn disease
Appendicitis
Pelvic inflammatory disease
Diabetes mellitus
- Any other source of infection, including dental
- Renal infection
- Infective spondylitis (vertebra)
- Osteomyelitis
- Sacroiliac joint infection

Anterior thigh pain is commonly disk related, resulting from L3–L4 disk herniation, and occurring most often in older clients with a previous history of lumbar spine surgery. The clinical presentation varies among affected individuals, but thigh pain alone is most common.

Systemic Presentation

The pain pattern for anterior thigh pain produced by systemic causes is often the same as that presented for pain resulting from neuromusculoskeletal causes. That is why it can be so difficult to know for sure that the problem being treated is within the scope of a PT's (and therefore PTA's) practice. For example, obstruction, infection, inflammation, or compression of the ureters may cause a pattern of low back and flank pain that radiates anteriorly to the ipsilateral lower abdomen and upper thigh.

? PICTURE THE PATIENT

The client with urologic-related thigh pain usually has a past history of similar problems or additional urologic symptoms such as pain with urination, urinary frequency, low-grade fever, sweats, or blood in the urine.

Retroperitoneal or intraabdominal tumor or abscess may also cause anterior thigh pain. A past history of reproductive or abdominal cancer, or the presence of any condition listed in Box 7.6, is a red flag that should be discussed with the therapist. The therapist will guide the PTA in knowing what to look for, ask about, and report during the episode of care.

Knee and Lower Leg

Pain in the lower leg is most often caused by injury, inflammation, tumor (malignant or benign), altered peripheral circulation, deep vein thrombosis, or neurologic impairment (Table 7.1).

Neuromusculoskeletal Presentation

Many musculoskeletal or neuromuscular conditions can cause generalized knee pain, including muscle spasm, strain, or tear; patellofemoral pain syndrome; tendinitis; ligamentous disruption, meniscal tear, or osteochondral lesion; stress fracture[42]; and nerve entrapment.[43,44] True knee pain or symptoms are often described as mechanical (local pain and tenderness with locking or giving way of the lower leg) or loading (poorly localized pain with weightbearing). The PTA should also remember that weakness in the muscles at the hip can be a factor for instability and pain at the knee.[45]

Degenerative joint disease of the hip[46] or other hip pathology can masquerade as knee pain in adults.[47] Neurologic problems, including spinal stenosis, complex regional pain syndrome (type 1), neurogenic claudication, and lumbar radiculopathy are common disorders that can produce knee pain. Isolated knee pain involving SI dysfunction has also been reported.[48]

Pain and impaired function from a variety of intraarticular or extraarticular sources can also develop following a total knee arthroplasty.[49,50] TrPs in the lower extremity can also refer pain to the knee.[51,52]

Systemic Presentation. Systemic or pathologic conditions presenting as *generalized knee pain* can include fractures, Baker cyst, tumors (benign or malignant), arthritis, infection, and/or deep venous thrombosis (DVT).[34] Other types of cancer such as lymphoma, leukemia, and myeloma can also cause knee pain.

▶ PTA ACTION PLAN
What to Report

Any unusual bleeding, easy bruising, unintentional weight loss, fatigue, fevers, worsening pain (duration and intensity), sweats, dyspnea, and patient report of swollen lymph nodes should be documented and reported to the therapist. Night pain, localized swelling or warmth, locking, and palpable mass with any of the other symptoms listed previously are considered additional red flags (e.g., of bone or soft tissue tumor).[53]

? PICTURE THE PATIENT

Burning and pain in the legs and feet at night are common in older adults; this is also a potential side effect of some chemotherapy drugs. The exact mechanism is often unknown; many red-flag risk factors can be discussed with the therapist, including allergic response to the fabric in clothing and socks, poorly fitting shoes, long-term alcohol use, adverse effects of medications, diabetes, pernicious anemia, and restless legs syndrome.

Leg cramps, especially those occurring in the lower leg and calf, are common in the adult population.[54,55] Older adults, athletes, and pregnant women are at increased risk.[56] The most common causes of leg cramps include dehydration, arterial occlusion from peripheral vascular disease, neurogenic claudication from lumbar spinal stenosis,[56] neuropathy, medications (diuretics, statins, beta blockers), metabolic disturbances, nutritional (vitamin, calcium) deficiency, and anterior compartment syndrome from trauma, hemophilia, sickle cell anemia, burns, casts, snakebites, or revascular perfusion injury.

Athletes often experience leg cramps preceded by muscle fatigue or twitching. Fractures and ligament tears can mimic a cramp. Cramping associated with severe dehydration may be a precursor to heat stroke.[57,58]

Heel pain is often a symptom of plantar fasciitis, heel spurs, nerve compression (e.g., tarsal tunnel syndrome), or stress fractures. Heel pain can also be a symptom of systemic conditions such as rheumatoid arthritis, seronegative arthrotides, primary bone tumors or metastatic disease, gout, sarcoidosis, Paget disease of the bone, inflammatory bowel disease, osteomyelitis, infectious diseases, sickle cell disease, and hyperparathyroidism.[59]

No matter what area of the lower extremity is affected, the PTA who asks about the presence of other signs and symptoms and identifies/reports these red flags will help the therapist in the clinical decision-making process.

▶ PTA ACTION PLAN
Follow-Up Questions

Remember to always ask:
* Are there any other symptoms of any kind anywhere else in your body we haven't talked about yet?

Even if the client says, "No," the PTA may want to ask some general questions, including questions about constitutional symptoms (i.e., presence of nausea, vomiting, unexplained sweating, fever, chills).

Failure to improve with physical therapy intervention may be part of the medical differential diagnosis and should be reported within a reasonable length of time, given the particular circumstances of each client.

TABLE 7.1   Symptoms and Differentiation of Leg Pain

	Vascular Claudication	Neurogenic Claudication	Peripheral Neuropathy	Restless Legs Syndrome
Description	Pain[a] is usually bilateral No burning or dysesthesia	Pain is usually bilateral but may be unilateral Burning and dysesthesia in the back, buttocks, and/or legs	Pain, aching, and numbness of feet (and hands) Motor, sensory, and autonomic changes: burning, prickling, or tingling may be present; extreme sensitivity to touch (or numbness); weakness, falling (foot drop), muscle atrophy; infection, ulcers, gangrene	Crawling, creeping sensation in legs; involuntary Involuntary contractions of calf muscles, occurring especially at night Pain[b] can be mild to severe, lasting seconds, minutes, or hours
Associated signs and symptoms	Decreased or absent pulses Color and skin changes in feet Normal deep tendon reflexes; may be absent in people older than 60 Sciatica possible (ischemia)	Normal pulses Good skin nutrition Depressed or absent ankle jerks Positive straight leg raise Sciatica Positive "shopping cart" sign (leaning forward on supportive surface; unable to straighten up because of painful symptoms)	Pulses may be affected, depending on underlying pathologic condition (e.g., diabetes) Deep tendon reflexes diminished or absent May have positive straight leg raise May have sciatica	Sleep disturbance, paresthesias
Location	Usually calf first but may occur in the buttock, hip, thigh, or foot	Low back, buttock, thighs, calves, feet	Feet and hands in stocking-glove pattern	Feet, calves, legs
Aggravating factors	Pain is consistent in all spinal positions; brought on by physical exertion (e.g., walking, positive van Gelderen bicycle test); increased by climbing stairs or walking uphill (increased metabolic demand)	Increased in spinal extension Increased with walking or by walking downhill (increased lumbar lordosis); less painful when walking uphill	Depends on underlying cause (e.g., uncontrolled glucose levels with diabetes; progressive alcoholism)	Caffeine, pregnancy, iron deficiency
Relieving factors	Relieved promptly by standing still, sitting down, or resting (1–5 min)	Pain decreased by sitting, lying down, bending forward, or flexion exercises (may persist for hours)	Relieved by pain medications and relaxation techniques; treatment of underlying cause	Eliminate caffeine; increase iron intake, movement, walking, moderate exercise; medications; stretching; maintain hydration; application of heat or cold
Ages affected	40–60+	40–60+	Varies depending on underlying cause	Variable
Cause	Atherosclerosis in peripheral arteries	Neoplasm or abscess Disk protrusion Osteophyte formation Ligamentous thickening	More than 100 causes: diabetes; medications; accidents; nerve compression; metal toxicity; nutritional deficiency; diseases such as rheumatoid arthritis, systemic lupus erythematosus, AIDS; cancer, hypothyroidism, alcoholism	Cause unknown; may be a sleep disorder, arterial disorder, or dysautonomic disorder of the autonomic nervous system; may occur with dehydration or as a side effect of many medications

[a]"Pain" associated with vascular claudication may also be described as an "aching," "cramping," or "tired" feeling.
[b]"Pain" associated with restless legs syndrome may not be painful but may be described as a "frantic," "unbearable," or "compelling" need to move the legs.
AIDS, Acquired immunodeficiency syndrome.

TRAUMA AS A CAUSE OF HIP, GROIN, OR LOWER EXTREMITY PAIN

Trauma, including accidents, injuries, and physical or sexual assault, can be the underlying cause of buttock, hip, groin, or lower extremity pain.

Stress Reaction or Fracture

An undiagnosed stress reaction or stress fracture is a possible cause of hip, thigh, groin, knee, shin, heel, or foot pain. A stress reaction or fracture is a microscopic disruption, or break, in a bone that is not displaced; it is not seen initially on regular x-rays. Exercise-induced groin, tibial, or heel pain are the most common stress fractures.

Two types of stress fractures can occur: *insufficiency* fractures are breaks in abnormal bone under normal force, whereas *fatigue* fractures are breaks in normal bone that has been put under extreme force. Fatigue fractures are usually caused by new, strenuous, very repetitive activities, such as marching, jumping, or distance running.

Fatigue fractures are more likely in distance runners, sprinters,[60] military recruits, or other high-intensity athletes affecting the pubic ramus, calcaneus, femoral neck, and anterior tibia most often.[61,62] Older adults are more likely to present with insufficiency hip fractures. Depending on the age of the client, the therapist should look for a history of high-energy trauma, prolonged activity, or abrupt increase in training intensity. Traction from attached muscles such as the adductor magnus on the inferior pubic ramus is a contributing factor to pubic ramus stress fractures.

Other risk factors include changes in running surface, use of inadequately cushioned footwear, and the presence of the female athlete triad of disordered eating, osteoporosis, amenorrhea and menopause.[63-65] Anything that can lead to poor bone density should be considered a risk factor for insufficiency stress fractures, including radiation and/or chemotherapy,[66] prolonged use of corticosteroids, renal failure, metabolic disorders affecting bone, Paget disease, and coxa vara.[67,68] A smaller cross-sectional diameter of the long bones of the leg in male distance runners is a unique risk factor for tibial stress fractures.[69]

Osteopenia or osteoporosis, especially in the postmenopausal female or older adult with arthritis, can result in injury and fracture or fracture and injury (Case Example 7.4). The client has a small mishap, perhaps losing her footing on a slippery surface or tripping over an object. As she tries to "catch herself," a torsional force occurs through the hip, causing a fracture and then a fall. This is a case of fracture then fall, rather than the other way around. Often, but not always, the client is unable to get up because of pain and instability of the fracture site.[70,71]

The PTA should stay aware of the following clues suggestive of hip, groin, or thigh pain caused by a stress reaction or stress fracture.

Clinical Signs and Symptoms of Stress Reaction/Stress Fracture

- Pain described as aching or deep aching in hip and/or groin area; may radiate to the knee
- Pain increases with activity and improves with rest
- Compensatory gluteus medius gait
- Pain localizing to a specific area of bone (localized tenderness)
- Possible local swelling
- Increased tone of hip adductor muscles; limited hip abduction
- Night pain (femoral neck stress fracture)

CASE EXAMPLE 7.4   Insufficiency Fracture

A 50-year-old White female was referred to physical therapy with a 4-year history of rheumatoid arthritis (RA). She had been taking prednisone (5–30 mg/day) and sulfasalazine (1 g twice a day).

She has a history of hypertension, smokes a pack of cigarettes a day, and drinks a six-pack of beer every night. She lives alone and no longer works outside the home. She admits to very poor nutrition and does not take a multivitamin or calcium. The client has multiple risk factors for osteoporosis, and surgical menopause took place 10 years ago.

Clinical Presentation/Initial Evaluation: Symmetric arthritis with tenderness and swelling of bilateral metacarpophalangeal joints, proximal interphalangeal joints, wrists, elbows, and metatarsophalangeal joints.

The patient reported "hip pain," which started unexpectedly 2 weeks ago in the right groin area. The pain went down her right leg to the knee but did not cross the knee. Any type of movement made it hurt more, especially on walking.

Hip range of motion was limited because of pain; formal range of motion (active, passive, accessory motions) and strength testing were not possible.

What are the Red Flags in this Case?
- Age
- Insidious onset with no known or reported trauma
- Cigarette smoking
- Alcohol use

- Poor diet
- Corticosteroid therapy

Clinical Presentation During Follow-Up Session With PTA: The patient was unable to stand on the right leg unsupported. She could not squat because of her arthritic symptoms and could not tolerate supine or side-lying positions for modality treatment.

Communication With the PT: The PTA reported the red flags and treatment intolerance to the physical therapist (PT) immediately. The PT referred the patient back to her rheumatologist with a request for a hip x-ray before any further physical therapy was provided. The therapist pointed out the risk factors present for osteoporosis and briefly summarized the client's current clinical presentation.

Result: The client was given a diagnosis of insufficiency fracture of the right inferior and superior pubic rami. An insufficiency fracture differs from a stress fracture in that it occurs when a normal amount of stress is placed on abnormal bone. A stress fracture occurs when an unusual amount of stress is placed on normal bone.

Conservative treatment was recommended with physical therapy, pain medications, and treatment of the underlying osteoporosis. The PT prescribed weight-bearing as tolerated, a general conditioning program, and an osteoporosis exercise program. Client education about managing active RA and synovitis was also included.

(From Kimpel DL: Hip pain in a 50-year-old woman with RA, *J Musculoskelet Med* 16:651–652, 1999.)

Clinical Signs and Symptoms of Assault

The client may not report assault as the underlying cause, or he or she may not remember any specific trauma or accident. If the PTA suspects domestic violence or assault of any kind as a potential cause of the person's symptoms, communication with the therapist is imperative. It may be necessary for the therapist to take a sexual history that includes specific questions about sexual activity (e.g., incest, partner assault or rape) or the presence of sexually transmitted infection.

RECOGNIZING RED FLAGS ASSOCIATED WITH SCIATICA

Sciatica, described as pain radiating down the leg below the knee along the distribution of the sciatic nerve, is usually related to mechanical pressure or inflammation of lumbosacral nerve roots (Fig. 7.3). *Sciatica* is the term commonly used to describe pain in a sciatic distribution without overt signs of radiculopathy.

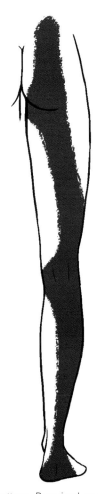

FIG. 7.3 Sciatica pain pattern. Perceived or reported pain associated with compression, stretch, injury, entrapment, or scarring of the sciatic nerve depends on the location of the lesion in relation to the nerve root. The sciatic nerve is innervated by L4, L5, S1, S2, and sometimes S3 with several divisions (e.g., common fibular [peroneal] nerve, sural nerve, tibial nerve).

Radiculopathy denotes objective signs of nerve (or nerve root) irritation or dysfunction, usually resulting from involvement of the spine. Symptoms of radiculopathy may include weakness, numbness, or reflex changes. Sciatic *neuropathy* suggests damage to the peripheral nerve beyond the effects of compression, often resulting from a lesion outside the spine that affects the sciatic nerve (e.g., ischemia, inflammation, infection, direct trauma to the nerve, compression by neoplasm or piriformis muscle).

The terms *radiculopathy, sciatica,* and *neuropathy* are often used interchangeably, although there is a pathologic difference.[72] Electrodiagnostic studies, including nerve conduction studies, electromyography, and somatosensory evoked potential studies, are used to make the differentiation.

Risk Factors

Sciatica has many neuromuscular causes, both diskogenic and nondiskogenic; systemic or extraspinal conditions can produce or mimic sciatica (Table 7.2). Risk factors for a mechanical cause of sciatica include previous trauma to the low back, taller height, tobacco use, pregnancy, and work and occupational-related posture or movement.[72,73]

Risk factors for systemic or extraspinal causes vary with each condition (Box 7.7). For example, clients with arterial insufficiency are more likely to be heavy smokers and to have a history of atherosclerosis. Increasing age, past history of cancer, and comorbidities such as diabetes mellitus, endometriosis, or intraperitoneal inflammatory disease (e.g., diverticulitis, Crohn disease, pelvic inflammatory disease [PID]) are risk factors associated with sciatic-like symptoms (Case Example 7.5).

Total hip arthroplasty is a common cause of sciatica because of the proximity of the nerve to the hip joint. Possible mechanisms for nerve injury include stretching, direct trauma from retractors, infarction, hemorrhage, hip dislocation, and compression. Sciatica referred to as sciatic nerve "burn" has been reported as a complication of hip arthroplasty caused by cement extrusion. The incidence of this complication has decreased with its increased recognition and the increasing use of cementless implants,[25] but even small amounts of cement can cause heat production or direct irritation of the sciatic nerve.[76]

Propionibacterium acnes, a cause of spinal infection, has been linked to sciatica.[77] Bacterial wound contamination during spinal surgery has been traced to this pathogen on the patient's skin. Minor trauma to the disk with a breach to the mechanical integrity of the disk may also allow access by low virulent microorganisms, thereby initiating or stimulating a chronic inflammatory response. These microorganisms may cause prosthetic hip infection but also may be associated with the inflammation seen in sciatica; they may even be a primary cause of sciatica.[73,74]

Anyone with pain radiating from the back and down the leg as far as the ankle has a greater chance that disk herniation is the cause of low back pain. This is true with or without neurologic findings. Unremitting, severe pain and increasing neurologic deficit are red-flag findings. Sciatica caused by extraspinal bone tumors, bone metastases, and soft tissue tumors can occur when a mass is present in the pelvis, sacrum, thigh, popliteal fossa, and calf.[78,79]

TABLE 7.2 Causes of Sciatica

NEUROMUSCULAR CAUSES

Disorder	Symptoms	Physical Signs
Diskogenic		
Disk herniation	Low back pain with radiculopathy and paravertebral muscle spasm; Valsalva maneuver and sciatic stretch reproduce symptoms	Restricted spinal movement; restricted spinal segment; positive Lasèque sign or restricted SLR
Lateral entrapment syndrome (spinal stenosis)	Buttock and leg pain with radiculopathy; pain often relieved by sitting, aggravated by extension of the spine	Similar to disk herniation
Nondiskogenic		
Sacroiliitis	Low back and buttock pain	Tender sacroiliac joint; positive lateral compression test; positive Patrick test
Piriformis syndrome	Low back and buttock pain with referred pain down the leg to the ankle or midfoot	Pain and weakness on resisted abduction/external rotation of the thigh
Iliolumbar syndrome	Pain in iliolumbar ligament area (posterior iliac crest); referred leg pain	Tender iliac crest and increased pain with lateral or side bending
Trochanteric bursitis	Buttock and lateral thigh pain; worse at night and with activity	Tender greater trochanter; rule out associated leg length discrepancy; positive "jump sign" when pressure is applied over the greater trochanter
Greater trochanteric pain syndrome	Mimics lumbar nerve root compression	Low back, buttock, or lateral thigh pain; may radiate down the leg to the iliotibial tract insertion on the proximal tibia; inability to sleep on the involved side[5]
Ischiogluteal bursitis	Buttock and posterior thigh pain; worse with sitting	Tender ischial tuberosity; positive SLR and Patrick tests; rule out associated leg length discrepancy
Posterior facet syndrome	Low back pain	Lateral bending in spinal extension increases pain; side bending and rotation to the opposite side are restricted at the involved level
Fibromyalgia	Back pain, difficulty sleeping, anxiety, depression	Multiple tender points

SYSTEMIC/EXTRASPINAL CAUSES[a]

Disorders

Vascular
- Ischemia of sciatic nerve
- Peripheral vascular disease
- Intrapelvic aneurysm (internal iliac artery)

Neoplasm (primary or metastatic)
Diabetes mellitus (diabetic neuropathy)
Megacolon
Pregnancy; vaginal delivery
Endometriosis
Infection
- Bacterial endocarditis
- Wound contamination[74,75]
- Herpes zoster (shingles)
- Psoas muscle abscess (see Box 7.6)
- Reactive arthritis syndrome

Total hip arthroplasty
Deep venous thrombosis (blood clot)

[a]Clinical symptoms of systemic/extraspinal sciatica can be very similar to those of sciatica associated with disk protrusion.
SLR, Straight leg raise.
(From Namey TC, An HC: Sorting out the causes of sciatica, *Mod Med* 52:132, 1984.)

BOX 7.7 Risk Factors for Sciatica

Musculoskeletal or Neuromuscular Factors
Previous low back injury or trauma; direct fall on buttock(s); gunshot wound
Total hip arthroplasty
Pregnancy
Work- or occupation-related postures or movements
Fibromyalgia
Leg length discrepancy
Congenital hip dysplasia; hip dislocation
Degenerative disk disease
Piriformis syndrome
Spinal stenosis

Systemic/Medical Factors
Tobacco use
History of diabetes mellitus
Atherosclerosis
Previous history of cancer (metastases)
Presence of intraabdominal or peritoneal inflammatory disease (abscess):
- Crohn disease
- Pelvic inflammatory disease
- Diverticulitis

Endometriosis of the sciatic nerve
Radiation therapy (delayed effects; rare)
Recent spinal surgery, especially with instrumentation

CASE EXAMPLE 7.5   Intermittent Claudication With Sciatica

A 41-year-old female who was referred by her primary care physician with a medical diagnosis of sciatica reported bilateral lower extremity (LE) weakness with pain in the left buttock and left sacroiliac (SI) area. She also noted that she had numbness in her left leg after walking more than half a block.

Symptoms are made worse by walking and better after resting or by standing still. Symptoms have been present for the last 2 months and came on suddenly without trauma or injury of any kind. No night pain was reported.

Past Medical History: Significant positive for family history of heart disease (both sides of the family); smoking history: one pack of cigarettes/day for the past 26 years. No medical tests or imaging studies have been done at this time.

Clinical Presentation During Initial Evaluation:

NeurologicScreeningExamination: Negative/within normal limits (WNL)

Neural Tissue Mobility: Tests were all negative; tissue tension WNL

Complete Lumbar Spine Examination: Unremarkable; ruled out as a source of client's symptoms

Diminished dorsalis pedis pulse on the left side

Clinical Presentation During Intervention/Follow-Up: The client reports to the physical therapist assistant (PTA) that both her legs felt like they were going to "collapse" after she walked a short distance and that her left leg would go "hot and cold" during walking. She also experiences cramping in her right calf muscle after walking more than half a block.

Symptoms are made worse by walking and better after resting or by standing still.

The physical therapist (PT) instructed the PTA to perform the bike test—used to stress the integrity of the vascular supply to the lower extremities—during the first follow-up appointment. The bike test showed that cycling in a position of lumbar forward flexion reproduced leg weakness and eliminated dorsalis pedis pulse on the left; no change was noted on the right.

The PTA Concluded the Red Flags to be the Following:

- LE weakness without pain accompanied by "giving out" sensation
- Symptoms brought on by specific activity, relieved by rest or standing still
- Significant family history of heart disease
- No known cause; onset of symptoms without trauma or injury
- Temperature changes in LEs
- Positive smoking history

PTA Action: Based on the results of the bike test and follow-up questioning, the PTA immediately reported the red-flag concerns and observations to the PT.

Result: Given the poor activity tolerance and severity of her family history of heart disease (sudden death at a young age was very common), she was sent back to the doctor immediately. The therapist briefly outlined the red flags and asked the physician to reevaluate for a possible vascular cause of symptoms.

Medical testing revealed a high-grade circumferential stenosis (narrowing) of the distal aorta at the bifurcation. The client underwent surgery for placement of a stent in the occluded artery. After the operation the client reported complete relief from all symptoms, including buttock and SI pain.

(From Gray JC: Diagnosis of intermittent vascular claudication in a patient with a diagnosis of sciatica: case report, *Phys Ther* 79:582–590, 1999.)

PICTURE THE PATIENT

Clinical signs and symptoms of sciatica/sciatic radiculopathy are variable and may include the following:

- Pain along the sciatic nerve anywhere from the spine to the foot (see Fig. 7.3)
- Numbness or tingling in the groin, rectum, leg, calf, foot, or toes
- Diminished or absent deep tendon reflexes
- Weakness in the L4, L5, S1, S2 (and sometimes S3) myotomes (distal motor deficits more prominent than proximal)
- Diminished or absent deep tendon reflexes (especially of the ankle)
- Ache in the calf

Sciatic Neuropathy

- Symptoms of sciatica as described above
- Dysesthetic* pain described as constant burning or sharp, jabbing pain
- Foot drop (tibialis anterior weakness) with gait disturbance

*Dysesthesia is the distortion of any sense, especially touch; it is an unpleasant sensation produced by normal stimuli.

PTA ACTION PLAN

Reporting Patient Progress to the Therapist

Given all of the possible reasons why sciatica may occur, the PTA is encouraged to observe patients with sciatica carefully and report any red flags, especially including if/when the patient is not progressing as expected. The PTA must also consistently document the intent to follow-up via verbal communication with the PT regarding any red-flag concerns discussed in this text.

RECOGNIZING ONCOLOGIC RED FLAGS IN THE LOWER EXTREMITY

Many clients with orthopedic or neurologic problems have a previous history of cancer. The therapist must be vigilant to observe for signs and symptoms of cancer recurrence and those associated with cancer treatment such as radiation therapy or chemotherapy. The effects of these may be delayed by as long as 10 to 20 years or more.

PTA ACTION PLAN

Reviewing Red Flags of Cancer With the Therapist

Whenever possible, it is a good idea for the PT and PTA to discuss potential red flags of cancer, especially with individuals who have a previous history of cancer. What to watch out for, what to report, and what to ask the patient are three areas of important communication between PT and PTA. The PTA can initiate this conversation by asking the therapist, "I want to be prepared to help you treat this client, so can we discuss some important areas that I should keep in mind?"

Until recently, the emphasis has been on advancing age as a key red flag for cancer. Anyone older than 50 years is more likely to develop systemic origin of symptoms mimicking a musculoskeletal or neuromuscular presentation. With cancer and, specifically, musculoskeletal pain caused by primary cancer or metastases to the bone, young age is a red flag as well. Primary bone cancer occurs most often in adolescents and young adults, hence the new red flag: age younger than 20 years, or bone pain in an adolescent or young adult.

Cancer Recurrence

Rehab staff is far more likely to encounter clinical manifestations of metastases from cancer recurrence than from primary cancer. Breast cancer often affects the shoulder, thoracic vertebrae, and hip first, before other areas. Recurrence of colon (colorectal) cancer is possible with referred pain to the hip and/or groin area.

Beware of any client with a past history of colorectal cancer and recent (past 6 months) treatment by surgical removal. Reseeding the abdominal cavity is possible. Every effort is made to shrink the tumor with radiation or chemotherapy before attempts are made to remove the tumor. Even a small number of tumor cells left behind or introduced into a nearby (new) area can result in cancer recurrence.

Spinal Cord Tumors

❓ PICTURE THE PATIENT

Spinal cord tumors (primary or metastasized) present as dull, aching discomfort or sharp pain in the thoracolumbar area in a beltlike distribution, with pain extending to the groin or legs. Depending on the location of the lesion, symptoms may be unilateral or bilateral with or without radicular symptoms.

Bone Tumors

Osteoid osteoma, a small, benign but painful tumor, is relatively common, with 20% of lesions occurring in the proximal femur and 10% in the pelvis. A great many varieties of benign and malignant tumors may appear differently, depending on the age of the client and the site and duration of the lesion.[80,81] Malignant lesions compressing the lateral femoral cutaneous nerve can cause symptoms of meralgia paresthetica, delaying diagnosis of the underlying neoplasm.

❓ PICTURE THE PATIENT

The client is usually in the second decade of life and complains of chronic dull hip, thigh, or knee pain that is worse at night and is alleviated by activity and aspirin and nonsteroidal antiinflammatory drugs. Usually, an antalgic gait is present, along with point tenderness over the lesion with restriction of hip motion.

▶▶ PTA ACTION PLAN
Red Flags to Report

- Bone pain, especially on weightbearing
- Antalgic gait
- Night pain (constant, intense; unrelieved by change in position)
- Pain relieved disproportionately by aspirin
- Fever, sudden and unexpected weight loss, unusual bleeding, skin lesions
- Painless, progressive enlargement of inguinal and/or popliteal lymph nodes

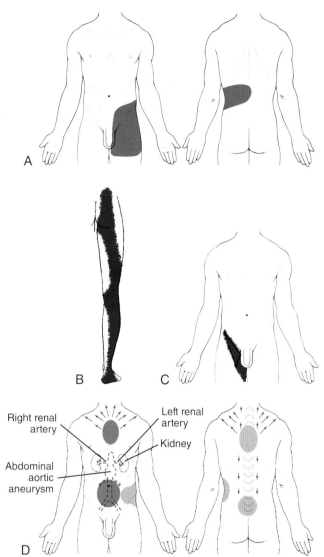

FIG. 7.4 Overview: composite figure. (A) Ureteral pain may begin posteriorly in the costovertebral angle, radiating anteriorly to the ipsilateral lower abdomen, upper thigh, or groin area. Isolated anterior thigh pain is possible, but uncommon. (B) Pain pattern associated with sciatica from any cause. (C) Pain pattern associated with psoas abscess from any cause. (D) Abdominal aortic aneurysm can cause low back pain that radiates into the buttock unilaterally or bilaterally (*not shown*), depending on the underlying location and size of the aneurysm.

▶▶ PTA ACTION PLAN
Follow-Up Questions

Whenever faced with a patient or client with a past medical history of (or currently in treatment for) cancer who now presents with new symptoms or a progression of the primary symptoms, the PTA can ask about associated signs and symptoms (e.g., constitutional symptoms, bleeding or discharge, swollen glands). The sooner any new information is communicated to the therapist, the sooner the affected individual will receive appropriate follow-up care.

RECOGNIZING UROLOGIC RED FLAGS IN THE LOWER EXTREMITY

Ureteral pain usually begins posteriorly in the costovertebral angle but may radiate anteriorly to the upper thigh and groin (Fig. 7.4), or it may be felt just in the groin and genital area.

These pain patterns represent the pathway that genitals take as they migrate during fetal development from their original position, where the kidneys are located in the adult, down the pathways of the ureters to their final location. Pain is referred to a site where the organ was located during fetal development. A kidney stone down the pathway of the ureters causes pain in the flank that radiates to the scrotum (male) or labia (female).

The lower thoracic and upper lumbar vertebrae and the SI joint can refer pain to the groin and anterior thigh in the same pain pattern that occurs with renal disease.[82,83] Irritation of the T10–L1 sensory nerve roots (genitofemoral and ilioinguinal nerves) from any cause, but especially from diskogenic disease, may cause labial (females), testicular (males), or buttock pain.[84-86]

▶▶ PTA ACTION PLAN
Communication With the Therapist

Any time a patient reports pain or other symptoms in the groin or genital area, the PTA should let the patient know these symptoms will be relayed to the therapist. The PTA should not try to explain the cause of the symptoms or conduct further assessment. The therapist can evaluate these conditions by conducting a neurologic screening examination. The PTA will need to make the clinical decision whether or not it is appropriate to contact the PT immediately or document the information and discuss as soon as the PT is available.

RECOGNIZING INFECTIOUS AND INFLAMMATORY RED FLAGS IN THE LOWER EXTREMITY

Anyone with joint pain of unknown cause who presents with current (or recent, i.e., within the past 6 weeks) skin rash or recent history of infection (e.g., hepatitis, mononucleosis, urinary tract infection, upper respiratory infection, sexually transmitted infection, streptococcus, dental infection)[87] must be referred to a health care clinic or physician for further evaluation.

Conditions affecting the entire peritoneal cavity such as PID or appendicitis may cause hip or groin pain in the young, healthy adult. Widespread inflammation or infection may be well tolerated by athletes, sometimes for up to several weeks (Case Example 7.6).

Clinical Presentation

The clinical presentation can be deceptive in young people. The fever is not dramatic and may come and go. The athlete may dismiss excessive or unusual perspiration ("sweats") as part of a good workout. Loss of appetite associated with systemic disease

---

CASE EXAMPLE 7.6 Dancer With Appendicitis

A 21-year-old dance major was referred to the physical therapy clinic by the sports medicine clinic on campus with a medical diagnosis of "strained abdominal muscle."

Clinical Presentation During Initial Evaluation: She described her symptoms as pain with hip flexion when shifting the gears in her car. Some dance moves involving hip flexion also reproduced the pain, but this was not consistent. The pain was described as "deep," "aching," and "sometimes sharp, sometimes dull."

Past medical history was significant for Crohn disease, but the client was having no gastrointestinal (GI) symptoms at this time. On examination, no evidence of abdominal trigger points or muscle involvement was found. The pain was not reproduced with superficial palpation of the abdominal muscles on the day of initial examination.

Clinical Presentation During Intervention/Follow-Up: Intervention with stretching exercises did not change her symptoms of pain during the first week. She reports to the physical therapist assistant (PTA) that she has had some "sweating" off and on during the past 2 weeks. The PTA assessed her vitals with all results showing normal values except the presence of a low-grade fever. These observations were reported to the physical therapist (PT) after the therapy session on a Friday afternoon, with a plan for the PT to examine the client during the next appointment.

Result: The client was a no-show for her Monday afternoon appointment, and the physical therapy clinic receptionist received a phone call from the campus clinic with information that the client had been hospitalized over the weekend with acute appendicitis and peritonitis.

The surgeon's report noted massive peritonitis of several weeks' duration. The client had a burst appendix that was fairly asymptomatic until peritonitis developed with subsequent symptoms. Her white blood cells were in excess of 100,000 at the time of hospitalization.

In retrospect, the client did relate some "sweats" occurring off and on during the last 2 weeks and possibly a low-grade fever.

What additional follow-up questions would have been appropriate for the PTA to ask this client?

1. Ask the client whether she is having any symptoms of any kind anywhere in her body. If she answers negatively, be prepared to offer some suggestions such as the following:
   - Any headaches? Fatigue?
   - Any change in vision?
   - Any fevers or sweats, day or night?
   - Any blood in your urine or stools?
   - Burning with urination?
   - Any tingling or numbness in the groin area?
   - Any trouble sleeping at night?
2. Even though she has denied having any GI symptoms associated with her Crohn disease, it is important to follow-up with questions to confirm this:
   - Any nausea? Vomiting?
   - Diarrhea or constipation?
   - Any change in your pattern of bowel movements?
   - Any blood in your stools? Change in color of your bowel movements?
   - Any foods or smells you can't tolerate?
   - Any change in your symptoms when you eat or don't eat?
   - Unexpected weight gain or loss?
   - Is your pain any better or worse during or after a bowel movement?
3. As part of the past medical history, it is important with hip pain of unknown cause to know whether the client has had any recent infections, sexually transmitted diseases, use of antibiotics or other medications, or skin rashes.
4. In a female of reproductive years, it may be important to take a gynecologic history:
   - Have you been examined by a gynecologist since this problem started?
   - Is there any chance you could be pregnant?
   - Are you using an intrauterine device?
   - Have you had an abortion or miscarriage in the last 6 weeks?
   - Are you having any unusual vaginal discharge?

PTA Action Plan: Any answer to the above questions that may lead the PTA to have a red-flag concern should be reported to the PT with ample opportunity for the PT to perform an immediate examination if warranted.

is often welcomed by teenagers and young adults and is not recognized as a sign of physiologic distress.

Psoas Abscess

Although uncommon, any infectious or inflammatory process affecting the abdominal or pelvic region can lead to psoas abscess and irritation of the psoas muscle. For example, lesions outside the ureter, such as infection, abscess, or tumor, or abdominal or peritoneal inflammation, may cause pain on movement of the adjacent iliopsoas muscle that presents as hip or groin pain.

Peritonitis as a result of any infectious or inflammatory process can result in psoas abscess. Besides the diseases and conditions mentioned here, peritonitis can occur as a surgical complication. Look for a history of abdominal surgery of any kind, especially the anterior approach to spinal surgery for disk removal, spinal fusion, and insertion of a cage or artificial disk implant.

The psoas muscle is not separated from the abdominal or pelvic cavity. Fig. 7.5 shows how most of the viscera in the abdominal and pelvic cavities can come into contact with the iliopsoas muscle. Any infectious or inflammatory process (see Box 7.6) can seed itself to the psoas muscle by direct extension, resulting in a psoas abscess—a localized collection of pus.[88]

🔎 PICTURE THE PATIENT

Hip pain associated with such an abscess may involve the medial aspect of the thigh and femoral triangle areas (Fig. 7.6). Soft tissue abscess may cause pain and tenderness to palpation without movement. Once the abscess has formed, muscular spasm may be provoked, producing hip flexion and even contracture. The leg may also be pulled into internal rotation. Pain that increases with passive and active motion can occur when infected tissue is irritated. Iliopsoas abscess can also masquerade as "sciatica."[89] Pain elicited by stretching the psoas muscle through extension of the hip, called the positive psoas sign, may be present.

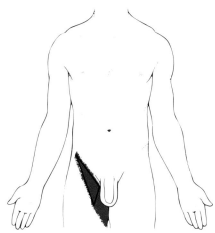

FIG. 7.6 Femoral triangle: referred pain pattern from psoas abscess. Hip pain associated with such an abscess may involve the medial aspect of the thigh and femoral triangle areas. The femoral triangle is the name given to the anterior aspect of the thigh formed as different muscles and ligaments cross each other, producing an inverted triangular shape.

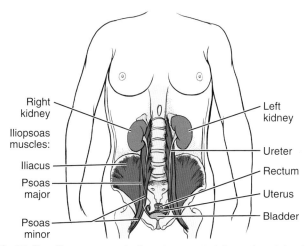

FIG. 7.5 The iliopsoas muscle is not separated from the abdominal or pelvic cavity. As this illustration shows, most of the viscera in the abdominal and pelvic cavities can come in contact with the iliopsoas muscle. Any infectious or inflammatory process present in either of these cavities can seed itself to the psoas muscle by direct extension.

Systemic causes of hip pain from psoas abscess are usually associated with loss of appetite or other GI symptoms, fever, and sweats. Symptoms from an iliopsoas TrP are aggravated by weight-bearing activities and are relieved by recumbency or rest. Relief is greater when the hip is flexed.[8,90] Clinical manifestations of a psoas or iliacus abscess can also include lower abdominal, pelvic, or back pain. The right side is affected most often when associated with appendicitis. An experienced PTA will see the unusual cases, making it necessary to know both the typical pain patterns associated with systemic disease, as well as the atypical presentations.

RECOGNIZING GASTROINTESTINAL RED FLAGS IN THE LOWER EXTREMITY

The relationship of the gut to the joint is well known but poorly understood. Intestinal bypass syndrome, inflammatory bowel disease, ankylosing spondylitis, celiac disease, postdysenteric reactive arthritis, bowel bypass syndrome, and antibiotic-associated colitis all share the fact that some "interface" exists between the bowel and the hip articular surface. It is possible that the clinical expression of immune-mediated joint disease results from an immunologic response to an antigen that crosses the gut mucosa with an autoimmune response against self.[91-98]

The PTA may treat a patient with joint or back pain with an underlying enteric cause before the therapist realizes what the underlying problem is. Palliative intervention can make a difference in the short term but does not affect the final outcome. Symptoms that are unrelieved by physical therapy intervention are always a red flag. Symptoms that improve after physical therapy but then get worse again are also a red flag, revealing the need for further evaluation.

Follow-Up Questions

For the client with hip pain of unknown cause, that does not respond to treatment, or that seems to improve but then gets worse, the PTA can ask whether any back or abdominal pain is ever present. Alternating abdominal pain with low back pain at the same level, or alternating abdominal pain with hip pain, is a red flag that requires reporting to the PT.

In the case of enterically induced joint pain the client will get worse without medical intervention. Without early identification and referral the client will eventually return to his or her gastroenterologist or primary care physician. Medical treatment for the underlying disease is essential in affecting the musculoskeletal component. Physical therapy intervention does not alter or improve the underlying enteric disease. It is better for the client if the PT/PTA team recognizes the need for medical intervention as soon as possible.

Crohn Disease

Anyone with hip or groin pain of unknown cause, a history of PID, Crohn disease (regional enteritis), ulcerative colitis, irritable bowel syndrome, diverticulitis, or bowel obstruction requires careful observation and evaluation by the PT/PTA team.

It is possible that new onset of low back, sacral, buttock, or hip pain is merely a new symptom of an already established enteric (GI) disease. Twenty-five percent of those with inflammatory enteric disease (particularly Crohn disease) have concomitant back or joint pain that are symptoms of spondyloarthritis/spondyloarthropathy.[97,99]

PTA ACTION PLAN

Follow-Up Questions

A skin rash that comes and goes can accompany enterically induced arthritis. A flat rash or raised skin lesion of the lower extremities is possible; it usually precedes joint or back pain. The client should be asked whether he or she has had skin rashes of any kind over the past few weeks.

Reactive Arthritis

In the case of reactive arthritis, joint symptoms occur 1 to 4 weeks after an infection, usually GI or genitourinary.[98] The joint is not septic (infected) but rather aseptic (not infected). Affected joints often occur at a site that is remote from the primary infection. Prosthetic joints are not immune to this type of infection and may become infected even years after the joint is implanted.

PICTURE THE PATIENT

Whether the infection occurs in the natural joint or in the prosthetic implant, the client is unable to bear weight on the joint. An acute arthritic presentation may occur, and the client often has a fever (commonly of low grade in older adults or in anyone who is immunosuppressed).

PTA ACTION PLAN

Follow-Up Questions

The PTA can ask if the individual has had a recent (last 30 days) infection of any kind that may have been missed as part of the past medical history. This type of question may be helpful for the client with joint pain of unknown cause or with an unusual presentation/history that does not fit the expected pattern for injury, overuse, or aging.

RECOGNIZING VASCULAR RED FLAGS IN THE LOWER EXTREMITY

Vascular pain is often throbbing in nature and exacerbated by activity. With atherosclerosis a lag time of 5 to 10 minutes occurs between when the body asks for increased oxygenated blood and when symptoms occur because of arterial occlusion. The client is older and often with a personal or family history of heart disease. Other risk factors include hyperlipidemia, tobacco use, and diabetes.

Peripheral Vascular Disease

Peripheral vascular disease (peripheral arterial disease; arterial insufficiency), in which the arteries are occluded by atherosclerosis, can cause unilateral or bilateral low back, hip, buttock, groin, or leg pain, along with intermittent claudication and trophic changes of the affected lower extremities.

PICTURE THE PATIENT

Peripheral vascular disease is a rare cause of lower extremity pain in anyone under the age of 65 years, but leg pain in recreational athletes caused by isolated areas of arterial stenosis has been reported.[100]

Intermittent claudication of vascular origin may begin in the calf and gradually make its way up the lower extremity. The client may report the pain or discomfort as "burning," "cramping," or "sharp." Pain or other symptoms begin several minutes after the start of physical activity and resolve almost immediately with rest. As discussed in Chapter 5, the site of symptoms is determined by the location of the pathology (see Fig. 5.6).

PTA ACTION PLAN

Patient Assessment and Observation

The therapist may direct the PTA to include assessment of vital signs along with observation and documentation of any trophic skin changes so often present with chronic arterial insufficiency. Pulse oximetry may be helpful when thrombosis is not clinically obvious; for example, pulses can be present in both feet with oxygen saturation levels at 90% or less.[101]

PICTURE THE PATIENT

DVT as a cause of lower leg pain may present as loss of knee or ankle motion or swelling of the knee, calf, or ankle, with calf tenderness and erythema. Increased local skin temperature, local edema, and decreased distal pulses in the lower extremity can also occur.[102]

Abdominal Aortic Aneurysm

AAA may be asymptomatic; discovery occurs on physical or x-ray examination of the abdomen or lower spine for some other reason. The most common symptom is awareness of a pulsating mass in the abdomen, with or without pain, followed by abdominal and back pain. Groin pain and flank pain may occur because of increasing pressure on other structures.

Be aware of the client's age. The client with an AAA can be of any age because this may be a congenital condition, but usually, he or she is over 50 years old and, more likely, is 65 years or older. The condition remains asymptomatic until the wall of the aorta grows large enough to rupture. If that happens, blood in the abdomen causes searing pain accompanied by a sudden drop in blood pressure.

PICTURE THE PATIENT

Symptoms of impending rupture or actual rupture of the aortic aneurysm include the following:
- Rapid onset of severe groin pain (usually accompanied by abdominal or back pain)
- Radiation of pain to the abdomen or to posterior thighs
- Pain not relieved by change in position
- Pain described as "tearing" or "ripping"
- Other signs, such as cold or pulseless lower extremities

An increasingly prevalent risk factor in the aging adult population is initiation of a weight-lifting program without prior medical evaluation or approval. The presence of atherosclerosis, elevated blood pressure, or an unknown aneurysm during weight training can precipitate rupture.

PTA ACTION PLAN

Communication With the Physical Therapist

The PTA should document and report directly to the PT any time patients report new or progression of previously present symptoms. For symptoms described here that are associated with aneurysms, immediate notification is required. In addition, anytime the patient or client is concerned about new symptoms or expresses alarm, immediate action is required.

REFERENCES

1. Hammond NA: Left lower-quadrant pain: guidelines from the American College of Radiology appropriateness criteria, *Am Fam Physician* 82(7):766–770, 2010.
2. Maccauro G, Liuzza F, Scaramuzzo L, et al: Percutaneous acetabuloplasty for metastatic acetabular lesions, *BMC Musculoskelet Disord* 9:66, 2008.
3. Lishchyna N, Henderson S: Acute onset-low back pain and hip pain secondary to metastatic prostate cancer: a case report, *J Can Chiropr Assoc* 48(1):5–12, 2004.
4. Wang CY: Comparison of distribution characteristics of metastatic bone lesions between breast and prostate carcinomas, *Oncol Lett* 5(1):391–397, 2013.
5. Sottnik JL: Integrin alpha (2) beta (1) (α2β1) promotes prostate cancer skeletal metastasis, *Clin Exp Metastasis* 30(5):569–578, 2013.
6. Legakis I, Syrigos K: Osteoporosis in patients with breast and prostate cancer. Effect of disease and treatment modalities, *Endocr Metab Immune Disord Drug Targets* 13(2):168–174, 2013.
7. Lachiewicz PF: Thigh mass resulting from polyethylene wear of a revision total hip arthroplasty, *Clin Orthop Relat Res* 455:274–276, 2007.
8. Browder DA, Erhard RE: Decision making for a painful hip: a case requiring referral, *J Orthop Sports Phys Ther* 35:738–744, 2005.
9. Lesher JM, Dreyfuss P, Hager N, et al: Hip joint pain referral patterns: a descriptive study, *Pain Med* 9:22–25, 2008.
10. Cibulka MT, Bloom NJ, Enseki KR, et al: Hip pain and mobility deficits—hip osteoarthritis: revision 2017, *J Orthop Sports Phys Ther* 47(6):A1–A37, 2017.
11. Bertot AJ, Jarmain SJ, Cosgarea AJ: Hip pain in active adults: 20 clinical pearls, *J Musculoskelet Med* 20:35–55, 2003.
12. Tortolani PJ, Carbone JJ, Quartararo LG: Greater trochanteric pain syndrome in patients referred to orthopedic spine specialists, *Spine J* 2:251–254, 2002.
13. Strauss EJ: Greater trochanteric pain syndrome, *Sports Med Arthroscop* 18(2):113–119, 2010.
14. Williams BS, Cohen SP: Greater trochanteric pain syndrome: a review of anatomy, diagnosis, and treatment, *Anesth Analg* 108(5):1662–1670, 2009.
15. Lyle MA, Manes S, McGuinness M, et al: Relationship of physical examination findings and self-reported symptom severity and physical function in patients with degenerative lumbar conditions, *Phys Ther* 85:120–133, 2005.
16. Greenwood MJ, Erhard RE, Jones DL: Differential diagnosis of the hip vs. lumbar spine: five case reports, *J Orthop Sports Phys Ther* 27:308–315, 1998.
17. Cyriax J: *Textbook of orthopaedic medicine*, ed 8, London, 1982, Bailliere' Tindall.
18. VanWye WR: Patient screening by a physical therapist for nonmusculoskeletal hip pain, *Phys Ther* 89(3):248–256, 2009.
19. Kurosawa D, Murakami E, Aizawa T: Groin pain associated with sacroiliac joint dysfunction and lumbar disorders, *Clin Neurol Neurosurg* 161:104–109, 2017.
20. Cibulka MT: Symmetrical and asymmetrical hip rotation and its relationship to hip rotator muscle strength, *Clin Biomech* 25(1):56–62, 2010.
21. Cuckler JM: Unexplained pain after THR: what should I do? *Orthopedics* 33(9):648, 2010.
22. Brown TE, Larson B, Shen F, et al: Thigh pain after cementless total hip arthroplasty: evaluation and management, *J Am Acad Orthop Surg* 10:385–392, 2002.
23. Horwood NJ, Nam D, Greco NJ: Reduced thigh pain with short femoral stem design following direct anterior primary total hip arthroplasty, *Surg Technol Int* 34:437–444, 2019.
24. Kim YH, Oh SH, Kim JS, et al: Contemporary total hip arthroplasty with and without cement in patients with osteonecrosis of the femoral head, *J Bone Joint Surg* 85:675–681, 2003.
25. Khanuja HS, Vakil JJ, Goddard MS, Mont MA: Cementless femoral fixation in total hip arthroplasty, *J Bone Joint Surg Am* 93(5):500–507, 2011.
26. Hair LC, Deyle G: Eosinophilic granuloma in a patient with hip pain, *J Orthop Sports Phys Ther* 41(2):119, 2011.
27. Zajick D, Zoga A, Omar I, et al: Spectrum of MRI findings in clinical athletic pubalgia, *Sem Musculoskelet Radiol* 12(1):3–12, 2008.

28. Sahrmann SA: *Diagnosis and treatment of movement impairment syndromes*, St. Louis, 2002, Mosby.

29. Sahrmann S: *Movement system impairment syndromes of the extremities, cervical, and thoracic spines*, St. Louis, 2010, Mosby.

30. Grumet RC: Lateral hip pain in an athletic population: differential diagnosis and treatment options, *Sports Health* 2(3):191–196, 2010.

31. Schilders E: Adductor-related groin pain in recreational athletes, *J Bone Joint Surg Am* 91A(10):2455–2460, 2009.

32. Kluin J: Endoscopic evaluation and treatment of groin pain in the athlete, *Am J Sports Med* 32(4):944–949, 2004.

33. Swan KG, Wolcott M: The athletic hernia: a systematic review, *Clin Ortho Rel Res* 455:78–87, 2006.

34. Larson CM: Athletic pubalgia: current concepts and evolving management, *Orthopedics Today* 31(2):46–52, 2011.

35. van Veen RN: Successful endoscopic treatment of chronic groin pain in athletes, *Surg Endosc* 21:189–193, 2007.

36. Kachingwe AF, Grech S: Proposed algorithm for the management of athletes with athletic pubalgia (sports hernia): a case series, *J Orthop Sports Phys Ther* 38(12):768–781, 2008.

37. Burnett SJ: Clinical presentation of patients with tears of the acetabular labrum, *J Bone Joint Surg Am* 88A(7):1448–1552, 2006.

38. Parvizi J: Femoroacetabular impingement, *J Am Acad Ortho Surg* 15(69):561–570, 2007.

39. Mcintyre J: Groin pain in athletes, *Curr Sports Med Report* 5(6):293–299, 2006.

40. Devin CJ: Hip-spine syndrome, *J Am Acad Orthop Surg* 20(7):434–442, 2012.

41. Mabry LM, Ross MD, Tall MA: Insufficiency fracture of the pubic rami, *J Orthop Sports Phys Ther* 40(10):666, 2010.

42. Rosenthal MD: Diagnosis of medial knee pain: atypical stress fracture about the knee joint, *J Orthop Sports Phys Ther* 36(7):526–534, 2006.

43. Constantinou M: Differential diagnosis of a soft tissue mass in the calf, *J Orthop Sports Phys Ther* 35:88–94, 2005.

44. Fink ML, Stoneman PD: Deep vein thrombosis in an athletic military cadet, *J Orthop Sports Phys Ther* 36(9):686–697, 2006.

45. Khayambashi K: The effects of isolated hip abductor and external rotator muscle strengthening on pain, health status, and hip strength in females with patellofemoral pain: a randomized controlled trial, *J Orthop Sports Phys Ther* 42(1):22–29, 2012.

46. Poppert E, Kulig K: Hip degenerative joint disease in a patient with medial knee pain, *J Orthop Sports Phys Ther* 41(1):33, 2011.

47. Dibra FF, Prieto HA, Gray CF, Parvataneni HK: Don't forget the hip! Hip arthritis masquerading as knee pain, *Arthroplast Today* 4(1):118–124, 2017.

48. Vaughn DW: Isolated knee pain: a case report highlighting regional interdependence, *J Orthop Sports Phys Ther* 38(10):616–623, 2008.

49. Gandhi R, Santone D, Takahashi M, et al: Inflammatory predictors of ongoing pain 2 years following knee replacement surgery, *Knee* 20(5):316–318, 2013.

50. Brown EC: The painful total knee arthroplasty: diagnosis and management, *Orthopedics* 29(2):129–138, 2006.

51. Cummings M: Referred knee pain treated with electroacupuncture to iliopsoas, *Acupunct Med* 21:32–35, 2003.

52. Roach S, Sorenson E, Headley B, San Juan JG: Prevalence of myofascial trigger points in the hip in patellofemoral pain, *Arch Phys Med Rehabil* 94(3):522–526, 2013.

53. Muscolo DL: Tumors about the knee misdiagnosed as athletic injuries, *J Bone Joint Surg Am* 85-A:1209–1214, 2003.

54. Berger D: Leg discomfort: beyond the joints, *Med Clin North Am* 98(3):429–444, 2014.

55. Butler JV: Nocturnal leg cramps in older people, *Postgrad Med J* 78:596–598, 2002.

56. Matsumoto M: Nocturnal leg cramps, *Spine* 34(5):e189–e194, 2009.

57. Steele MK: Relieving cramps in high school athletes, *J Musculoskelet Med* 20:210, 2003.

58. Hausfater P: Serum sodium abnormalities during nonexertional heatstroke: incidence and prognostic values, *Am J Emerg Med* 30(5):741–748, 2012.

59. Lui E: Systemic causes of heel pain, *Clin Podiatr Med Surg* 27:431–441, 2010.

60. Krause DA, Newcomer KL: Femoral neck stress fracture in a male runner, *J Orthop Sports Phys Ther* 38(8):517, 2008.

61. Thelen MD: Identification of a high-risk anterior tibial stress fracture, *J Orthop Sports Phys Ther* 40(12):833, 2010.

62. Duquette TL, Watson DJ: Femoral neck stress fracture in a military trainee, *J Orthop Sports Phys Ther* 40(12):834, 2010.

63. Kline PW, Williams DSB:3rd, Effects of normal aging on lower extremity loading and coordination during running in males and females, *Int J Sports Phys Ther* 10(6):901–909, 2015.

64. Seidenberg PH, Childress MA: Managing hip pain in athletes, *J Musculoskelet Med* 22:246–254, 2005.

65. Kelly AK, Hame SL: Managing stress fractures in athletes, *J Musculoskelet Med* 27(12):480–486, 2010.

66. Cho CH, Mathis JM, Ortiz O: Sacral fractures and sacroplasty, *Neuroimaging Clin N Am* 20(2):179–186, 2010.

67. Gurney B, Boissonnault WG, Andrews R: Differential diagnosis of a femoral neck/head stress fracture, *J Orthop Sports Phys Ther* 36(2):80–88, 2006.

68. Carpintero P: Stress fractures of the femoral neck and coxa vara, *Arch Orthop Trauma Surg* 123(6):273–277, 2003.

69. Tommasini SM: Relationship between bone morphology and bone quality in male tibias: implications for stress fracture risk, *J Bone Min Res* 20(8):1372–1380, 2005.

70. Barron RL, Oster G, Grauer A, Crittenden DB, Weycker D: Determinants of imminent fracture risk in postmenopausal women with osteoporosis, *Osteoporos Int* 31(11):2103–2111, 2020.

71. Coughlan T, Dockery F: Osteoporosis and fracture risk in older people, *Clin Med (Lond)* 14(2):187–191, 2014.

72. Valat JP: Sciatica, *Best Pract Res Clin Rheumatol* 24(2):241–252, 2010.

73. Jewell DV, Riddle DL: Interventions that increase or decrease the likelihood of a meaningful improvement in physical health in patients with sciatica, *Phys Ther* 85(11):1139–1150, 2005.

74. Yuan Y, Chen Y, Zhou Z, Jiao Y, et al: Association between chronic inflammation and latent infection of *Propionibacterium acnes* in non-pyogenic degenerated intervertebral discs: a pilot study, *Eur Spine J* 27(10):2506–2517, 2018.

75. McLorinn GC, Glenn JV, McMullan MG, et al: *Propionibacterium acnes* wound contamination at the time of spinal surgery, *Clin Orthop Rel Res* 437:67–73, 2005.

76. Martin WN, Dixon JH, Sandhu H: The incidence of cement extrusion from the acetabulum in total hip arthroplasty, *J Arthroplasty* 18:338–341, 2003.

77. Carricajo A: *Propionibacterum acnes* contamination in lumbar disc surgery, *J Hosp Infect* 66(3):275–277, 2007.

78. Bickels J, Kahanvitz N, Rubert CK, et al: Extraspinal bone and soft-tissue tumors as a cause of sciatica: clinical diagnosis and recommendations: analysis of 32 cases, *Spine* 24:1611, 1999.

79. Chin KR, Kim JM: A rare anterior sacral osteochondroma presenting as sciatica in an adult: a case report and review of the literature, *Spine J* 10(5):e1–e4, 2010.

80. Arromdee E, Matteson EL: Bursitis: common condition, uncommon challenge, *J Musculoskelet Med* 18:213–224, 2001.

81. Magee DJ: *Orthopedic physical assessment*, ed 5, Philadelphia, 2008, WB Saunders.

82. Oikawa Y: Lumbar disc degeneration induces persistent groin pain, *Spine (Phila Pa 1976)* 37(2):114–118, 2012.

83. Kim DS: Clinical features and treatments of upper lumbar disc herniations, *J Korean Neurosurg Soc* 48(2):119–124, 2010.

84. Doubleday KL, Kulig K, Landel R: Treatment of testicular pain using conservative management of the thoracolumbar spine: a case report, *Arch Phys Med Rehabil* 84:1903–1905, 2003.

85. Yu Y: Diagnosis of discogenic low back pain in patients with probable symptoms but negative discography, *Arch Orthop Trauma Surg* 132(5):627–632, 2012.

86. Takasaki H: Nucleus pulposus deformation following application of mechanical diagnosis and therapy: a single case report with magnetic resonance imaging, *J Man Manip Ther* 18(3):153–158, 2010.

87. Keulers BJ, Roumen RH, Keulers MJ, et al: Bilateral groin pain from a rotten molar, *Lancet* 366:94, 2005.

88. Le Pennec V: Imaging in infections of the left iliac fossa, *Diagn Interv Imaging* 93(6):466–472, 2012.

89. Shields DW, Robinson PG: Iliopsoas abscess masquerading as 'sciatica', *BMJ Case Rep* 2012, 2012. bcr2012007419

90. Williams K: Direct extension of a psoas muscle abscess leading to spinal cord compression, *Am J Phys Med Rehabil* 92(4):370, 2013.

91. Gaston JSH, Lillicrap MS: Arthritis associated with enteric infection, *Best Pract Res Clin Rheumatol* 17(2):219–239, 2003.

92. Townes JM: Reactive arthritis after enteric infections in the United States: the problem of definition, *Clin Infect Dis* 50(2):247–254, 2010.

93. Gran JT, Husby G: Joint manifestations in gastrointestinal diseases. 1. Pathophysiological aspects, ulcerative colitis and Crohn's disease, *Dig Dis* 10:274–294, 1992.

94. Gran JT, Husby G: Joint manifestations in gastrointestinal diseases. 2. Whipple's disease, enteric infections, intestinal bypass operations, gluten-sensitive enteropathy, pseudomembranous colitis and collagenous colitis, *Dig Dis* 10:295–312, 1992.

95. Keating RM, Vyas AS: Reactive arthritis following *Clostridium difficile* colitis, *West J Med* 162:61–63, 1995.

96. Tu J: Bowel bypass syndrome/bowel-associated dermatosis arthritis syndrome postlaparoscopic gastric bypass surgery, *Australas J Dermatol* 52(1):e5–e7, 2011.

97. Brakenhoff LK: The joint-gut axis in inflammatory bowel disease, *J Crohns Colitis* 4(3):257–268, 2010.

98. Prati C: Reactive arthritis due to *Clostridium difficile*, *Joint Bone Spine* 77(2):190–192, 2010.

99. Huang V: Patient awareness of extraintestinal manifestations of inflammatory bowel disease, *J Crohns Colitis* 7(8):e318–e324, 2013.

100. Lundgren JM, Davis BA: End artery stenosis of the popliteal artery mimicking gastrocnemius strain, *Arch Phys Med Rehabil* 85:1548–1551, 2004.

101. Brau SA, Delamarter RB, Schiffman ML, et al: Vascular injury during anterior lumbar surgery, *Spine J* 4:409–441, 2004.

102. Fink ML, Stoneman PD: Deep vein thrombosis in an athletic military cadet, *J Orthop Sports Phys Ther* 36(9):686–697, 2006.

INDEX

Page references followed by an "*f*" indicate figures, by "*b*" indicate boxes, and by "*t*" indicate tables.